6/10

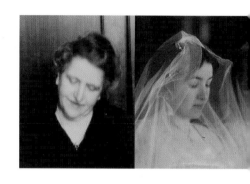

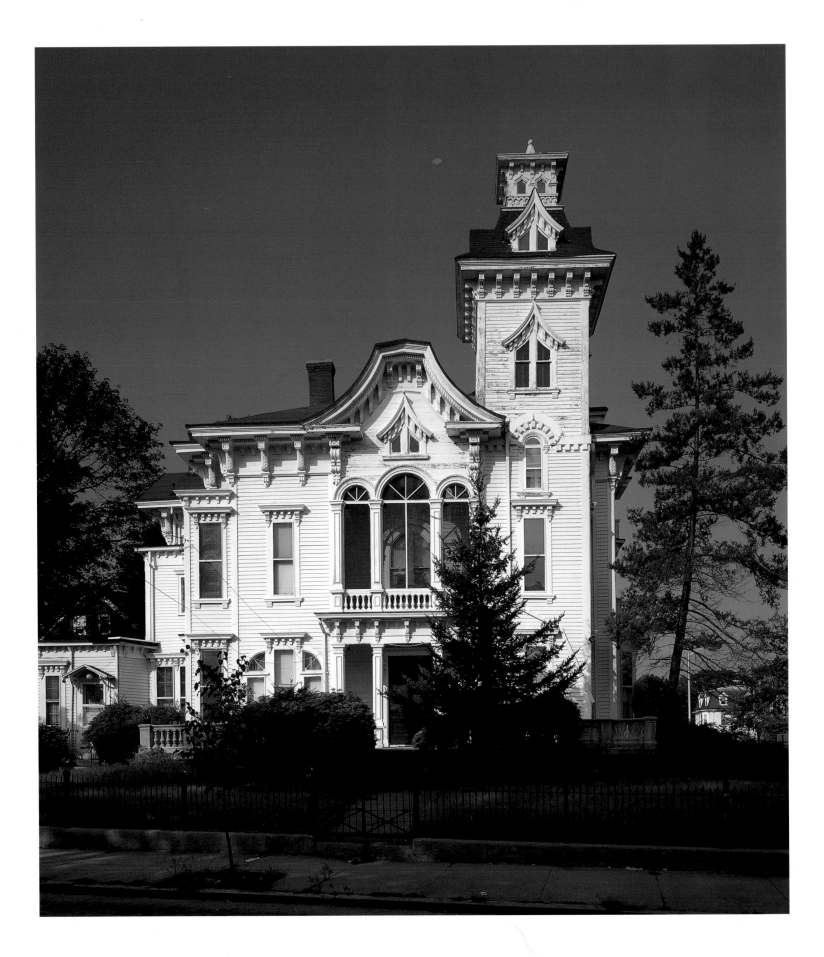

From Paris *to* Providence

Fashion, Art, and the Tirocchi Dressmakers' Shop, 1915–1947

SUSAN HAY, *Editor*

MUSEUM OF ART
RHODE ISLAND SCHOOL OF DESIGN
PROVIDENCE, RHODE ISLAND
2000

CONTRIBUTING
AUTHORS

Susan Porter Benson

John W. Briggs

Susan Hay

Pamela A. Parmal

Madelyn Shaw

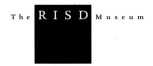

The RISD Museum

Published in conjunction with the exhibition *From Paris to Providence: Fashion, Art, and the Tirocchi Dressmakers' Shop, 1915–1947*, Museum of Art, Rhode Island School of Design, Providence; January 12 – April 8, 2001.

This project was made possible in part by research and publication grants from the National Endowment for the Humanities, dedicated to expanding American understanding of history and culture; and by funds from the RISD Museum Associates.

Edited by Judith A. Singsen, Museum of Art, Rhode Island School of Design, Providence
Designed by Gilbert Design Associates, Inc., Providence
Printed in Hong Kong

COVER:
Silk textile with metallic silver threads and cubist pattern, probably French; ca. 1926. Museum of Art, RISD, gift of Dr. Louis J. Cella, Jr.

FRONTISPIECE:
The Prentice Mansion at 514 Broadway, Providence, site of the shop operated by sisters Anna and Laura Tirocchi from 1915 to 1947; front view, 1999. Tirocchi Archive.

CONTENTS

PHILLIP M. JOHNSTON
Director
Museum of Art, Rhode Island School of Design

A long-term project requires the collaboration of many friends and colleagues. When curators from the Museum of Art at Rhode Island School of Design (RISD) went to the Tirocchi dressmakers' shop at the end of 1989, they had no idea that twelve years later they would still be working on the objects and documents found there, nor that the project of sorting through the shop's contents would result in a dramatic exhibition showcasing this unique collection. Nowhere else is to be found such a complete record of a dressmaking shop, a rare survival and a veritable time capsule of its era. With generous support from the National Endowment for the Humanities, curators and consultants have turned these records into a history of the shop and of early twentieth-century Providence. In the process, an intriguing picture has formed of the way fashion reflected art in this period.

In addition to the refining of hundreds of pages of data based on the textile and paper records of the Tirocchi shop, a curriculum has been developed for eighth-graders studying American history, immigration, and art; and a Tirocchi website will extend knowledge of the project beyond Providence, beyond the dates of the exhibition, and beyond the readers of the catalogue.

It would take a book twice the length of this one to list all those who have contributed to the endeavor over the years. First and foremost, the RISD Museum is indebted to the donors of the Tirocchi shop contents, Dr. Louis J. Cella, Jr., and his sons L. J. Cella III and Edward Cella of California. They have closely followed the reconstruction of their family history and have assisted with support both moral and financial. The Museum is particularly grateful to Dr. Louis J. Cella, Jr., whose idea it was to offer the collection to RISD. N. David (Nino) Scotti of Providence was instrumental in bringing about this proposed end. The Tirocchi family in Rhode Island, including Louisa Furia D'Amore, Emily Valcarenghi Martinelli, Anthony Tirocchi, Joseph Tirocchi, Lisa Tirocchi, Primrose Tirocchi, and Vincenzo (Jimmy) Tirocchi, were very gracious in providing information, photographs, and encouragement. To Anthony and Lisa we owe special thanks for making available their extensive genealogical research on the family back to its roots in Italy.

Panfilo Basilico, Dr. Louis J. Cella, Jr., Emily Valcarenghi Martinelli, Primrose Tirocchi, and Mary Rosa Traverso also willingly agreed to be interviewed and thereby contributed much to our knowledge of the past. Mrs. Charles (Ruth Trowbridge) Smith III, client of Anna and Laura Tirocchi, offered us her memories and was interviewed by John and Mary Wall. Ann Holst lent us materials about the Junior League during the early part of the twentieth century. Ginny McQueen, Saundra Verri, and Mary Wall of the Museum Associates energetically supported the project in many ways. While the curators were taking inventory in the early 1990s of all that was in the shop, Rodney Andrews and Charlene Webb provided invaluable assistance. We are also grateful to William McCue of New York for financial support.

Our consultants were Dr. Susan Porter Benson, University of Connecticut, Storrs; Dr. John W. Briggs, Syracuse University; archivist Dr. Suzanne Etherington of the New York State Archives, Binghamton; Betty Kirke of New York; and Dr. Valerie Steele, Fashion Institute of Technology, New York. They added immeasurably to the interpretation of the data contained in the records of the Tirocchi shop, to the mounting of the exhibition, and to the production of the catalogue. Drs. Margaret Ordoñez and Linda Welters of the University of Rhode Island, Kingston, contributed their talents, and Dr. Ordoñez assembled a team of staff, student workers, and conservators who ably researched, photographed, and prepared garments and textiles for the documentation and exhibition phases of the project. Members of this team were Cathy Coho, Cynthia Cooper, Elizabeth Dubrovsky, Elizabeth Eubanks, Rebecca Faria, Tess Fredette, Mary Beth Gale, Rebecca Hall, Kate Irvin, Natasha Kelly, Amy Lund, Willow Mullins, Cressie Murphy-David, Melanie Sanford, Deborah Saville, Katie Schelleng, Eileen Stack, and Sarah Stevens. Karen Conopask also aided us in these labors.

Michelle Tolini, while a student at Providence College, was especially helpful during the inventory phase of the process. Former Museum staff member Paul Harmon entered the data developed through the inventory into a computer data base of more than five thousand entries. University of Rhode Island graduate student Diane Joyce Montenegro did important research on Tirocchi clients and workers. Julia Turner, while a student at Brown University, volunteered her time to complete the data base of clients and wrote her senior thesis on the Tirocchi shop. Many students from RISD and Brown University have assisted in all parts of the project: Kimberly Becker, Susan Becker, Paige Berrien, Kathleen Blair, Scott Bodenner, Bridget Camp, Linda Dunn, Elizabeth Enck, Amy Fields, Sarah B. Forbes, Xochitl Gonzales, Phillip Iain Huynh, Christina Liu, Amy Lund, Paul Mann, Claudia Mendes-Martí, Kim Merriman, Sonali Patel, Pia Restina, Paula M. Sibson, Regina Smith, Susannah Strang, Cheryl Taylor, Arlene Wilson, Mary Ann Wong, and Sarah Woodard. While Mellon fellows, RISD students Sarah Dinger and Chu-Ying J. Hu respectively wrote a family guide to the Tirocchi exhibition and researched and catalogued Tirocchi jewelry. RISD Museum Docent Christine Williams also contributed to the process.

Curators, librarians, and friends in the United States and in Europe have been of assistance throughout the research phase of this project: Odile Blanc, Guy Blazy, Catherine Calba, Audrey Mathieu, and Pierre Verrier of the Musée des Tissus de Lyon; Jacqueline Jacqué, Musée de l'Impression sur Étoffes, Mulhouse; Bernard Jacqué, Musée des Papiers Peints, Rixheim; Pamela Golbin, Marie-Hélène Poix, and Emanuelle Montet, Musée de la Mode et du Textile, Paris; Liliane Schildge, Musée des Arts Décoratifs, Paris; and Valérie Guillaume, Musée de la Mode et du Costume, Palais Galliéra, Paris. Pierre Vernus graciously shared his newly produced Ph.D. thesis on Bianchini-Férier for the Université Lumière Lyon II. Florence Charpigny of Université Lumière Lyon II contributed her insights. We also thank François Férier of Lyon; Pierre Fraction of Bianchini-Férier, Lyon; Titi Halle of Cora Ginsburg, New York; Isabelle Hiffler of the Fondation Angladon-Dubrujeaud, Avignon; Martin Kamer of Paris and New York; and Giles Kotcher of Massachusetts. For information on fashion in Italy, we extend our gratitude to Dr. Luigi Ballerini, Stanford University; Dr. Gloria Bianchino, Director, Centro Studi e Archivio della Communicazione, Università di Parma; Enrica Morini, Instituto di Communicazione, Milan; Dr. Alessandra Mottola Molfino, Museo Poldi Pezzoli, Milan; and Tony Shugaar of Paracultur. Linda Parry of the Victoria and Albert Museum, London, and Nathalie Rothstein of London were also most helpful; as were Maris Heller, Fashion Institute of Technology, New York; and staff at the Rhode Island Historical Society, Providence, including Jennifer Bond, Alison Cywin, Al Klyberg, Rick Stattler, and Madeleine Telfian. We also extend our thanks to Father Robert Hayman of Providence College; Diane Fagan Affleck and Karen Herbaugh, American Textile History Museum, Lowell (Massachusetts); Cynthia Amneus, Cincinnati Art Museum; Dilys Blum, Philadelphia Museum of Art; Anne Clark, Brookline Public Library; Victoria Hamilton, Arizona State University, Phoenix; Jamelle Tanous Lyons, Fall River Hisorical Society; Paul Miller, Preservation Society of Newport County, Newport; Susan Newkirk, Providence Athenaeum; Henry Orzechowski of North Kingstown; and Marian Sachs, Providence Art Club.

Laureen Cervone of Brown University wrote the aforementioned eighth-grade history curriculum. Website author Margaret Weaver of Baltimore was an important advisor to the project, over and above her herculean task of turning the Tirocchi story into a fascinating script. We are grateful to John S. Nordyke for his beautiful preliminary designs for the Web pages and to our Website consultants, Brown University's Scholarly Technology Group, particularly Sara Grady, Claire Iltis, Allen Renear, David Reville, Giovanna Roz, and Jacque Russom. We also wish to thank Paul Kahn and Krzysztof Lenk of Dynamic Diagrams for their help. We much appreciate Sarah Buie's graceful design for the exhibition, for which David Clinard and David Harvey of New York made initial suggestions. Our community advisory committee provided welcome input: Marjorie Catanzaro, Deborah DeCarlo, Marie DiBiasio, Joseph Fuoco, Gail Fowler Mohanty, Leo Narducci, Margaret Ordoñez, Tom Roberts, Daniel A. Romani, Jr., Susan Smulyan, and Linda Woods. Joseph Gilbert and Maureen Daniels of Gilbert Design Associates, Providence, are responsible for the elegant look of this volume.

At the RISD Museum, we wish to thank past Museum Directors Doreen Bolger and Frank Robinson and Acting Directors Thomas Leavitt and Margaret Weaver, who supported the project strongly during their tenures; David Stark, formerly the RISD Museum's Curator of Education, now at the Art Institute of Chicago; Christopher Monkhouse, formerly the Museum's Curator of Decorative Arts, now at the Minneapolis Institute of Arts; David Henry, Head of Education, and Susan B. Glasheen and Deborah Wilde of that department; curators Thomas Michie, Maureen O'Brien, and Jayne Stokes; administrative staff members Judy Amaral, Carol Anderson, Melody Ennis, Tracy Jenkins, Angela Kondon, Glenn Stinson; past curatorial secretaries Laurel Barker, Raquel Benros, Ann LaVigne, and Debra Pezzullo; Registrar Ellie Vuilleumier, Associate Registrar Tara Emsley, and past Registrar Louann Skorupa; and Conservator Margaret Leveque. Assistant Director Lora Urbanelli and her predecessor Richard Benefield, now at the Harvard University Art Museums, both deserve special recognition for their part in the supervision of this project. Carole Villucci of the Museum's Education Department, played important roles in both curriculum and website development; interviewed several of the surviving Tirocchi workers; and made major contributions as part of the planning team.

Museum photographer Erik Gould took many of the splendid photographs that appear in this catalogue. Erik's father, David R. Gould of Schenectady, was able to provide important information about the railroads for which male members of the Tirocchi family worked, an example of the wonderful serendipity that has marked the development of this project. The Museum's Paper Conservator, Linda Catano, assisted with design and mounting of the exhibition; and Stephen Wing and his crew did a superb job of installing it. The catalogue could not have been completed without the expert editing and organization of Judith A. Singsen, the Museum's Publications Coordinator. We are most grateful to Jean Lewis Keith, who volunteered her time to edit the catalogue in its early state, to improve and fine-tune the finding aid for the Tirocchi Archive, and to help proofread all of the various versions. We thank her for these and numerous other contributions, not the least of which were her enthusiasm and moral support. We are grateful to Laurie Whitehill Chong, Gail Geisser, Ellie Nacheman, and Carol Terry of the RISD Library; RISD Development staff Cheryl Comai, Elizabeth Edsall, Ronn Smith, and Deborah Tobey; RISD Communications staff Ann Hudner and Monica Smith; and RISD Publications Director Elizabeth O'Neil. We also wish to thank RISD Professor Emerita Lorraine Howes and former Professor Andrew Maske (now at the Peabody Essex Museum).

Special thanks go to Susan Hay, curator of the Museum's Department of Costume and Textiles, who has directed all phases of this complex and long-running project from its initial day of discovery in 1989 to its culmination in the exhibition and accompanying catalogue. She has been assisted throughout by her associate curators, past and present: Pamela A. Parmal, now at the Museum of Fine Arts, Boston; Blenda Femenias, who graciously filled the interim after Pam's departure; and Madelyn Shaw. All have made important contributions. Blenda wrote a preliminary version of the website script. Pam and Madelyn each wrote an essay for the catalogue, and Pam served as Project Co-Director for many years. They and authors Susan Porter Benson and John W. Briggs are to be praised for their accomplishments. Susan joins me in recognizing the work of these four scholars who were contributing authors.

Without the support of the National Endowment for the Humanities (NEH), the Tirocchi project could never have been undertaken in the first place. The Museum received generous NEH grants for documentation, planning, and implementation. Public Programs Officer Clay Lewis was most helpful. We are also grateful to the Rhode Island Committee for the Humanities and to Jane Civins, Joe Finkhouse, and Drake Patten in particular for supporting the writing of the website script. To the RISD Museum Associates we express our deep appreciation for their gift of funds to forward this project.

Because of the efforts of all those involved, the Museum has been able to preserve, study, interpret, and now disseminate the remarkable legacy of Anna and Laura Tirocchi.

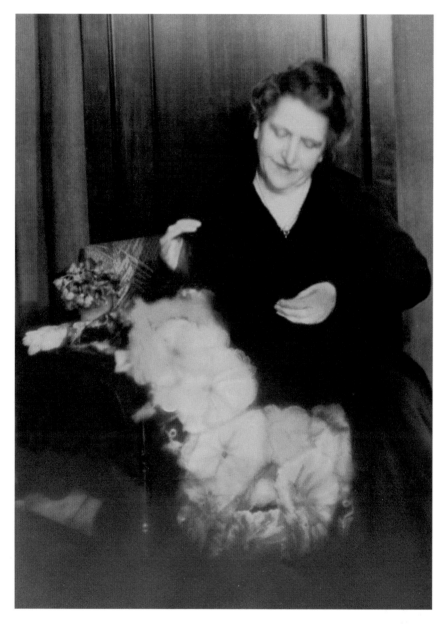

Fig. 1
Anna Tirocchi sewing; ca. 1915. Tirocchi Archive.

SUSAN HAY
Curator of Costume and Textiles
Museum of Art, Rhode Island School of Design

A. & L. Tirocchi:

A Time Capsule Discovered

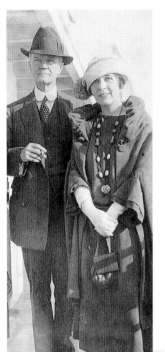

Fig. 2
Mrs. Ashbel T. (Lucy) Wall, a Tirocchi client, and her husband; ca. 1924. Private collection.

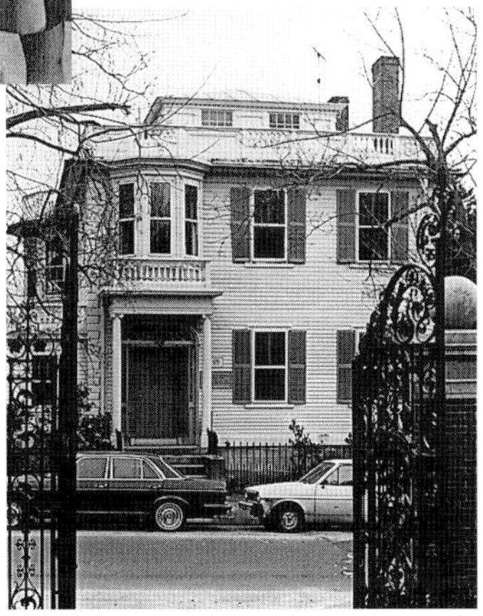

Fig. 3
The Ashbel T. Wall house on George Street, East Side, Providence. Courtesy Brown University Archives, Providence.

"My dress made a great hit – and one lady said 'Oh – that's Paris, all right,'" wrote Lucy Wall to Anna Tirocchi [fig. 1] around 1920. "I said 'Our Anna made it for me.' It made a great sensation and I love it myself."[1]

The writer of the letter was Mrs. Ashbel T. Wall [fig. 2], who lived in a large mansion on George Street across from the pastoral green of Brown University on Providence's historic East Side [fig. 3]. The sensational dress in question was possibly the "black silver pocadots evening gown" trimmed with silver ribbon, half-ball jet for the neck, and steel tassels for the back; or the black and gold brocaded evening gown with jet, two dress ornaments for the shoulders, and fringe front and back; both of which she had ordered from the dressmaking shop of the Tirocchi sisters in 1920 and which she had worn during the winter social season.

The recipient of this letter was Miss Anna Tirocchi – Madam Tirocchi, as she was called – proprietress, with her sister Laura Tirocchi Cella [fig. 4], of A. & L. Tirocchi. Many fashionable women besides Mrs. Wall came to order their exclusive clothing from this Providence establishment, located in an elaborate Victorian Italianate house on fashionable Broadway [frontispiece]. A. & L. Tirocchi operated there between 1915 and 1947, catering to wealthy clients, many of whom, like Lucy Wall, were wives and daughters of newly successful industrialists from Providence, Rhode Island, and Fall River, Massachusetts. This shop and its unusual owners bridged three socio-cultural groups: their employees (from southern Italy), themselves (from near Rome), and their powerful and wealthy clients, such as Mrs. Wall, whose husband ran a company that manufactured gold and silver plate for Providence's burgeoning jewelry industry.

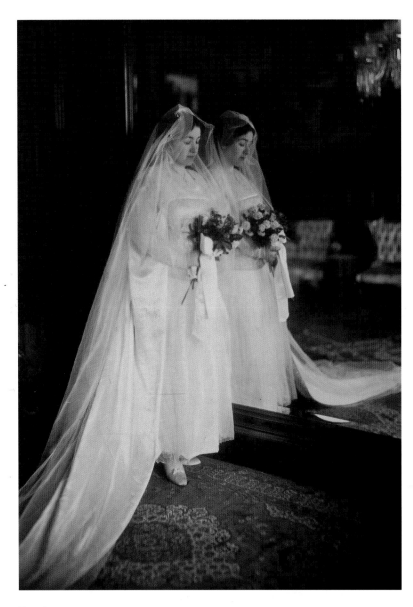

Fig. 4
Laura Tirocchi at the time of her marriage to Dr. Louis J. Cella; 1915. Tirocchi Archive.

This book and the exhibition it accompanies are based on a unique collection in the Museum of Art, Rhode Island School of Design (hereafter referred to as RISD), of early twentieth-century textiles and garments selected from the Tirocchi shop, along with all of the shop's records. When Anna Tirocchi died in 1947, Laura Tirocchi Cella wrapped everything in tissue paper and carefully put it all away, together with the business papers. These were not to be disturbed until 1989, when curators from the RISD Museum were invited by Laura's son, Dr. Louis J. Cella, Jr., inheritor of the house, to make their choice of objects for the Museum.

When RISD's Susan Hay and Pamela Parmal, curators of costume and textiles, entered the house at 514 Broadway, they stepped back into the world of the 1920s and 1930s. There, preserved as in a life-size time capsule, were textiles and garments from every period of the shop's operation [fig. 5], sewing machines and tools, notions and trims, bottles of perfume, imported linens, costume accessories, and an encyclopedic collection of early twentieth-century lace, both hand- and machine-made. Eighteen cubic feet of archival materials were also identified: business correspondence, business papers, ledgers, daybooks, check registers, employee time books, client books and bills, suppliers' bills and receipts, programs from couture showings at Paul Poiret and Lucien Lelong in Paris during the 1920s, photographs, and personal correspondence. The Museum accessioned more than three hundred garments and textiles and a few pieces of the ornate furniture that served to show off the fine textiles. At the curators' suggestion, Dr. Cella, Jr., gave about two thousand additional objects (including one-yard lengths of all the fabrics and samples of all the trims) to the University of Rhode Island for the collection of the Department of Textiles, Fashion Merchandising, and Design. In order to make a permanent record of the shop and its operations, the Museum curators, with the assistance of students and staff from RISD and the University of Rhode Island, inventoried everything in the shop and transferred the information to various data bases (see "Note on the A. & L. Tirocchi Archive, Collection, and Catalogue," p. 23).

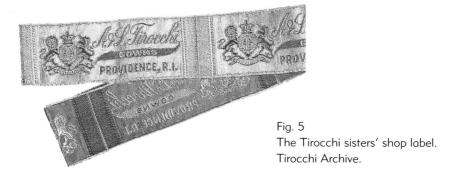

Fig. 5
The Tirocchi sisters' shop label.
Tirocchi Archive.

Such complete documentation of an historical dressmaking business exists nowhere else in the United States. Individual dressmakers are known from many cities, but other museums and archives do not contain similar riches of original source material. The Tirocchi collection is an unparalleled resource for understanding many wide-ranging historical issues, including Italian immigration, women as workers and consumers, and the transition from hand production of garments to ready-to-wear clothing. Because both clientele and workers are identified, the collection also illuminates the lives of actual individuals in history, people who were experiencing the impact of many social changes and responding to them in diverse ways. These choices are expressed in decisions about the production and appearance of clothing. The business records describe the texture of the daily lives of Italian immigrant women, a segment of the population that is barely recorded elsewhere, and thus provide an unusual opportunity to show the particular way in which Italian American women integrated their work in the Tirocchi shop into their lives.

As a study in material culture, the profusion of textiles, articles of clothing, and accessories – many purchased by the Tirocchis in Paris or made by them from Paris designs and fine French fabrics imported by New York suppliers – illustrates the close connection between fashion and art in the early twentieth century, when the birth of modernism spawned experimentation in all media and when artists approached dress as a decorative art form. Simply arranging the costumes and textiles by date makes clear the assimilation into design of abstraction, cubism, futurism, exoticism, and other trends in modern art as they were developing in the first decades of the twentieth century. By the 1920s, the American "machine age" was also influencing fashion. Many garments in the Tirocchi collection reflect the taste for streamlined purity of line and shiny materials that permeated all areas of design.

The shop of Anna and Laura Tirocchi was located on the second and third floors of an historic 1860s mansion at 514 Broadway, on the edge of Providence's thriving Italian neighborhood on Federal Hill. The house also served as the office of Laura Tirocchi's husband, Dr. Louis J. Cella, an American-born physician. The third floor of the house served as the workshop, where "the girls," as they were called, fabricated, decorated, beaded, altered, and tailored clothing to the desires of the clientele. The essay by Pamela Parmal, "Line, Color, Detail, Distinction, Individuality: A. & L. Tirocchi, Providence Dressmakers" (chapter one of this book), explores the operations of the shop itself as clients came and went, studied the design books, and, with the valued advice of Anna and Laura Tirocchi, decided on the fashionable Paris clothes that they would order.

The women who were clients of the shop are known not only from the shop's written records enumerating the textiles and garments they used and preferred, sometimes over the span of twenty years, but also from their letters to Anna, photographs they sent to the Tirocchi sisters, and newspaper clippings that the Tirocchi sisters carefully saved in boxes. Then, as now, women were important consumers. This economic role has often been ignored or belittled, along with fashion itself, as

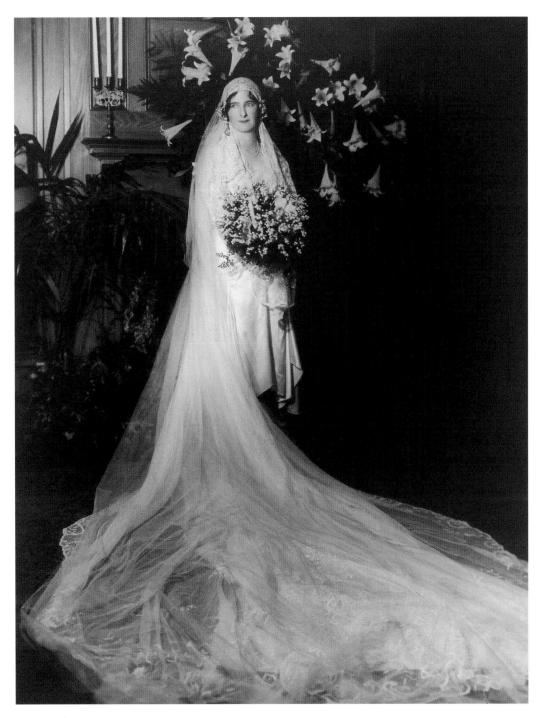

Fig. 6
Louise Aldrich in her Tirocchi-made wedding gown, worn at her marriage to
Wallace Hoge; 1931. Tirocchi Archive (photograph by Toshiba Studios, Providence).

feminine frivolity. In point of fact, women's decisions about their clothing and personal appearance document the culture of early twentieth-century America, including the female role of social arbiter, the emergence of women as community leaders in their own right, and their participation in the working world. The city of Providence, rich in traditional aspects of American culture, presented many opportunities for women of the new elite to become involved in the community through institutions such as the Providence Art Club, the Rhode Island Historical Society, and Rhode Island School of Design and its Museum of Art. RISD was itself founded by women of the Metcalf family, whose descendents still maintain a leadership role in all of these institutions. At least one member of the Metcalf family was a Tirocchi client. So were Mrs. Stuart (Martha L.) Aldrich and her daughter Louise, respectively the daughter-in-law and granddaughter of U.S. Senator Nelson Aldrich, sometimes referred to in his heyday at the turn of the century as "the Boss of the Senate." Louise, who became Mrs. Wallace Hoge in a Tirocchi wedding gown in 1931 [fig. 6], was a lifelong friend and substantial donor to the RISD Museum before her death in 1996.

All three daughters of Republican U.S. Senator LeBaron B. Colt – brother of Colonel Samuel Colt, owner of the vastly successful United States Rubber Company – were Tirocchi clients. A lawyer and jurist, LeBaron Colt served in the Rhode Island legislature from 1879 to 1881 and was elected to the United States Senate in 1913, two years after Nelson Aldrich resigned his Senate seat. LeBaron Colt's eldest daughter, Theodora, arrived on the Tirocchis' doorstep in June 1926, shortly after her divorce from Edwin A. Barrows of Providence, the president of Narragansett Electric Lighting Company. A year later, her youngest sister Elizabeth followed Theodora to her dressmakers' showroom. In 1929, the middle sister, Mary, wife of insurance tycoon Harold J. Gross of Providence, first appeared in the Tirocchi records.

Harriet Sprague Watson Lewis [fig. 7], a Tirocchi client in the late 1920s at the same time as the Colt sisters, kept a lifelong diary that happily allows

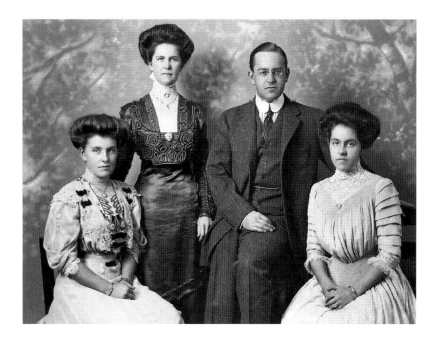

Fig. 7
The Watson siblings: (left to right) Mary D. Watson (married Freeman Cocroft), Harriet Sprague Watson (married Jack Lewis), Byron Watson (whose wife Isabel Loomis was a long-term Tirocchi customer), and Annie Watson (married Charles Fletcher); ca. 1917. Courtesy Rhode Island Historical Society, Providence.

a glimpse into the lives of these women and suggests why they purchased so many outfits from the Tirocchi shop.[2] Fifty-two years of age in 1926, Mrs. Lewis and her husband Jack, a successful shoe manufacturer, were members of a particular Providence social set made up of old families and newly wealthy industrialists. Harriet Lewis had been a friend of Theodora Colt since before her marriage, and Mary Colt Gross was among the women Harriet regularly met for "luncheon." According to Harriet's diary and to her scrapbook containing newspaper clippings of social events such as the "Welsh rarebit" parties surrounding her marriage in 1898, Harriet was also a friend of Abby Aldrich. Abby, in 1898, was being courted by John D. Rockefeller, Jr., then a student at Brown University (they were married in 1901). Abby's sister Lucy Truman Aldrich was also a friend. Lucy would later collect a superb group of Asian textiles, many of which she donated to RISD's Museum during her lifetime, with more entering the Museum holdings at her death. Both Abby and

Lucy were sisters-in-law of the aforementioned Mrs. Stuart Aldrich, the wife of their youngest brother and one of the most faithful Tirocchi clients.

Over the years, Harriet Sprague Watson Lewis mentions at least ten women who were Tirocchi clients, including Helen Merriman (listed as Mrs. Bruce Merriman in the Tirocchi records), Ella Fielding-Jones, Mrs. Harry Horton, Mrs. Frank D. Lisle, Mrs. Henry Lampher, Ann Kilvert (who married Howard Merriman in a Tirocchi wedding gown in 1931), and even one of the Daley sisters – Anna and Mary, nurses dressed by the Tirocchis – who attended Harriet Lewis after her husband died suddenly in 1930. Annie Watson Fletcher, Harriet's sister and the wife of Charles H. Fletcher, was a customer in the late 1920s. Isabel Watson, wife of Harriet's brother Byron S. Watson, had been patronizing the Tirocchi shop since 1918 at least and was one of the most fashionable clients until Anna Tirocchi became too ill to work in the early 1940s.

Harriet Sprague Watson Lewis lived in a whirlwind of social activity. In 1926, when she started coming to the Tirocchi shop, Harriet and Jack Lewis began the year with the Aldrich's dance at the Biltmore Hotel in downtown Providence. Every evening in early January a dinner party was scheduled at a home of one of their friends. Later in the winter season, there were dinner dances, birthday parties, luncheons at the Providence Art Club, Bridge Club and Junior League meetings, theater parties, movie-goings, friends to dinner, and evenings of poker and "auction" (bridge). All required particular clothing. Harriet Lewis's favorite charity was the Providence Lying-In Hospital, which she served as a Board member through many hours of meetings yearly. For each she would have worn a different "good" outfit. Often in March or April, the Lewises as a couple or Harriet alone would travel to Europe (in 1926 she went with friends to Spain, Monte Carlo, and Cannes) or south to the Caribbean: special traveling clothes were considered necessary. Summers were spent at the Lewis farm in Narragansett, where the social calendar continued full tilt with dinners and poker parties. The house was always full of people, either friends of the Lewises or of their three boys, then in their teens and twenties. It was a rare evening when there was quiet time at home together for the Lewis family.

This life was shared by a number of Tirocchi clients, many of whom are mentioned in Harriet Lewis's diary as participants in these same events. The 1920 census reveals that these women, friends and members of a very social coterie, were East Side neighbors as well. Harriet Lewis lived at 2 Benevolent Street; her sister-in-law Isabel Watson resided at number 20. Backing up to these houses was "Clients' Row" on George Street, where, in large mansions [figs. 8–9] opposite the entrance to the main green at Brown University, lived Lucy Wall, Edna Miller, and May Nicholson. May was the wife of Samuel Mowry Nicholson, President of Nicholson File, one of the largest companies in Rhode Island and one of the most successful machine toolmakers in the country. One block away across the Brown green on Waterman Street was the Providence residence of Senator LeBaron Colt, father of Theodora Colt Barrows, Mary Colt Gross, and Elizabeth Colt Anthony.

The exquisite textiles and clothing found in the Tirocchi shop are examples of what these women, who wielded considerable social and financial power, thought appropriate for their own active lives and circumstances. The profusion of client ledgers, correspondence, bills, clippings, and photographs reveal vital women with lives rich in social contacts and artistic interests who also had the time, motivation, and opportunity to move into active roles in their communities, all the while managing their elaborate homes, staffs of servants, and complicated household routines.

Many details relating to the rites of passage and pursuits of these women are illuminated by the records and by the garments made in the Tirocchi shop for confirmations, weddings, and other festivities. For example, shop records list the garments sewn for brides and their wedding parties: in the case of Ann Kilvert for her marriage to Howard Richmond Merriman in 1931, the purchase of an imported gown by the fashionable English designer Lucile and its alteration with long train and "special made sleeves by Mr. John's in N.Y." at a cost of $288. The Tirocchi Archive also includes photographs and clippings of this wedding party. Ann Kilvert Merriman (now deceased) gave the still-cherished wedding dress to the Museum when the Tirocchi shop came to light.

Susan Porter Benson's essay (chapter two), "Clients and Craftswomen: The Pursuit of Elegance," discusses the relationship between the workers in the shop, many of whom were Italian or of Italian descent, and the wealthy American-born clients for whom they performed the delicate work of sewing, embroidery, and beadwork. Providence city records show that employees of A. & L. Tirocchi were women from thriving Italian American families. Many came to the shop already in command of considerable needle skills. Annual city directories, marriage and death records, and the 1920 federal census reveal that at least some (and probably most) of the families of the women who worked in the Tirocchi shop had come to Providence at least ten years previously and already were entrepreneurs and homeowners, both traditional goals of Italian immigrants.[3] Some were related to the Tirocchi sisters, such as Emily Valcarenghi Martinelli, who worked in the shop at various times throughout its existence and who was the daughter of Anna and Laura's sister, Eugenia Tirocchi Valcarenghi.

Workers in the shop drew weekly wages, and Anna and Laura gave close attention to the hours and productivity of their employees, as detailed by the pay books.[4] For the young Italian American workers in the Tirocchi shop, this was still appropriate "women's work," not the kind of work in a factory setting that other Italian women in Rhode Island were entering.[5] The sewing rooms in the Tirocchi house were safe areas where women were sheltered from exploitation and bad behavior and were under the supervision of two female members of their own community. Interviews recorded with surviving workers indicate that, in the employees' minds, the Tirocchi establishment was far from a sweatshop, in contrast to the situations of many workers in the garment industry at that time, or indeed in the early twenty-first century. Those interviewed regarded it as a family, and they loved the beautiful fabrics with

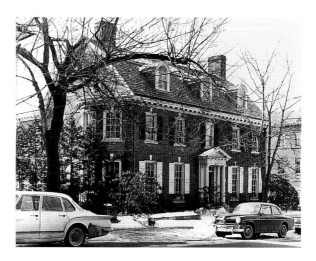

Fig. 8
The Pardon Miller house, Edna Miller's home on George Street, East Side, Providence. Courtesy Brown University Archives, Providence.

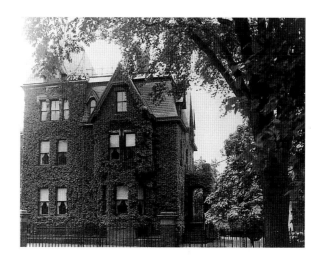

Fig. 9
The Samuel Mowry Nicholson house, May Nicholson's home on George Street, East Side, Providence; ca. 1958. Courtesy Brown University Archives, Providence.

which they worked. Their reactions to the some-times peremptory clientele were another story.

When the Tirocchi sisters first arrived in Providence, they settled into a neighborhood in the Silver Lake section, composed of interrelated families mostly from southern Italy. Much of the shop's eventual work force also lived in Silver Lake and had themselves adjusted from the economy and environment of a traditional Italian society to that of modern America. In this book's third chapter, "Strategies for Success: The Tirocchis, Immigration, and the Italian American Experience," John Briggs recounts the story of the Tirocchi family's arrival in America as part of a chain migration partially financed by several of the earliest immigrants, who earned enough to summon their families by laying railroad track in northern New England and Canada or by working as laborers in Providence, as documented by personal papers, including correspondence with family members in Italy; family photographs; and the oral histories of surviving family members.

Anna and Laura Tirocchi at first glance seem unlikely candidates for fashion advisers to very wealthy, very social, and very American clients. The sisters were born before 1890 in Guarcino, Italy, a tiny town in the hills southeast of Rome. In the early years of this century, Guarcino was still isolated from the outside world. Only when the sisters revisited the town in the 1930s did they find a narrow-gauge railway connecting the town to the provincial capital of Frosinone.[6] According to family legend, the sisters were taught the dressmaking trade in Rome before coming to the United States and settling in Providence. Their first shop was located in the Butler Exchange building on Westminster Street, where they employed eleven young women between ca. 1911 and 1915. In 1915, Laura Tirocchi married. In the same year, Anna purchased the house on Broadway and opened the shop on its second floor. By this time, the sisters had already developed their wealthy clientele.

Tirocchi customers demanded copies of couture clothing from Paul Poiret, Lucien Lelong, Jeanne Paquin, Redfern, and other Parisian cou-turiers. In the first years after the business was moved to Broadway, these garments continued to be constructed on the premises by Anna, Laura, and their workers, using fabric purchased in New York. Made-to-order dresses, coats, blouses, and petticoats were patterned on sketches of French designs published in magazines such as *Harper's Bazaar* or were taken from design books distributed by the fabric suppliers. With the advent of ready-to-wear clothing in the early 1920s, the shop underwent a thorough transformation. By 1926, the sisters were buying garments directly from the Parisian ateliers of Poiret, Lelong, and others, then altering them for customers or selling them directly, while also purchasing from suppliers in New York many ready-made models based on Paris designs. Madelyn Shaw documents in chapter four the American fashion scene, supplying the context within which the sisters carried on their trade.

What was the fascination that French couture held for American women? Part of it was the fantasy of Paris, the cultural capital of Europe, the apex of luxury, art, and fine living, home to *cordon bleu* cuisine, promenades in the Bois de Boulogne, fine architecture and grand boulevards, the newly constructed Opéra, and the venerable Comédie Française and Musée du Louvre. From the early nineteenth century, magazines, newspapers, and novels were more and more inclined to present Paris as the source of all that was best in women's fashion, that exquisite and frivolous art of decoration used not only to make women attractive and seductive, but also, as Anne Hollander has pointed out, to enhance their roles as transmitters of tradition, imagination, and emotion.[7]

When Charles Frederick Worth descended on Paris from London in the 1850s, he was quick to take advantage of this reputation. Building on the idea that Paris fashion was superior, he declared himself to be the most talented of its dressmakers. With a flair for publicity and the ego of an artist who brooked no disagreement, Worth added to the Paris mystique the certainty that the name of the designer of a woman's toilette was all-important to her image and allure. American women such as

Mrs. Potter Palmer, Edith Wharton, and Isabella Stewart Gardner became Worth's clients, bringing Paris fashion home to America and expanding its reputation still further.

By the end of the nineteenth century, Paris had also garnered a reputation as the capital of modernity with its new city plan of wide avenues according to Baron Haussmann and its profusion of recently constructed beaux-arts buildings. In the American mind, Paris was the site where the most rich and well-born from all over the world came to enjoy the high life, an experience that only Paris could provide in full measure. American dancer Isadora Duncan, welcomed into the salons of the intellectual and artistic elite after she arrived in Paris at the turn of the century, thought that "Paris…stands in our world, for our times, for what Athens was in the epoch of the glory of 'ancient Greece.'"[8] Even during the First World War, Americans still thought of Paris as "the permanent rendez-vous of aristocracy – an aristocracy formed of the diplomates [sic] of all the great Empires, historical families, renowned and glorious intellects, celebrated beauties, illustrious artists, eloquent ministers – born in every part of the world," even as the elite were fleeing to Deauville and Biarritz.[9]

Paris had another aspect: a slightly sinister, even shocking cast, with its demimondaines luxuriously dressed by Worth, Jacques Doucet, Paul Poiret, and Jeanne Paquin. Actresses like Sarah Bernhardt and Réjane were veritable advertisements for the fashions created by these designers, and through photographs, Americans followed their visits, along with those of the titled and wealthy, to the races at Longchamps or to the Paris Opéra.

The cultural sophistication and piquant worldliness of Paris in the early part of the century appealed to the American woman in a way that New York or London could not. Ordering and wearing a dress from Paris meant that a woman could have as her own a small bit of the unique life of the world's most distinguished elite in the world's most exciting city. In America, Paris fashion ensured that others would recognize a woman's status as a cultivated and wealthy person, perhaps able to travel to Paris, but certainly able to afford the best that her own locale had to offer. For the Tirocchi clientele – active and intelligent wives and daughters of wealthy industrialists in a thriving city of long history and old money   nothing short of Paris couture would do.

In many ways, the fantasy of Paris was true. Paris *was* modern. It was a time of cultural ferment in Europe and particularly in Paris, which was giving birth to recognizably twentieth-century visual and performing arts and literature. The world of fashion and textiles was closely connected with these developments. As the French recognized, "The decorative and industrial arts are, like all the forms of art, an expression of life: they evolve from era to era with the needs, moral or material, to which they must respond."[10]

Paris fashion *was* artistic. The designers and couturiers of the early years of the twentieth century were part of the art world. They moved in "artistic circles." Even though they did not socialize with their elite clients, who regarded them as mere dressmakers, they shared their clients' tastes for theater and gallery, lavish entertaining, and elegant display. They sent models, dressed in their very latest creations, to Longchamps and the Bois de Boulogne, where they could be sure that the elite would see them. They knew well, traveled, and socialized with artists of every stripe, from fauvist painters to avant-garde writers. They collected art and collaborated with artists in theater and interior-design projects. They belonged to the same organizations. Interconnections between painters, decorative artists, and couturiers were so common as to be institutionalized: for example, in the Société des Artistes Décorateurs, which promoted French design and broached the idea for the famous Exposition des Arts Décoratifs et Industriels Modernes of 1925, the source for the term "Art Deco."

The clothing and textiles found in the Tirocchi shop point directly to these connections. In this book's fifth and sixth chapters, Susan Hay discusses how the developing aesthetic of modernism may be followed in the progression of fashion design. Heavily corseted s-curved dresses that show an art-nouveau interpretation of the female silhouette at the beginning of the century had given way to the first simplified, uncorseted, tubular silhouettes before the Tirocchi shop opened on Broadway. The shop contained many of the newly fashionable chemises, which dominated in the 1920s, to be followed by the streamlined, body-hugging dresses of the 1930s. The luxurious textiles used by the Tirocchis also reflected the adoption of an international modernist aesthetic influenced by cubism, the German and Austrian *werkbund* movements, the *"moderne"* style, and its 1930s outgrowth, "machine-age" design, a cultural progression that was appearing worldwide, but especially in Paris.

Thanks to Anna and Laura Tirocchi's ability to adapt to changing circumstances in the fashion world and to interpret Paris fashion artistically for their American clientele, they continued to maintain their business at a time when their craft was under assault from all sides. "That's Paris," said Lucy Wall's friend of Lucy's garment, and many others must have agreed. The Tirocchi sisters were able to wrest their fashionable customers from other dressmakers in Providence, despite speaking almost no English at first and having few contacts among the wealthy. Their success may be attributed to their sewing skills, their creative talents, and their great fortitude in the face of overwhelming challenges. The sisters had cachet as Italians, trained, as they were said to have been, in the salons of Rome, and perhaps their charming accents actually helped, rather than hindered, their success. Judging from their long tenure at 514 Broadway and the enduring loyalty of their most faithful clients, their success was great, perhaps as great as any dressmaking establishment of their era. Among Italian immigrant women, they were very unusual indeed. The Tirocchi shop is an important historical record of aspiring women, their work, and their times.

1. Lucy Wall to Anna Tirocchi, n.d.

2. Harriet Sprague Watson Lewis diary, 1926; collection of the Rhode Island Historical Society, Providence.

3. Virginia Yans-McLaughlin, *Family and Community: Italian Immigrants in Buffalo, 1880–1930.* Ithaca: 1997, pp. 44–47.

4. Shop pay books; Tirocchi Archive.

5. Judith E. Smith, *Family Connections: A History of Italian and Jewish Immigrant Lives in Providence, Rhode Island 1900–1940.* Albany: 1985, p. 10.

6. Karl Baedeker, *Central Italy and Rome: Handbook for Travellers.* Leipzig, London, New York: 1909, frontispiece; and *Rome and Central Italy: Handbook for Travellers.* Leipzig, London, New York: 1930, pp. 525, 530.

7. Anne Hollander, *Sex and Suits.* New York: 1994, p. 81.

8. Isadora Duncan, *My Life.* New York: 1927, p. 87.

9. *The 1915 Mode as Shown by Paris. Panama Pacific International Exhibition.* New York: 1915.

10. "Evolution of decorative and industrial art," in *Encyclopédie des arts décoratifs et industriels modernes au XXième siècle, en douze volumes,* vol. 1. New York: 1977 (reprint), p. 9.

Note on the A. & L. Tirocchi Archive, Collection, and Catalogue

The contents of the A. & L. Tirocchi shop, gift of Dr. Louis J. Cella, Jr., to the RISD Museum, were inventoried during the years 1990–92. The shop was in operation between 1915 and 1947. Its business records, related papers, and the interviews conducted by Museum curators with surviving members of the family and/or the shop's seamstresses form the core of the A. & L. Tirocchi Archive. An extensive finding aid lists the various vendor records; customer records; employee records; banking and financial records; documents pertaining to business trips; personal, family, and other nonbusiness papers; and printed materials, including issues of fashion magazines, manufacturer and importer catalogues, etc. Among these materials are newspaper and magazine clippings, photographs, correspondence, and other ephemera. References in the essays to these primary sources do not contain specific locations within the Archive, as this information is readily available in the finding aid mentioned above. Discrete categories of information were compiled and entered into several data bases, for example, a list of all client names and addresses.

The interviews are herewith listed:

Panfilo Basilico, interviewed by Pamela A. Parmal and Carole Villucci, December 29, 1997; tape recording and transcript. Mr. Basilico is the husband of Mary Riccitelli Basilico, one of the longtime workers in the shop.

Dr. Louis Cella, Jr., interviewed by Susan Hay and Pamela A. Parmal, October 28, 1992; tape recording and transcript. Dr. Cella, Jr., inherited the A. & L. Tirocchi shop and is the son of Laura Tirocchi Cella and Dr. Louis J. Cella.

Emily Valcarenghi Martinelli, interviewed by Susan Hay and Pamela A. Parmal, March 23, 1993; tape recording and transcript. Mrs. Martinelli (now deceased) was the daughter of Anna and Laura's sister Eugenia Tirocchi Valcarenghi and Luigi Valcarenghi and was another longtime worker at A. & L. Tirocchi.

Ruth Trowbridge Smith (Mrs. Charles Smith III), interviewed by Mary and John Wall, May 1998; written notes. Mrs. Smith was a longtime client.

Primrose Tirocchi, interviewed by Carole Villucci and Pamela A. Parmal, December 30, 1997; tape recording, transcript, and videotape. Ms. Tirocchi is the daughter of Anna and Laura's brother Frank Tirocchi and Maria Del Signore Tirocchi.

Mary Rosa Traverso, interviewed by Carole Villucci and Pamela A. Parmal, November 5, 1997; tape recording, transcript, and videotape. Ms. Traverso was also a worker in the shop.

The many articles of clothing and accessories (jewelry, purses, scarves, etc.), as well as bolts, lengths, and smaller swatches of fabric; laces; trims; and other textiles have been accessioned into the Museum's holdings in the Department of Costume and Textiles.

In addition, the Museum's Department of Costume and Textiles maintains a department library, which contains books and bound volumes of magazines; a sizable clipping file; and a collection of ephemera, including loose magazines.

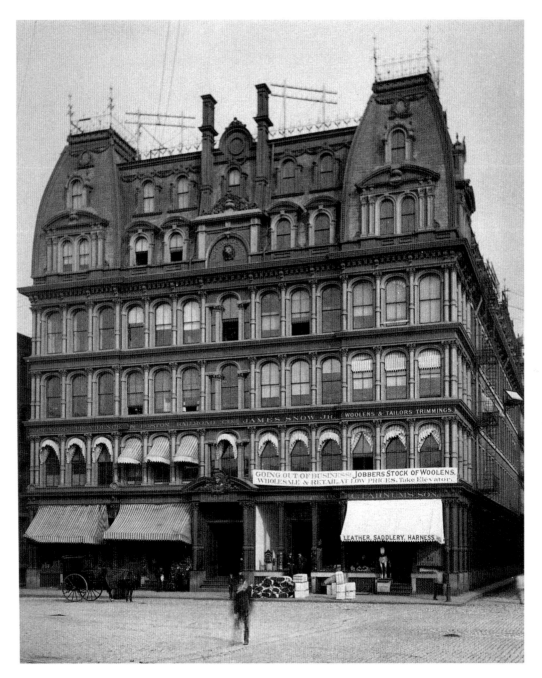

Fig. 10
The Butler Exchange, Westminster Street, downtown Providence, first site of the
A. & L. Tirocchi shop; ca. 1915. Tirocchi Archive, gift of Pamela A. Parmal.

PAMELA A. PARMAL
Curator, Department of Textile and Fashion Arts
Museum of Fine Arts, Boston

Line, Color, Detail, Distinction, Individuality:

A. & L. Tirocchi, Providence Dressmakers

In 1906, the *Providence City Directory* listed 890 dressmakers. By 1920, that number had decreased by half. Among those who continued to stay in business were Anna and Laura Tirocchi. The sisters' struggle to satisfy customers whose lifestyles were changing significantly during the early decades of the twentieth century is documented in the A. & L. Tirocchi Archive. The accelerating pace of life, due to improved transportation (automobiles, airplanes) and communication (telephone and radio); the increasing number of working women in a booming economy; and the growing availability of women's ready-to-wear were crucial factors to be taken into account. By 1911, when Anna and her younger sister Laura established their downtown Providence business [fig. 10], the descending spiral in the number of dressmakers had already begun; however, the sisters' skill, creativity, and adaptability gained them a large, loyal, and wealthy clientele that remained with them throughout the 1910s, 20s, and into the 30s.

When Anna and Laura Tirocchi opened their shop, Providence – and the entire nation – was enjoying a period of great prosperity. The city was still the United States' primary manufacturer of worsted textiles and the secondary maker of woolens,[1] despite the fact that its previous industrial base of cotton manufacturing had already begun to relocate in the South. Fruit of the Loom underwear and J. P. Coat's thread were manufactured in the Providence area, which was also home to Nicholson File Company; Brown & Sharpe Manufacturing Company, tool and die makers; American Screw Company; office suppliers Boston Wire Stitch Company and Loose Leaf Manufacturing Company; Gorham Manufacturing Company, silver makers; and an increasing number of costume jewelry firms and rubber manufacturers. The women

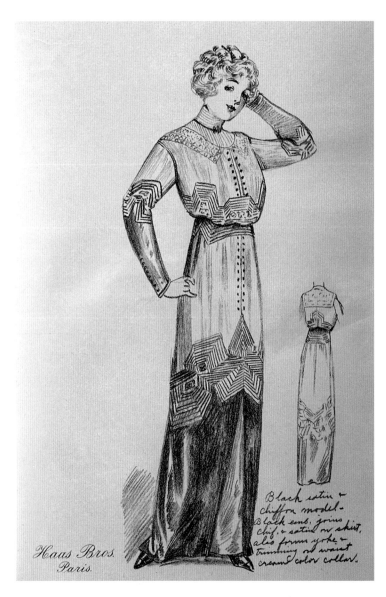

Fig. 11
Design that could serve as inspiration to dressmakers and clients, published in *Haas Brothers Book of Model Gowns* (1917), no. 374. Tirocchi Archive.

who frequented Anna and Laura Tirocchi's business were the wives and daughters of company owners and executives. These women's attire was an indicator of their husbands' economic success.

Custom-made clothing was still the rule for women at a time when the ready-to-wear trade had already become established for men's and children's apparel. The proper fit over a tightly corseted body could only be achieved through the services of a dressmaker; likewise, the complex draping of fabric and the disposition of elaborate trims and ornaments considered necessary for female attire. The custom process also enabled the buyer to enjoy a level of creativity and the ability to express her individuality. Clients chose their own fabrics, trims, and ornaments and worked with their dressmakers to produce the one-of-a-kind garments that suited their tastes, figures, and budgets.

Anna Tirocchi was well trained in custom dressmaking, and, most likely, her sister Laura was also. According to family tradition, they worked in Rome for one of the dressmakers to Queen Margherita of Italy. Although the only evidence for this is oral family history (interviews with Dr. Louis J. Cella, Jr., and Primrose Tirocchi), Anna certainly seems to have been familiar with the demands of a wealthy and discriminating clientele. Upon coming to Providence, both Anna and Laura were employed for a short time in the shop of one of the city's leading seamstresses, Rose Carraer-Eastman.[2] According to niece Primrose Tirocchi, Anna arrived in the United States with the determination to cater to American women of high social standing. The client ledgers show that she achieved just that, although her Providence customers were members of a plutocracy rather than an aristocracy. Anna certainly was the prime mover behind the opening of the sisters' business.

The success of the A. & L. Tirocchi shop was due not only to Anna's training and experience, but also to her commitment to her profession, which extended to the exclusion of marriage. Research on dressmakers and milliners from nineteenth-century Boston indicates that the trade was dominated by maiden ladies who had mastered their craft through years of dedication.[3] The situation of Anna's sister Laura is a case in point. Laura had followed Anna into the business and, according to Primrose Tirocchi, also had learned her craft in Italy. Laura's son, Dr. Louis J. Cella, Jr., described his mother Laura's role in the household as a difficult one, for her marital responsibilities often conflicted with those of the business. Her loyalties to her husband and sister were often at odds, and Anna's demands on her sister's time eventually resulted in a household divided between male and female spheres. After Anna's death in 1947, Laura and her husband reestablished a closer relationship. Dr. Cella, Jr., recalled that his mother gradually replaced the many pictures of his aunt on display at 514 Broadway with those of his father.

Marriage was not an issue when A. & L. Tirocchi opened at the Butler Exchange. Anna was about thirty-seven years old and had more than twenty years of experience in the dressmaking business. Laura was thirteen years younger and as yet unmarried. The work experience of both sisters and their training in Italy, with its reputation for craftsmanship of "quality and distinction," would have given A. & L. Tirocchi the advantage of a certain "chic appeal" in acquiring the high-end clientele Anna sought.[4] Aside from the focus on fine work, the dressmaking skills Anna and Laura had been taught in Italy were not dissimilar to those practiced throughout the rest of Europe and the United States at the end of the nineteenth century.

About fifty percent of the sisters' business was work for clients who desired that their clothes be altered, made over, repaired, cleaned, and pressed. The remaining fifty percent involved creating garments with fabric and ideas provided by the client or inspired by French styles. This tradition emerged in France during the eighteenth century at a time when dressmakers, unlike today's designers or couturiers, were considered to be craftspeople, not style makers. Fashion, until the middle of the nineteenth century, was measured by the choice of textiles and trims used to make up a garment. This was the province of the mercer, or his female counterpart, the *marchande des modes*, the purveyors of fashion-

able fabrics and trims from which clothing was made. The mercer's establishment was the first stop for the well dressed. There, one could discuss and examine the latest materials, which would then be taken to the dressmaker or tailor, who made the garments in consultation with the client. The cut or style of the dress was less important then, as it varied little from season to season. By the mid-nineteenth century, the mercer had lost his dominance, and women began to look to the rising star of French fashion: the couturier. The couturier combined the work of the mercer with that of the dressmaker, offering original designs along with the fabrics and trims from which the garments would be custom-made for the client.

Englishman Charles Frederick Worth is considered to be the first great couturier of Paris, where in 1858 he opened Worth et Bobergh with Swedish partner Otto Gustav Bobergh. Worth's timing was superb, as the debut of the business coincided with the establishment of Napoleon III's Second Empire and the creation of a fashionable court styled after that of Napoleon I and presided over by the Empress Eugénie. Within a decade, Worth was designing for the Empress and the other women at court. Unlike dressmakers and tailors before him, he did not create garments in consultation with his clients. Worth considered himself an artist: he designed new styles of dress, which he promoted to his customers. Instead of working with his clients, he dictated to them, originating "couture" and placing it atop the fashion pyramid.

By the end of the nineteenth century, the dressmaking profession – and eventually the women's ready-to-wear trade – was almost completely dependent upon French couture. Most high-end dressmakers copied Paris designs, altering them to suit their clients. Anna and Laura Tirocchi were no different. They purchased many fashion magazines, including *Vogue, Harper's Bazaar*, and *Les Créations Parisiennes*. As early as 1917, Anna ordered from Haas Brothers (one of the New York importers/ready-to-wear manufacturers) a "model book" illustrating copies of Paris designs [fig. 11]. These were published each fall and spring by importers and department stores, among them B. Altman & Company. Anna and her clients often referred to such volumes for inspiration. The client day book for the years 1917 and 1918 records many transactions in which customers ordered garments inspired by designs from both magazines and model books. On November 22, 1917, Mrs. R. W. Blanding requested that Anna and Laura make over one of her gowns. The neckline was to be fashioned after an illustration of a Worth creation that appeared in the magazine *Les Élégances Parisiennes*, (figs. 555 and 551 *bis* in the publication), while the back and front of the gown were to follow the design of a Bulloz garment (no. 91), illustrated in the model book of the New York manufacturer E. L. Brady Company.[5]

A. & L. Tirocchi stocked fabrics, trims, and notions, and if a woman so desired, she could take advantage of the fact that Anna would design original garments using them, just as a French couturier would do. In later years, also following the couturier's practice, every spring and fall Anna would invite her clients to visit the shop to view her current line. Two announcements of Anna's collections survive in the Tirocchi Archive. A handwritten note from the Butler Exchange years (around 1911 to 1915) emphasizes the Tirocchi offerings of fabric and trims:

> *Anna and Laura Tirocchi*
> *Beg to advise you that they are in New York*
> *selecting new Imported Materials and Trimmings*
> *for the Spring Season*
> *They cordially invite you to inspect*
> *their new stock at their parlors*
> *Butler Exchange, March 15th*

By the fall of 1926, Anna was distributing printed announcements that advertised their fashions for the winter season. By this time she was using the name Di Renaissance for the shop, perhaps to add the cachet of Italian craftmanship, and listing herself as manager. In the announcement, she offers her clients "Line, Color, Detail, Distinction, Individuality," stressing the unique look and quality of garments made by a custom dressmaker [fig. 12]:

"Distinction" and "Individuality" that could not be found in the mass-produced goods of a department store. Anna's emphasis on individual attention and service – the hallmark of a successful dressmaker – made her a leader in her chosen profession.

In 1915, after a few years in business, Anna and Laura's success gave them the wherewithal to move the business from its original location in the Butler Exchange (in downtown Providence, directly across the street from the historic Arcade) to their new home at 514 Broadway on Providence's West Side [see frontispiece]. The 1915 *Providence City Directory* shows that there were already eleven dressmakers and seven tailors on the street, with an even larger concentration of men's and ladies' tailors at work a

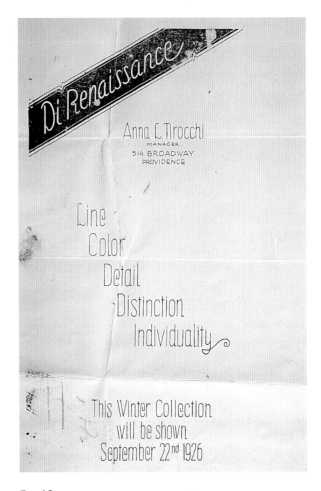

Fig. 12
Announcement of the 1926 winter collection of Di Renaissance, Anna and Laura Tirocchi's recently renamed shop. Tirocchi Archive.

few blocks south on Broad Street. The presence of dressmaking establishments in the area, along with the proximity of Broadway to downtown Providence and the fashionable East Side, where most of Anna and Laura's local clients lived, made the neighborhood a suitable place for the business. The Prentice mansion, bought in Anna's name, was one of the largest and most ornate on Broadway. The decision to move the business coincided with Laura's marriage to Dr. Louis J. Cella. On arriving in Providence, Anna and Laura had lived with their sister Eugenia Valcarenghi and her family on Pocasset Avenue in the Silver Lake area and then for a short time with their brother Frank's family at 39 Bradford Street on Federal Hill. Laura and Louis were married on June 30, 1915. Dr. Cella, Laura, and Anna moved into the Broadway address and set up a household that would accommodate under one roof Laura's responsibilities as a wife, dressmaker, and mother. In this domestic arrangement, the shop resembled those of other dressmakers at the turn of the century, most of whom worked out of their homes, thus saving time and money and allowing the women to remain on the site of family responsibilities.[6] Each of the eleven dressmakers located on Broadway was living at her business address, while four of the tailors lived elsewhere and three worked out of their homes.

The first floor at 514 Broadway housed Dr. Cella's medical offices and the formal family rooms, while the dressmaking business occupied all of the second floor and part of the third. The remainder of the third floor was set aside for the family living quarters. Upon entering the house, Anna's clients would be ushered past the formal parlor/music room and up a flight of stairs. The second floor – housing showroom, fitting rooms, office, and stock rooms – was the public face of the shop, where customers interacted with Anna, Laura, and, less often, their employees. Anna filled the showroom/billiard room with her precious silk velvets, brocaded lamés, and laces [fig. 13]. The billiard table was often covered with artistically draped bolts of fabric for customers to admire. Husbands would also wait in this room and, according to Dr. Cella, Jr., would at times

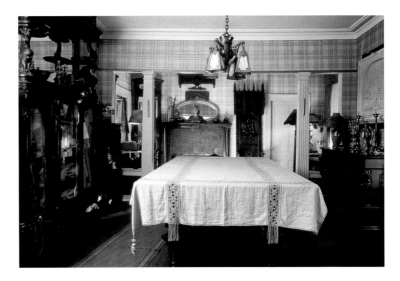

Fig. 13
The second-floor billiard room of the Prentice mansion (514 Broadway): it was used as a waiting room, showroom, and storage area for the A. & L. Tirocchi shop's silk brocades and laces; 1989. Tirocchi Archive (photograph by Cathy Carver).

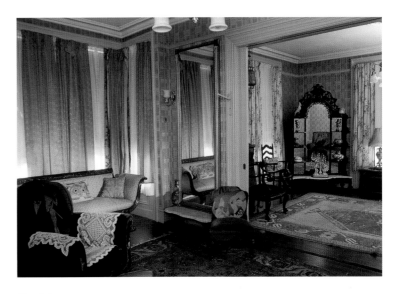

Fig. 14
The Prentice mansion's two upstairs parlors, called the "red" and the "blue" rooms (each named for the color of its carpet), where the Tirocchis' clients were fitted; 1989. Tirocchi Archive (photograph by Cathy Carver).

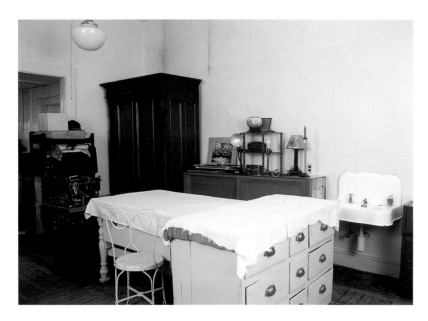

Fig. 15
The Prentice mansion's third-floor sewing room (the family living quarters were also located on this floor), where most of the handwork was accomplished; 1989. Tirocchi Archive (photograph by Cathy Carver).

machines located in one of the rooms to accomplish quick repairs.

The third floor of the house contained the workrooms and the family living quarters. Two rooms at the front were occupied by the shop [fig. 15]. A large closet off the larger of the two rooms served as storage for Anna's dress forms, sized to the most loyal customers. The workrooms were furnished with tables, one in the smaller room and three in the larger. A sizable table in the bigger room was used to lay out and cut fabric. A small chest/table placed at one end of the large table was heavily padded and used for ironing. In the middle of the chest/table sat a gas burner on which the irons were heated. Fine handwork was done in each room at a table under a window. A low cabinet with four large drawers occupied the space along the north wall of the large room. Anna stored bolts of fabric in these drawers – chiffons, georgettes, nets, laces, and crepes – and on top of the cabinet were placed on end the brocaded silks, velvets, and lamés that were too wide to fit in the drawers and so were rolled on tubes. At night the rolls were covered to keep off the dust, but during day they must have created a luxurious atmosphere in which to work.

Between the years 1915 and 1931, Anna employed an average of twelve to sixteen "girls," as they referred to themselves. At peak times the girls would spread out through the entire third floor. Dr. Cella, Jr., remembered going into his bedroom on the third floor and finding someone sitting in front of his window sewing. The girls who worked in the shop were assigned tasks according to their abilities and experience. Those who had been there longest did the more complicated work, while the less skilled were accorded the simpler jobs. Mary Rosa Traverso worked for Anna as a sewer between 1932 and 1936. She executed relatively easy needlework such as basting and overcasting seams, stitchery that would not have been visible on the face of the finished garment. The more experienced girls would take on exacting tasks that probably included the pressing and preparation of delicate fabrics or those difficult to work with, such as chiffon and velvet; the actual sewing together of the garment; and decorative needlework. Traverso recalled that the compli-

uncover the table and pass the time using it for its intended purpose. The two fitting rooms, called the "red" room and the "blue" room after the colors of the carpets [fig. 14], were more comfortably furnished than the billiard room and were probably where clients discussed their orders with Anna and/or had their fittings. The office and stock rooms occupied the back of the second floor. Anna employed a secretary/bookkeeper, who corresponded with suppliers and billed clients. It was also in the office that Anna would meet with the traveling salesmen, called "drummers," sent by the many New York importers and manufacturers from whom she purchased her stock. During the early years of the business, the drummers spread their textiles, laces, and trims on a large table in one corner of the office. Later, they tempted Anna and Laura with model dresses, ready-to-wear, and accessories. Dr. Cella, Jr., remembered hiding under this big oak table with its thick spiral legs during such visits and listening to his aunt and mother "Ooh" and "Aah" over the offerings. The remainder of the floor was used to house stock, with a few sewing cated procedure of steaming velvet was done by the more experienced girls, whom she assisted. Mary Rosa would hold upside-down an iron covered with a damp cloth to create steam. The velvet would be held above it and the pile of the velvet carefully brushed down. Laura's role in the shop was similar to that of the other girls, according to Traverso, but Laura also joined Anna during fittings and participated in the design process. She appears to have been the more practical of the two sisters and provided commentary and suggestions relative to the appropriateness or flattering qualities of Anna's designs, according to Emily Valcarenghi Martinelli.

During its early years, the day-to-day business of A. & L. Tirocchi may be reconstructed fairly well through the customer ledgers and day books. The chart below shows the breakdown of the transaction types for the years 1915–24, based on the customer ledgers. The business of the shop was split evenly between repairs, alterations, and make-overs on the one hand and custom work on the other until 1924, when Anna began to sell ready-to-wear. Unfortunately, the records are not always detailed enough to distinguish between the sale of a custom- or ready-made garment after 1924.

The emphasis on restyling and altering older apparel was typical of the period prior to the introduction of women's mass-market ready-to-wear. Custom-made clothing was expensive in terms of both money and time. The client needed to search out fabrics and trims; decide on the desired style; and be available for fittings. Garments were often restyled and altered to keep up with fashion and to prolong their useful life.

A. & L. Tirocchi Business Transactions 1915–24
(compiled from client ledgers)

	TOTAL TRANSACTIONS	MAKING AND FURNISHING	MAKING	MAKING OVER	FIXING OVER	ALTERATIONS	REFRESHING/ WASHING/ PRESSING	READY-MADE†	FURNISHING ACCESSORIES	FURNISHING FABRICS, ETC.	FURNISHING LINENS
1915*	173	75 (43.5%)	8 (4.5%)	46 (26.5%)	8 (5.5%)	22 (13%)	7 (4%)	7 (4%)	0	0	0
1916	490	212 (43.5%)	20 (4%)	51 (10.5%)	4 (0.8%)	144 (29%)	12 (2.5%)	32 (6.5%)	1 (0.2%)	14 (3%)	0
1917	433	228 (53%)	6 (1.5%)	28 (6.5%)	0	124 (28.5%)	21 (4.8%)	7 (1.5%)	1 (0.2%)	18 (4%)	0
1918	424	184 (43.5%)	20 (5%)	49 (11.5%)	1 (0.2%)	127 (30%)	28 (6.4%)	0	0	15 (3.4%)	0
1919	303	191 (63%)	12 (4%)	27 (9%)	0	64 (21%)	5 (1.5%)	0	4 (1.5%)	0	0
1920	336	165 (49%)	11 (3.3%)2	7 (8%)	3 (1%)	86 (25.6%)	5 (1.5%)	16 (4.8%)	2 (0.6%)	21 (6.2%)	0
1921	265	90 (34%)	30 (11.3%)	39 (15%)	1 (.4%)	77 (29%)	12 (4.5%)	1 (0.4%)	4 (1.5%)	11 (4%)	0
1922	280	158 (56.5%)	8 (2.8%)	17 (6%)	4 (1.5%)	64 (23%)	6 (2%)	17 (6%)	2 (0.7%)	4 (1.5%)	0
1923	281	141 (50%)	10 (3.5%)	29 (10.5%)	1 (0.3%)	48 (17%)	9 (3.2%)	15 (5.5%)	4 (1.5%)	3 (1%)	21 (7.5%)
1924	534	67 (12.5%)	8 (1.5%)	30 (5.6%)	1 (0.2%)	53 (10%)	18 (3.4%)	284 (53.2%)	38 (7.1%)	2 (0.3%)	33 (6.2%)

*Partial year account.
†This category includes "robes" and ready-made garments.

Anna and Laura's clients placed orders for evening, afternoon, and morning dresses, along with simpler dresses that were less occasion-specific. Suits were also commissioned, although not as often, since they were usually made by ladies' tailors, many of whom worked a few blocks away on Broad Street and in downtown Providence. Women would have their blouses, known as "waists," made by Anna and Laura. The shop's day books and correspondence indicate that most of the orders for custom garments were collaborations between Anna and her clients. A customer would choose the fabrics and trims from which the dresses would be made and discuss the style with Anna. In a letter dated December 30, 1919, Mrs. E. G. Butler of Rockville, Connecticut, wrote to Anna regarding an order for a coat and dress. The letter is fairly detailed with regard to the style of the coat, and Mrs. Butler is quite clear about what she wants it to look like. "I would like more of a dolman than a coat, but want more of a sleeve than many of them have. I would like a nice cloth, perhaps Duvetyn or something similar in a taupe shade. Of course, it would have to be made warm with wool padding or anything you thought best." In her letter she also requests Anna to make a dress for her, but is less certain about its style. In the end she decides that she will wait to see Anna so that they may discuss it together.

Mrs. Butler's letter helps to illuminate the process by which dresses were created during the early twentieth century. In the second paragraph, she refers to the completion of the lining of the dress by the next time she will visit. Until the early 1920s, the lining of the garment was the foundation on which the dress was built. Custom dressmakers, like Anna, carefully fitted the linings to their customer's measurements using dress forms padded out to the client's size. The lining was cut, most often by Anna, and the pieces pinned to the form and basted together. The client would then try on the lining to make sure the fit was proper. When this was achieved, the more costly satin or velvet fabric would be draped to form the skirt, and the bodice created using net, lace, and beaded trims. Most often a girdle or belt cinched the waist.

A photo from about 1914 of the shop at the Butler Exchange shows Anna adjusting a flower at the waist of an evening dress, the proverbial final touch [fig. 16]. The garment has a floral damask skirt drawn up at the side with a decorative band. The material used in the bodice cannot be identified, but it appears that Anna and her client had decided on an embroidered net or lace for the garment's kimono sleeves. Dressmakers, including Anna, did not focus on the cut of the garment as a fashion designer does today. Anna's creativity rested in the way that she combined fabrics and trims – satins, velvets, nets, laces, and jet and other beads – to create a whole. Anna, and often Laura, would work with the client to design the garment by actually taking the client's chosen fabric and draping it on the dress form. "They'd…put it this way, or put it this other way, and we'd do this on the back with a train or whatever," according to Anna and Laura's niece, Emily Valcarenghi Martinelli, who worked in the shop from the period when it was located at the Butler Exchange (ca. 1911–15) until 1932.

At times, clients looked to French designs for inspiration. The most detailed of the shop's day books, that for 1916 to 1919, is filled with examples of orders in which clients request Anna to copy from various sources. Sometimes the customers' wishes are quite clear, as in Mrs. Barnes Newberry's order of 1919. She requests a henna-colored chiffon evening gown based on the sketch of a garment published by B. Altman & Company under the name "Tosca" [fig. 17]. Other clients, such as Mrs. William Ely, requested that Anna combine elements of various garments to get the look that they wanted. In March 1917, Mrs. Ely ordered a gray-and-blue foulard gown using a variety of sketches as inspiration. The front of the waist was based on an illustration of a French design by the house of Premet, published by importer William H. Taylor. The Spring 1917 Harry Angelo Company's *Book of Models* provided the idea for the rest of the garment: the sleeves were taken from design no. 2, the back of the waist from design no. 28, and the front of the skirt from no. 13. Some clients were more vague about their desires. Anna was left to interpret

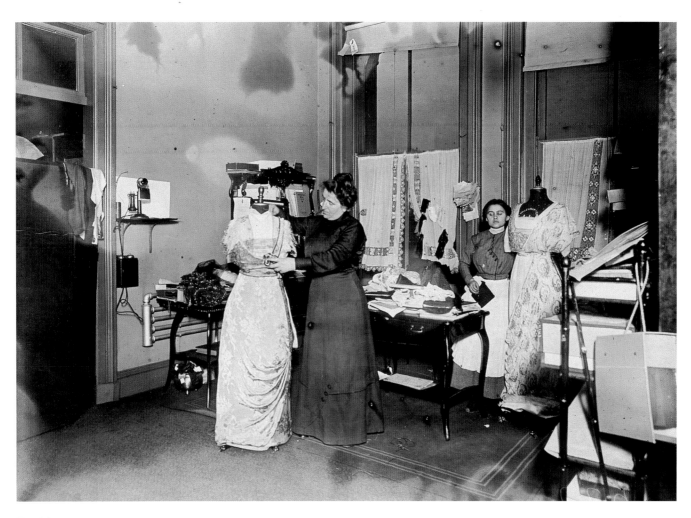

Fig. 16
Anna Tirocchi in the Butler Exchange workroom, making the
final adjustments to a dress; ca. 1914. Tirocchi Archive.

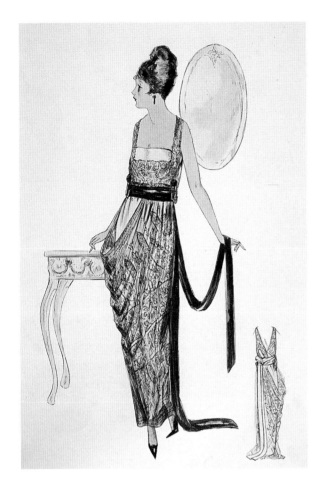

Fig. 17
B. Altman & Company model gown, "Tosca," 1919,
which served as inspiration for the creation of a garment
for Mrs. Barnes Newberry. Tirocchi Archive.

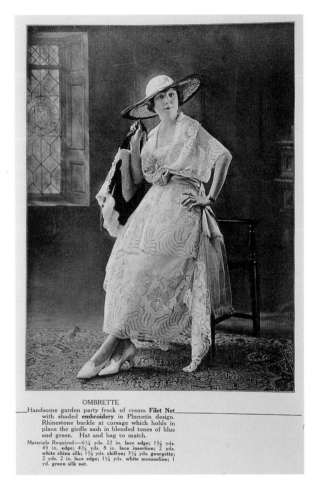

OMBRETTE
Handsome garden party frock of cream **Filet Net**
with shaded **embroidery** in Plumetis design.
Rhinestone buckle at corsage which holds in
place the girdle sash in blended tones of blue
and green. Hat and bag to match.
Materials Required:—6¼ yds. 22 in. lace edge; 1⅝ yds.
45 in. edge; 4¾ yds. 8 in. lace insertion; 2 yds.
white china silk; 1⅝ yds. chiffon; 3¼ yds. georgette;
2 yds. 2 in. lace edge; 1¼ yds. white mousseline; 1
yd. green silk net.

Fig. 18
B. Altman & Company model gown, "Ombrette," 1918,
which could be made by dressmakers with fabrics, laces,
and trims available from B. Altman, *Advance Styles for
Spring and Summer* (1918), n.p. Tirocchi Archive.

the instructions of Mrs. Brigham, who ordered a black satin evening dress that she wished to look like something between Haas Brothers's sketch no. 379 and Harry Angelo Company's no. 40, designed by Agnès.[7]

Although model books were available to tailors and dressmakers and were often used for design inspiration, they were published with another purpose in mind. American dry-goods importers and department stores produced model books semiannually and used them as sales catalogues in conjunction with week-long showings of their spring and fall models from Paris. With the model books, dressmakers from throughout the United States could acquire the textiles, trims, and notions needed to make true Paris designs. The majority of model books were illustrated with sketches of the designs or with photographs. In B. Altman's *Advance Styles for Spring and Summer*, 1918, photographs of the models are accompanied by detailed descriptions of the many materials available to create the gown. Of course, all of these components could be purchased from Altman's. Altman's model *Ombrette*, [fig. 18] could be constructed using "6¼ yds. 22 in. lace edge; 1⅝ yds. 45 in. edge; 4¾ yds. 8 in. lace insertion; 2 yds. white china silk; 1⅝ yds. chiffon; 3¼ yds. georgette; 2 yds. 2 in. lace edge; 1¼ yds white mousseline; 1 yd. green silk net."[8]

Importers and department-store buyers traveled to France at least twice a year to acquire the rights to Paris couture designs. Each design was accompanied by a list of the materials used in its creation, along with sources of supply. The American firm would acquire the materials used in the originals or make substitutions. The American showings included both the actual Paris models and the importer's versions of the designs, along with the fabrics from which they were constructed.[9] In 1918, the Harry Angelo Company acquired a dinner dress from the Parisian couturiere Jeanne Paquin and offered their interpretation of it in the 1918 spring model book [fig. 19]. The original dress was illustrated in *Vogue*, June 1, 1918 [fig. 20]. Although the dresses are similar, the lace used in the Harry Angelo Company model is of a more traditional design, giving the dress a somewhat conservative look. The

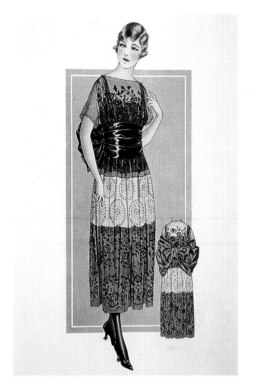

Fig. 19
Gown after a Paris original designed by Jeanne Paquin, as it appeared in Harry Angelo Company, *Illustrations for the Model Gowns...* (March 1918), no. 25. Tirocchi Archive.

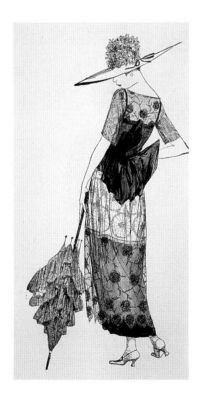

Fig. 20
Gown designed by Jeanne Paquin, Paris (after which the Harry Angelo Company garment in fig. 19 was modeled), as the original appeared in *Vogue,* vol. 51, no. 11 (June 1, 1918), p. 43 (reproduced by permission). Tirocchi Archive.

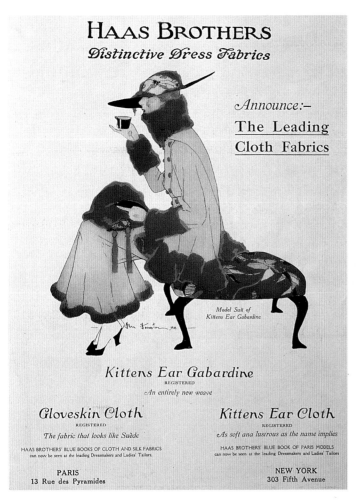

Fig. 21
Haas Brothers advertisement; published in *Vogue,* vol. 46, no. 7
(October 1, 1915), p. I (reproduced by permission).

Angelo lace would also have been less expensive, as
it lacked the scalloped lower edge. Very few
importers actually advertised in *Vogue.* One of them
was Haas Brothers, who announced in the magazine that their "Blue Book of Paris Models can now
be seen at the leading Dressmakers and Ladies'
Tailors" [fig. 21].

As the twentieth century progressed, manufacturers and importers introduced time- and labor-
saving innovations to enable dressmakers to more
easily reproduce model gowns. Decorated skirt panels, lace flounces, and pre-embroidered and orna-
mented lengths of fabric, called "robes," were made
available to dressmakers. The "robe's" embroidery
was usually worked to conform to the shape of the
finished garment, and pattern edges were clearly
indicated so that the dressmaker could easily cut
out and assemble the pattern's pieces with reference to the individual customer's measurements.
Model books – those of the Harry Angelo Company
form the most complete set in the Tirocchi Archive
– illustrate the evolution toward these time-saving
materials. Between 1918 and 1924, Harry Angelo's
model books increasingly offered embroideries,
"robes," and finally, "model sets" that included
everything needed to complete the garment, in
order to simplify the dressmaker's task. Anna took
advantage of these materials. During the early years
of the shop, she ordered a large number of embroidered and decorated panels. Dressmakers stitched
together the large panels to make overskirts, while
smaller panels could be adapted to create bodices
and kimono sleeves. Figure 22 shows a skirt panel
and matching border probably dating close to 1911
or 1912, when A. & L. Tirocchi opened for business
at the Butler Exchange. The panel and border have
been embroidered in the art nouveau taste popular
during the first decade of the twentieth century.
Lace flounces and borders were also available.

Cabinets full of lace and embroidered panels
remained in the shop on Broadway at the time of
Anna's death in 1947. Their survival was probably
due to a change in style that occurred between 1918
and 1924, when the bodice, skirt, and waist girdle typical of the 1910s and earlier gave way to the simple

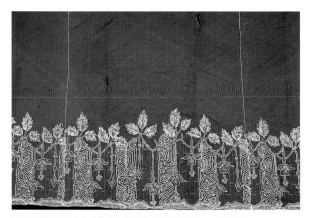

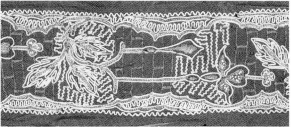

Fig. 22
Lace panel and border intended for use in the creation of a skirt and/or bodice; ca. 1911–12. Museum of Art, RISD, gift of Dr. Louis J. Cella, Jr.

chemise shape of the 1920s. The many varieties of laces, embroideries, trims, and panels offered during the 1910s and into the early 1920s did not suit this new conception, which lent itself to a different kind of overall decoration. The existing Tirocchi stock quickly went out of fashion, accounting for the large amount of material remaining in the house: goods that could not be returned to manufacturers or importers. The Tirocchis were not the only ones affected by the radical shift in fashion, for the industry as a whole suffered. In 1922, the *New York Times* reported on the effect of the new fashion on Paris industry: "…Paris modes are causing an annual loss to French commerce of 500,000,000 francs. The exportation of 'articles de modes' and dress accessories – laces, embroideries, feathers, etc. – is that much less now. The situation is attributed…to present feminine fashions which are characterized by an absence of practically all trimmings and ornaments."[10] To make up for the loss of interest in laces and embroideries, importers began offering more

"robes," which perfectly suited the changing fashion needs because they arrived with their ornament complete and integrated into the overall design. Figure 23 shows a "robe" purchased by Anna during a trip to Paris in 1926. The simple chemise shape allowed the embroidery designer to approach the garment as an overall canvas and create a design suited to it, such as these Kandinsky-inspired motifs.

The idea for "robes" was not new. It evolved naturally from the technique of embroidery, which was executed not on the finished garment, but on a length of fabric stretched over a hoop or frame. The same idea had been used in the eighteenth century for the creation of elaborately embroidered men's vests and waistcoats and had also been adapted to the drawloom for the production of "engineered" fabric, which was patterned with woven designs to the shape of the finished garment. Mercers sold these previously embroidered or brocaded lengths to their clients, who took them to tailors to be made up in the appropriate size. Although lavishly embroidered silk and velvet suits for men were replaced by those made of dark wool early in the nineteenth century, "robes" continued in use, particularly for women's dresses. Embroiderers employed them in

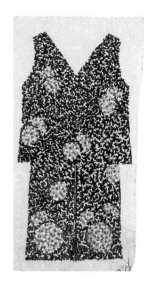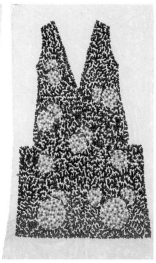

Fig. 23
Embroidered net "robe" purchased from Maurice Lefranc, Paris, by Anna Tirocchi during her European trip of 1926–27. Museum of Art, RISD, gift of L. J. Cella III.

the creation of the intricately embellished gowns of the Napoleonic era and revived them when elaborate ornament again became fashionable during the 1850s and 1860s. Mercers such as La Compagnie Lyonnaise and Gagelin-Opigez et Compagnie carried "robes" along with their other dry goods. A dress made from a "robe" of about 1855 in green taffeta brocaded with white silk to resemble lace has survived in the collection of the Brooklyn Museum, along with a picture of the skirt and a list of the materials needed to complete the dress.[11] An uncut embroidered "robe" in the RISD Museum from around 1865 provides evidence of the complexity and richness of such designs [fig. 24].

"Robes" resembling the RISD Museum example were expensive and not always appreciated by the fashion press. In 1869, *La Mode Illustrée* contained a remark that they were not worth the cost of plain silk, as they paralyzed the imagination of the dressmaker.[12] Despite such criticism, the use of "robes" during the early twentieth century helped dressmakers like Anna to survive the radical changes in the fashion industry that occurred after World War I, including the emergence of ready-to-wear. Like their nineteenth-century ancestors, the twentieth-century

"robes" arrived ready to cut and sew, often with a picture attached so that there could be no question about the look of the finished garment. [figs. 25–26]. Anna would often show the pictures to her clients when they were considering their orders for the season, so that she would not have to handle the delicate embroidered "robes," according to Emily Valcarenghi Martinelli.

The model books and the availability of "robes" not only saved Anna time and labor, but helped her in another less obvious way. After World War I, a new focus on youth culture emerged. The garments Anna had produced prior to and during the War were seen as old fashioned by the daughters of her loyal clients. Ruth Trowbridge Smith remembered that her mother loved going to visit the shop, but that she "couldn't wait to get out."[13] Alice Trowbridge, Ruth's mother, had been Anna's client since at least 1915 and had begun taking her daughter to the shop when she was a girl of sixteen.[14] In October 1922, Anna made Ruth's wedding dress and trousseau. Ruth made good use of the convenience of the

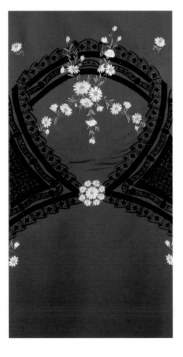

Fig. 24
Detail of a purple silk "robe," probably French, ca. 1865, embroidered with silk and black jet. Museum of Art, RISD, gift of Arthur B. DuBois, Mildred H. Rutter, Carl DuBois, and Rebeckah DuBois Glazebrook.

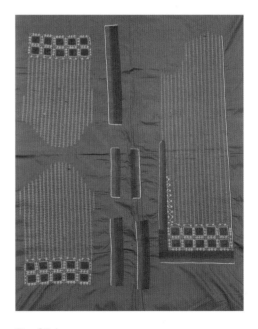

Fig. 25
Taffeta "robe" for a green embroidered coat of 1926, supplied by Harry Angelo Company, New York. Museum of Art, RISD, gift of L. J. Cella III.

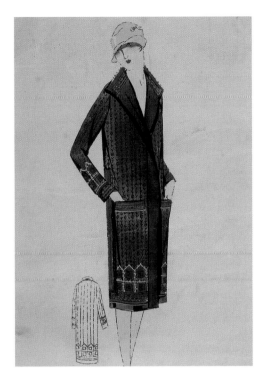

Fig. 26
Harry Angelo Company sketch for the green coat
assembled from the "robe" of fig. 25: such images
allowed dressmakers and their clients to view the
finished garments that could be made from particular
"robes." Museum of Art, RISD, gift of L. J. Cella III.

model books and had two of her dresses constructed
from "robes" provided by the Harry Angelo Company. A cerise velvet evening gown designed by
Miler Sœurs was probably made from embroidery
no. 4928 [figs. 27–28], while a chocolate-brown
afternoon dress, designed by Drécoll, was made
from embroidery no. 4930 [fig. 29]. The pieces for
both of these are referred to as "model sets" in the
Harry Angelo Company invoice and would have
provided Anna with all of the materials needed to
recreate the garments as they were pictured in
Harry Angelo Company's Fall 1922 book of model
gowns. By ordering her dresses in this manner,
Ruth was assured of the latest Paris styles and did
not have to rely on Anna or her mother's taste. Ruth
Trowbridge's parents spent $160 for their daughter's
evening gown and $98 for the afternoon dress, not
an insignificant amount at the time and almost
equal to the cost of custom-made gowns.

Clients like the Trowbridges paid dearly to purchase dresses created by the Tirocchis. Anna's prices
were significantly above those of ready-made dresses
offered in American catalogues, but her clients were
willing to pay for the privilege of having their gowns
custom made from the finest materials Anna could
obtain. A few of the entries in the customer ledger
include very detailed accounts of the materials
used and show that they were a significant aspect of
the final cost. In February 1920, Mrs. A. T. Wall had
an evening gown of black-and-gold brocaded fabric
made. The total cost came to $195.75 and was bro-
ken down as follows:[15]

5½ yds brocade @ $20.00	$110.00
Jet for neck and front	16.00
2 ornaments for shoulder @ $5.00	10.00
Fringe for front and back	3.75
Lining	10.00
Gold ribbon 42" and tulle for top	6.00
Labor	40.00

In contrast, an embroidered chiffon evening
dress from B. Altman's *Book of Styles*, the Spring/
Summer 1923 catalogue of ready-mades, was selling
for $42 and a silk afternoon dress for $44.50.[16] Sears,
Roebuck and Company was offering an all-silk can-
ton crepe afternoon dress for $15.95.[17]

A dress for day wear was as complicated as an
evening gown. There was little change in the cut or
construction of the basic garment to differentiate
one from the other. The main difference was in the
materials used, as may be seen in the record of a
day dress ordered by Mrs. Wall in the winter of
1916–17 for a total cost of $118:[18]

7 yds blue satin @3.00	$21.00
Blue embroidered garniture	40.00
Lining	10.00
7 yds silver ribbon	2.00
Findings	8.00
Labor	27.00

The fabrication of new garments was one
aspect of Anna's work. More challenging, perhaps,
was the making over and alteration of older garments

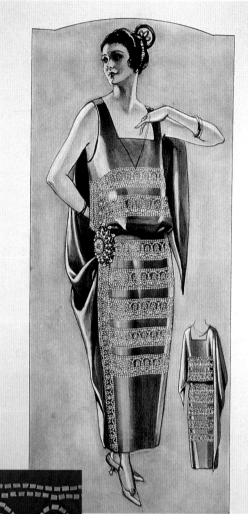

Fig. 27
Illustration of the dress originally designed by Miler Soeurs, Paris, that could be made from embroidery no. 4928 in Harry Angelo Company, *Model Book* (Fall 1922): it was chosen by Ruth Trowbridge for her wedding trousseau. Tirocchi Archive.

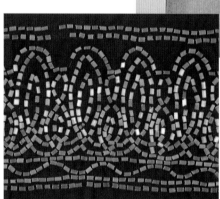

Fig. 28
Fragment of the embroidered velvet used in Ruth Trowbridge's dress; found in the Tirocchi shop, 1990. Courtesy University of Rhode Island, Kingston, Historic Costume and Textile Collection, gift of Dr. Louis J. Cella, Jr.

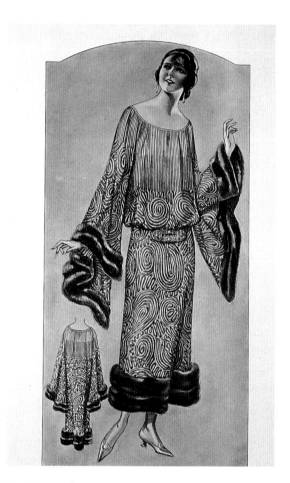

Fig. 29
Illustration of an afternoon dress originally designed by Drécoll that could be made from embroidery no. 4930 in Harry Angelo Company, *Model Book* (Fall 1922). chosen by Ruth Trowbridge for her wedding trousseau. Tirocchi Archive.

to keep them in style. This work was usually commissioned after women reviewed their wardrobes for the coming season. A look at the transactions of one of the Tirocchis' most loyal customers, Mrs. Charles B. Luther, shows that she had her clothing restyled often. In January of 1917 she was billed for the making and furnishing of a velvet evening dress with black and blue stripes. In November 1917, she returned and paid $2 to have a new collar put on it, and in November 1918, she brought the dress back again and had it remade for afternoon wear at a cost of $40. Between the years 1916 and 1920, Mrs. Luther had fifty-six business transactions with A. & L. Tirocchi: thirty-one involved the creation of new clothes and twenty-five the remaking or altering of the old. Clients also relied on A. & L. Tirocchi for the upkeep of their wardrobes. Women would bring to the shop clothing that was difficult to clean and press, particularly the elaborate evening gowns made by Anna early on. The delicate net sleeves of many of these appear to have been a constant problem, and women often brought back their dresses to have the sleeves repaired or replaced. Between 1917 and 1922, Mrs. Luther had Anna put new sleeves on at least six dresses. Later in the 1920s, as fashion moved away from the elaborately constructed garments of the 1910s, new difficulties arose, and many of the clients returned to have their velvet evening dresses steamed and the beads on their gowns resewn or replaced.

Custom-made garments and the restyling and upkeep of older garments formed the core of Anna's trade; however, as early as 1914 she had begun to offer her clients ready-made clothing. In the summer of 1914, she sold Mrs. A. T. Wall some ready-made lingerie and by the winter of 1915 was offering a selection of ready-made waists and blouses. The earliest surviving record of Anna's purchase of wholesale ready-to-wear is a September 1915 order. She received two waists and four dresses on approval from H. J. Gross Company, New York. Anna often ordered fabrics, laces, and nets from this company, but the supply of ready-to-wear appears to have been a new endeavor. Anna was pleased with the waists, but the dresses would not do and were returned on the same day. On November 20, 1915,

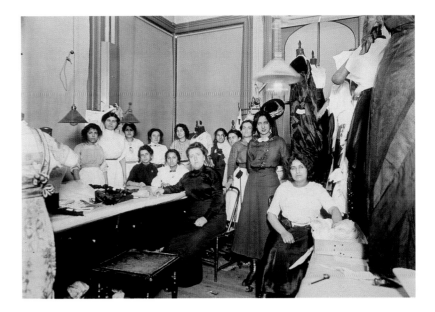

Fig. 30
Anna Tirocchi and her employees at the Butler Exchange shop wearing shirtwaists and skirts, the working woman's uniform at the turn of the century; ca. 1912. Tirocchi Archive.

she received another shipment of seven waists from Durante Brothers of New York, and in December Anna sold three of them: to Mrs. Erling Ostby, Mrs. A. T. Wall, and Mrs. Charles D. Owen, Jr. The acceptance of ready-made waists by Anna and her clients is easy to understand. Shirtwaists were widely manufactured in many styles and price ranges by the end of the nineteenth century. They had become an important part of American women's wardrobes, especially for those who, in unprecedented numbers, had started working outside the home in the garment industry, in department stores, and in offices as typists and secretaries. The shirtwaist, coat, and skirt became the professional working woman's uniform [fig. 30]. These three garments, the first women's separates, suited an increasing interest in practical clothing that could be worn daily on the job.

The shirtwaist and skirt also matched women's growing interest in a more active lifestyle and athletic pursuits. During the last half of the nineteenth century, the number of women participating in gymnastics and bicycling expanded, and by the end of the century women were also playing tennis, golf, and field hockey. This active, health-conscious American woman became the fashionable ideal and was personified in the illustrations of Charles Dana Gibson for *Life* magazine. The Gibson girl with her tall, athletic figure and her shirtwaist and skirt was illustrated in innumerable pictures and postcards and was known in both the U.S. and Europe.[19]

Ready-made dresses took a bit longer to catch on with Anna's customers, and when they did, it was the younger clients who first accepted them. In May 1916, Miss Lola Robinson purchased a ready-made dress for $50. In June, Miss Maude Martin purchased a ready-made evening dress for $60. Until 1924, ready-mades represented only a small percentage of Anna's business, ranging from no sales to about six percent in any given year (see chart on p. 31). It appears that in fall 1923, Anna was forced to confront the fact that since the 1915 move to 514 Broadway, her business had steadily declined. Almost every year saw a decrease in the number of client transactions, from a total of 490 in 1916 to 281 in 1923. The increasing availabilty of high quality and stylish women's ready-to-wear had seriously affected her business.

Providence Clothing Suppliers

(Compiled from Providence City Directories, *1906–35)*

	MEN'S CLOTHING DEALERS	DEPARTMENT STORES	LADIES' GARMENTS, RETAIL*	DRY GOODS RETAILERS	DRESSMAKERS	LADIES' TAILORS	MEN'S TAILORS
1906	55	4		76	890	31	219
1910	69	4		93	754	40	256
1915	84	4	2	112	727	40	331
1920	78	4	12	114	466	34	272
1925	84	7	16	133	322	17	302
1930	71[†]	10	58	134	245	11	274
1935	62	7	64	84	177	14	238

*This includes stores that also retailed children's wear. The number does not reflect those dressmakers, like Anna Tirocchi, who sold ready-to-wear in their shops.

†This number includes men's second-hand clothing dealers.

Anna was not the only Providence dressmaker to feel the effects of the introduction of better quality women's ready-to-wear. A study of the dressmakers listed in the *Providence City Directories* indicates a rapid decline in the number of dressmakers between 1915, when 727 were listed, and 1920, when that total decreased to 466. Concurrently, the directories show an increase in the number of ready-to-wear establishments from two to twelve. This trend continues during the next five years with an increase in ready-to-wear stores to sixteen and in department stores to four from seven.

The chart to the left is a comparison between the total number of ladies'-wear and menswear retailers, dressmakers, and tailors taken from the *Providence City Directories*. The explosion in the number of retailers of ladies' ready-to-wear is marked, as is the decrease in the number of dressmakers and ladies' tailors.

In 1923, the *New York Times* reported on the decline of the dressmaking business brought about by the increasing popularity of women's ready-to-wear. David N. Mosessohn, Executive Chairman of the Associated Dress Industries of America, was interviewed, and he spelled out the change in women's buying habits. According to Mosessohn, it was no wonder that women preferred shopping for ready-made clothing. For a custom-made garment, women had to acquire the fabrics, trims, and notions used to make it; then find the time to work out the design of the garment with the dressmaker and to attend several fittings and alteration sessions; and she might still end up with a garment that "just screams 'home-made,' and does not bear that chic, natty air of a garment designed, cut and tailored by experienced craftsmen and artists." A woman buying a ready-made dress had her choice of hundreds of garments in a variety of colors and sizes. She could try the garment on before committing to it, and there was no waiting or delay. "The dress is either carried out by the customer or it is delivered the same day to her home. It is ready to wear."[20] Anna's clients were not immune to the appeal of this growing trade. Manufacturers, primarily located in New York, invested heavily in turning out fashionable garments based on the latest styles from Paris. The simpler chemise dress, introduced as early as 1918, was relatively easy to size and produce, and by 1919, New York was home to more than eight thousand firms providing women's ready-to-wear.[21]

In the fall of 1923, Anna made a critical business decision and began to offer her clients a wide range of ready-made garments and accessories, while continuing to provide the traditional custom dressmaking services.[22] The vendor accounts show that her investment in ready-made goods increased substantially. Between 1922 and 1923, Anna's purchase of wholesale ready-made garments totaled thirteen dresses, two suits, one blouse, one sweater, and one negligée. In the spring of 1924, her investment jumped significantly when she returned from a trip to Paris with twenty-three dresses, seven knit sport suits, two coats, and five blouses. In addition, she purchased one hundred and fifty-eight dresses, two sweaters, a coat, and a wrap from American importers and manufacturers of ready-to-wear.[23]

Most of Anna's early suppliers of ready-mades were merchants and importers from whom she had been purchasing many of her textiles, laces, and trims for some years: H. I. Gross Company, Inc.; Sidney J. Stern Company, Inc.; Harry Angelo Company; and Maginnis & Thomas Importers. These large firms were also feeling competitive pressure from the growing ready-to-wear industry and were attempting to adjust. From the biggest to the smallest businesses, all were redefining their roles as the world of fashion spun faster to keep up a twentieth-century pace. Wholesalers in the millinery trade went through a similar transition, first offering clients labor-saving innovations such as prefabricated shapes (similar to the panels and "robes" of the dressmaker's wholesaler) and gradually moving into the sale of ready-made hats.[24]

The suppliers and manufacturers previously patronized by Anna and the new companies with whom she eventually established business relationships – among them the Misses Briganti, Traina Gowns, Inc., and Monte Sano and Pruzan – were instrumental in the development of upscale ready-to-wear, sometimes called "wholesale couture" or "middle-class fashion."[25] This level of ready-made manufacturing was suited to Anna's discriminating

clientele. These importers and manufacturers placed more importance on stylish design for their garments, looking to Paris for inspiration, while fit was of less concern with the newly fashionable, looser, chemise dresses. Manufacturers could more easily produce such garments in standard sizes that would satisfy women accustomed to clothing made to their measurements.

Among the first women's ready-to-wear garments, dating to the early nineteenth century, were coats, cloaks, and mantles, which did not rely on close fit. By the mid-nineteenth century, European and American ready-made manufacturers were seeking Paris cachet. The tradition of Paris fashion sold abroad through models was easily adapted to the developing ready-to-wear trade. The emergence and success of this industry was recognized in the French jury report for the Exposition Universelle of 1855. With true Gallic pride in their fashion superiority, the French jury claimed, "Women's ready-to-wear is done everywhere today,…but everywhere they work after Parisian designs or models, and foreign manufacturers know very well we have no interest in their sending us their products, more or less happily copied from ours."[26] As the early twentieth century progressed, concerns like the Harry Angelo Company, Maginnis & Thomas Importers, and H. J. Gross Company, Inc., began to offer more ready-to-wear, capitalizing on their Parisian connections. Some companies, like Harry Angelo, grew to specialize in the import of French ready-made goods, while others, like Maginnis & Thomas, gradually developed into manufacturers and made and sold copies of French models. Within the French fashion establishment, some of the young designers – among them Jean Patou and Lucien Lelong – catered to this growing and important aspect of their trade and helped to usher in the new era of couture after World War I. Subordinating the art of dressmaking to the business of fashion, Patou took advantage of the increasing use of advertising to market his gowns; he offered them at low prices; and he organized his shop like an assembly line. Lelong did the same. He was interested in the scientific management of his business and discouraged the usual adjustments and alterations to his models requested by clients, so that his shop could maintain peak efficiency.[27] Lelong and especially Patou were popular with the Seventh Avenue New York manufacturers. The Frenchmen's economical use of fabric and their attempts to streamline the manufacturing process were goals Americans could appreciate.

Oddly enough, Anna's clients occasionally requested that ready-made garments be copied for them. There are probably a number of reasons for this. Many of Anna's older clients would have been accustomed to having more creative input into the choice of fabric, trim, cut, and fit. If not satisfied with a ready-made's fabric or sleeve shape, the customer could easily have Anna duplicate the overall style while adjusting the particulars to the individual. The Tirocchi "merchandise received and returned" ledgers record that on September 2, 1927, Anna ordered from Maginnis & Thomas a Jean Patou transparent black velvet evening dress trimmed with a rhinestone buckle. The ledger notes that the gown was copied for Mrs. William Hoffman in the original transparent black velvet, a shiny thin fabric made of rayon,[28] and for Mrs. A. Burns Smythe in a more traditional black silk velvet. A few days earlier, on August 31, Anna had received a black georgette dress trimmed with velvet to be worn with a peach-colored vestee with rhinestone buttons from A. Traina. Before the dress was sold to Mrs. H. S. Lampher, it was copied in blue for Mrs. Charles MacKinney.[29]

The client day books indicate that Anna did not stock all of the ready-to-wear sold in the shop. Her customers first looked at the model books, then offering ready-mades instead of "robes" and "model sets," before placing their orders. Manufacturers sometimes customized orders, as a small group of surviving Maginnis & Thomas order slips in the Tirocchi Archive reveals. A slip dated January 11, 1926, requests five garments. Two were listed with no changes, but no. 1728D was ordered in black with two specifications: instead of fur trimming elsewhere, exactly the same trim that appeared at the hem was to be used, and a new price was to be quoted for approval before production. The fourth and fifth garments were to be made of fabrics that matched samples sent in with the order.[30] RISD Museum curators found in the shop a fashion illus-

tration meant for clients to use in the selection of garments. A very similar dress, but with a different skirt, was also found, the sort of garment that might have been requested by a client using a skirt from a different model. By contrast, a dress identical to the illustration exists in the Philadelphia Museum of Art, the gift of a Philadelphia woman who must have ordered it locally [figs. 31–33].

When the finished garments arrived, customers could keep or reject them. The client day book for 1924–25 records that Mrs. E. A. Loomis placed an order on October 10, 1924, for a black satin and velvet dress with black fur bands. This was probably Maginnis & Thomas no. 1103B, designed by Premet. The dress was ordered, received by Anna on October 23, and sent to Mrs. Loomis on November 13.[31] In an order of sixteen dresses in April 1925, a black lace evening dress by Lucien Lelong arrived for Mrs. A. T. Wall, who, upon seeing the garment, must not have found it to her liking. Anna eventually sent back this dress and three others.

Returned orders were a serious problem for manufacturers. Almost twenty percent of the garments ordered by Anna were eventually returned. In the spring of 1925, Anna ordered approximately one hundred dresses and returned at least seventeen.[32] Anna was not the only retailer to manage her inventory in this way, causing major losses for the manufacturers. When a garment was sent back, the manufacturers' profits often decreased by fifty percent, because by the time the merchandise was received, it would be too late in the season to sell it to another retailer except at a large discount. The Associated Dress Industries tried valiantly to stop returns, estimated at ten percent of all sales. In 1925, the Association put aside $40,000 of its own funds to hire staff to investigate cancellations and returns. Manufacturers found guilty of sending inferior goods would be expelled from the organization, and retailers abusing the return policy were to be tried in local courts to expose unfair business practices.[33] In a letter to the New York Times, a Kansas City retailer claimed that frequently the garments did not arrive in the correct sizes, could not be sold to the customers who ordered them in the first place, and had to be returned, causing a loss to both the manufacturer and retailer.[34] According to articles published in the *New York Times*, the most common complaint manufacturers received from retailers was that the garments were not as good as the samples, the fabrics were flawed, the wrong thread was used, or the fabric was sewn on the wrong side.[35]

After her decision to offer ready-to-wear to her clients, Anna's business flourished. By 1927, customer billings were triple what they had been in 1923, rising from $22,706 to $62,221. In addition to selling ready-to-wear from New York, Anna also journeyed to Europe in 1924, 1926–27, 1931, and 1938 to select garments and accessories for her clients. These trips are documented in the business records, although more frequent travel was cited by Tirocchi family members in their interviews. The many invoices and papers from her trips in the 1920s paint a picture of her purchasing patterns. Anna visited many couture houses and saw a number of model shows, which were held daily in this period.[36] Business cards from Paris couturiers Lucile, Lucien Lelong, Jean Patou, Martial & Armand, Drécoll, and the fur salons of Philippe & Gaston and Chanel bear witness to her interest. Invoices also survive, revealing that she did not buy much directly from the couturiers and that her purpose may have been largely to seek inspiration. On her 1924 trip, Anna purchased four dresses and a coat from Lucile: two of the dresses and the coat were on sale. She purchased a gown, "Coquillage," and a coat, "Méduse," from Philippe & Gaston. While there are two invoices and a receipt for a deposit on dresses from Martial & Armand, it appears from a company letter that she did not return to pick them up.

Other invoices from her 1924 trip reveal that Anna spent most of her money buying accessories from Mayer Frères; laces and embroideries from H. Béquet Rabin, Helliot & Cherrier; and fabrics from E. Meyer, Rodier, and the department stores Galeries Lafayette and Magasins du Louvre. She also visited the shops of Ernest Lévy and Bernard & Compagnie, buying a number of ready-made garments. From Lévy she purchased five blouses and eighteen dresses, while from Bernard & Compagnie she bought seven knit garments. The merchan-

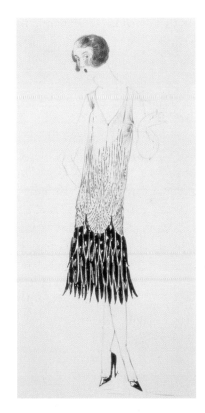

Fig. 31

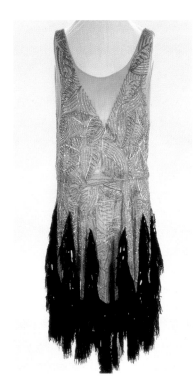

Fig. 32

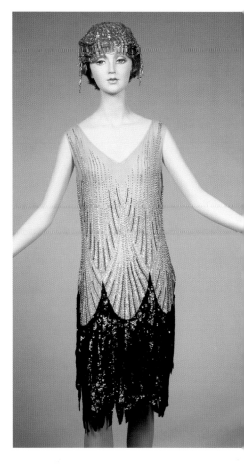

Fig. 33

Fig. 31.
Sketch for a dress by an unknown artist. Tirocchi Archive.

Fig. 32.
Dress very similar to fig. 31, but with slight differences in decoration and skirt style, perhaps illustrating how a design could be customized by the manufacturer. Museum of Art, RISD, gift of L. J. Cella, III.

Fig. 33
Dress identical to fig. 31 with beaded patterning and skirt cut in petals. Courtesy Philadelphia Museum of Art, gift of Mrs. Basil Beltran.

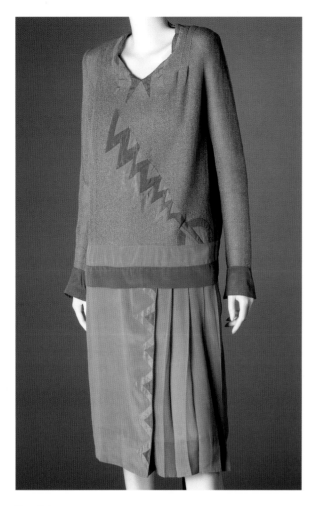

Fig. 34
Sport suit with a Paris label, "Robes de Paris," imported by W. H. Taylor, New York, and purchased by Anna Tirocchi in 1929: the casual ensemble of a knit sweater and silk bodice with matching skirt or underdress became popular in 1920 and remained fashionable into the early 1930s. Museum of Art, RISD, gift of Dr. Louis J. Cella, Jr.

dise she acquired during this trip to Paris characterizes the dual nature of the A. & L. Tirocchi shop at this time of transition to ready-mades. Anna continued to offer her clients custom-made clothing, so she purchased the necessary materials from some of the leading French houses. Meanwhile, her new interest in ready-to-wear and accessories led her to Ernest Lévy and Bernard & Compagnie, along with the couture houses and Mayer Frères, where she purchased thirty-six handbags on sale. Anna used French-made garments and accessories to great

advantage as she refocused her attention on ready-to-wear. There was a rush to her doors in April of 1924, shortly after her French goods must have arrived. Many of her best clients made purchases that month and brought their daughters, who also selected a number of ready-made garments. Six of the seven knits from Bernard sold and proved popular among the younger women. Hope Watson, Dorothy Newton Leech, Elizabeth Newton, and Maud Gardner, all second-generation clients, purchased knit ensembles called sport suits for casual wear [fig. 34].

Along with ready-to-wear, Anna expanded her business in other ways, offering a range of personal accessories and goods following the example set by the French couturiers. During the post-World War I period, the cachet of a designer's name was strong, and Paris couturiers like Poiret, Patou, and Chanel took advantage of their renown to begin marketing their own perfumes. By the 1920s, designers were also selling lingerie, hair ornaments, fans, handbags, and scarfs. At times, even household linens were available. Anna offered her clients the same. She recognized the convenience of one-stop shopping at department stores, and to retain her customers, she began in 1923 to offer linens, followed by a selection of handbags, scarves, and shawls that she brought back from France in early 1924. A few jewelry sales appear in the summer of 1924, and she continued to sell bags and scarves throughout 1924 and 1925. In 1926, she broadened her stock further, adding hats, boas, feathers, and a larger selection of jewelry [fig. 35].

Anna's business decisions proved sound, and A. & L. Tirocchi continued to be strong into the early 1930s. Her most loyal clients continued to visit 514 Broadway even after the stock market crash of 1929. By 1933, the number of clients was beginning to decline steadily, along with the amount of money they were spending. From 1931 to the spring of 1933, Anna listed sixty clients in her ledger; the 1933–34 ledger listed forty-four; the 1934–35 ledger listed thirty-eight; and the number continued to decline until 1938, when twenty-eight clients remained. Mrs. Harold J. (Mary Colt) Gross, who had become friendly with Anna and sent her photographs of herself wearing Anna's clothing, continued to purchase the majority of her wardrobe at the Tirocchi shop throughout the 1930s, although after 1931, she was seriously in arrears with her bills. In fact, all three Colt sisters had been good long-term customers, placing hundreds of dollars worth of orders, but they seem to have suffered financial reverses during the Depression. Theodora Colt Barrows left the Tirocchi fold in 1931, and Elizabeth Colt Anthony placed her last order in 1936. In 1933, Mary Colt Gross stopped making new orders and began to slowly pay off her balance of $1,219. In a letter dated June 11, 1934, she writes that she regrets "very much my delay in settling my account with you. As you know nothing like this has happened during all my business relations with you until the last year…I dislike very much to ask your further forbearance because

I realize your need of money in these times." By 1935, her financial situation must have improved, since orders for imported suits, hats, blouses, and dresses reappear. Perhaps this was because she had gone to work as the manager of the Good Luck Tea and Coffee Shop. At the beginning of the next decade, however, she ceased coming altogether. The end was amicable, for Anna enjoyed one of her greatest successes in 1939, when Mrs. Gross entrusted her with the cleaning of an heirloom handmade lace wedding veil that had been wrapped in blue paper and stored in the vault of a Providence bank. During the legendary hurricane of 1938, downtown Providence was flooded by more than seven feet of water, and the veil became hopelessly stained with blue dye from the paper. Anna asked Mrs. Gross for payment in advance for this task, despite being none too sure that she could remove the stains. She

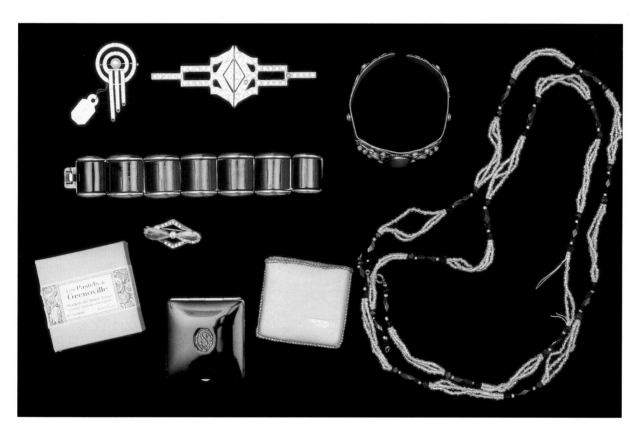

Fig. 35
Selection of jewelry and cosmetics available from A. & L. Tirocchi, as found in the shop, 1990.
Tirocchi Archive (photograph by Cathy Carver).

washed the veil in Ivory Soap Flakes, then sun-bleached it several times and was successful. Never one to miss a chance for self-promotion, Anna wrote a testimonial about the effectiveness of this method to the Ivory Soap Flakes Company.[37]

In the late 1930s, the shop's business correspondence is full of comments regarding Anna's state of health. By 1939, Anna had closed the shop to all but her favorite customers, employing two girls to help with the work. Letters, such as one dated July 26, 1939, from Mrs. Frederick S. Peck, one of her most loyal clients, must have been extremely disheartening. Mrs. Peck complains about a mistake on her bill, about high prices, and cancels an order, then goes on to request that Anna clean a piece of Brussels lace that her granddaughter wishes to use on her wedding gown. She finishes the letter by saying, "I am sorry she has decided to order her dress from someone else." By 1940, when she would have been around sixty-seven years old, Anna could no longer keep up with the pace of fashion and let the two remaining girls go. The last ledger in the archive covers the years 1941 to 1947. Anna continued to sew for only eight women: Mrs. Stuart Aldrich, Mrs. Edgar Brunschwig, Mrs. Fred Campbell, Mrs. H. A. DuVillard, Mrs. Harold J. Gross, Mrs. William Hoffman, Mrs. Frederick S. Peck, and Mrs. David A. Seaman. Most of these women had found other dressmakers by 1942, except for Mrs. Peck, who stayed with the Tirocchi shop until Anna's death from coronary thrombosis on February 26, 1947.

Through hard work, determination, and flexibility, Anna and Laura had managed to prolong the life of their business, despite the crippling effect of the introduction of women's ready-to-wear, the competition from proliferating department stores and specialty shops, and the economic effects of the Great Depression. While many dressmakers failed, A. & L. Tirocchi began to sell ready-to-wear, fashion accessories, perfumes, and even household linens and maintained an edge by offering the same individual attention to their clients that had always been expected of good dressmakers. Unfortunately, their energy and strategic readjustment could not stay the passage of time. After her death, Anna's family carefully packed all of the business records, wrapped the fabrics, laces, ribbons, and trims in tissue, stowed them away in the shop, and closed the doors on A. & L. Tirocchi. Laura and her husband continued to live in the house, but Laura's attention now turned to her family. Anna bequeathed the house to Laura's only daughter, Beatrice, on condition that she care for her mother. At Beatrice's death in 1990, her younger brother and only sibling, Dr. Louis J. Cella, Jr., inherited the property. When he opened its doors to the curators from RISD's Museum, the world of two early twentieth-century dressmakers and their clients, and indeed of the apparel industry itself, was called up from the dust of many years.

The interviews referred to and quoted in this essay are to be found in the A. & L. Tirocchi Archive, Museum of Art, Rhode Island School of Design, Providence [hereafter, Tirocchi Archive]. Such references have not been footnoted. All letters sent or received by Anna or Laura Tirocchi are understood to be found in the Tirocchi Archive. See "Note on the A. & L. Tirocchi Archive, Collection, and Catalogue," p. 23.

1. George H. Kellner and J. Stanley Lemons, *Rhode Island: The Independent State.* Woodland Hills (California): 1982, p. 66.

2. In their interviews, Dr. Louis J. Cella, Jr., and Primrose Tirocchi both mentioned Rose Carraer-Eastman as the early employer of Anna and Laura. Born in Providence in 1872, Rose was the daughter of Irish immigrant parents. Her birth name, Rose Carragher, appears among the practicing Providence dressmakers by 1896. The 1900 *City Directory* indicates that she had set up shop in downtown Providence and had anglicized her name to Rose Carraer. She often moved her business and eventually settled into Room 901 in the Lapham Building on Westminster Street, home to many other dressmakers and women's tailors. In 1905, she married and added her husband's name to her own. Rose Carraer-Eastman carried on her trade until the early 1940s with many changes along the way. She incorporated in 1924, after she began to sell women's ready-to-wear, and in the late 1920s remarried and changed the name of the business to Zarr, Inc., taking on her new husband's name.

3. Wendy Gamber, *The Female Economy: The Millinery and Dressmaking Trades, 1860–1930.* Urbana: 1997, p. 32.

4. Ornella Morelli, "The International Success and Domestic Debut of Postwar Italian Fashion," in Gloria Bianchini, *et. al.,* trans. Paul Blanchard, *Italian Fashion.* New York: 1987, p. 58.

5. Customer day book, 1916–19, p. 1; Tirocchi Archive.

6. Gamber, *op. cit.*, p. 100.

7. Customer day book, 1916–19; Tirocchi Archive.

8. B. Altman & Co., *Advance Styles for Spring and Summer*, 1918; Tirocchi Archive.

9. The *New York Times* headlined Haas Brothers' spring collections in 1921, 1922, and 1925, describing the fabrics in great detail. See "Some New Silk Weaves; They Are Shown Here in Attractive Imported Model Gowns," *New York Times* (March 3, 1921), p. 3; "New Coat Dress Popular in Paris," *New York Times* (March 2, 1922), p. 22; "New Dress Trend in French Models," *New York Times* (March 4, 1925), p. 19.

10. "New Paris Styles Cost France Dearly," *New York Times* (October 2, 1922), p. 4.

11. Elizabeth Ann Coleman, *The Opulent Era: Fashions of Worth, Doucet, and Pingat*. Brooklyn: 1989, p. 11, figs. 1.2, 1.3.

12. Françoise Tétart-Vittu, *Au Paradis des dames: nouveautés, modes et confections, 1810–1870*. Paris: 1992, p. 34, n. 10.

13. Ruth Trowbridge was born on July 7, 1899.

14. The first garment made for Ruth Trowbridge was a spotted foulard model gown from Sidney J. Stern. Her mother, Alice E. Trowbridge, was billed $40 for the gown in April 1917. See client ledger, Spring 1917; Tirocchi Archive.

15. Customer ledger, 1919–21, p. 29; Tirocchi Archive.

16. B. Altman & Company, *Book of Styles*, Spring and Summer 1923, p. 10; Tirocchi Archive.

17. Stella Blum, ed., *Everyday Fashions of the Twenties*. New York: 1981, p. 70.

18. Customer ledger, 1916–17, p. 57; Tirocchi Archive.

19. Elizabeth Ewing, *History of 20th Century Fashion*. London: 1992 (3rd ed.), p. 22. For more information on the development of women's sportswear during the late nineteenth and early twentieth centuries, see Elizabeth Wilson, *Adorned in Dreams*. Berkeley and Los Angeles: 1985, pp. 160–62.

20. "Are Dressmakers Becoming Fewer?," *New York Times* (June 21, 1923), sect. II, p. 7.

21. Philip Scranton, "The Transition from Custom to Ready-to-Wear Clothing in Philadelphia, 1890–1930," *Textile History*, vol. 25, no. 2 (Autumn 1994), p. 258.

22. Anna's former employer and main competitor, Rose Carraer-Eastman, also re-established her dressmaking business as a ready-to-wear concern sometime in 1923. In that year's *Providence City Directory*, she is listed as "Rose Carraer-Eastman, dressmaker." In 1924, she incorporated the business as "Rose Carraer, Inc. Gowns" and was no longer listed under dressmakers in the directory, but could be found among the women's clothing retailers.

23. Vendor accounts books, 1919–22, 1923–24, and 1924–25; Tirocchi Archive.

24. Gamber, *op. cit.*, p. 158.

25. E. Wilson, *op. cit.*, p. 77.

26. Tétart-Vittu, *op. cit.*, p. 42 (translation by Pamela A. Parmal).

27. For an interesting look at the Paris fashion industry of 1924 from a male perspective, see Robert Forrest Wilson, *Paris on Parade*. New York: 1932 (3rd ed.). For a discussion of Jean Patou and Lucien Lelong, see *ibid.*, pp. 71–75.

28. Caroline Milbank, *New York Fashion: The Evolution of American Style*. New York: 1996, p. 75.

29. Merchandise received and returned ledger, Fall 1927, pp. 38–39; Tirocchi Archive.

30. Maginnis & Thomas, order no. 11, January 11, 1926; Tirocchi Archive.

31. Customer day book, 1924–25, p. 3; vendor accounts book, 1924–25, p. 34; customer ledger, 1924–25, p. 69; Tirocchi Archive.

32. Vendor accounts book, 1924–25; Tirocchi Archive.

33. "Intend to War on Some Trade Evils," *New York Times* (March 17, 1924), p. 25.

34. Letter, *New York Times* (March 29, 1925), sect. II, p. 15.

35. "Seeking to Reach Dodging Buyers," *New York Times* (April 30, 1922), sect. II, p. 11.

36. According to R. F. Wilson, *op. cit.*, p. 50, public shows of couturiers' lines were held every afternoon in Paris.

37. This transaction appears in the customer ledger from the 1940s; however, Anna was quite proud of her ability to bring the veil back to life, and in June of 1940 used the story of its cleaning to enter a contest held by the Ivory Soap Flakes Company. Contestants were asked to express in twenty-five words or less why they used Ivory Soap Flakes. Anna sent along an additional letter explaining, at length, the story of the veil (letters of June 3 and 4, 1940). Textile conservators now know that even brief exposure to sunlight is damaging to fiber and discourage such practices as sun-bleaching.

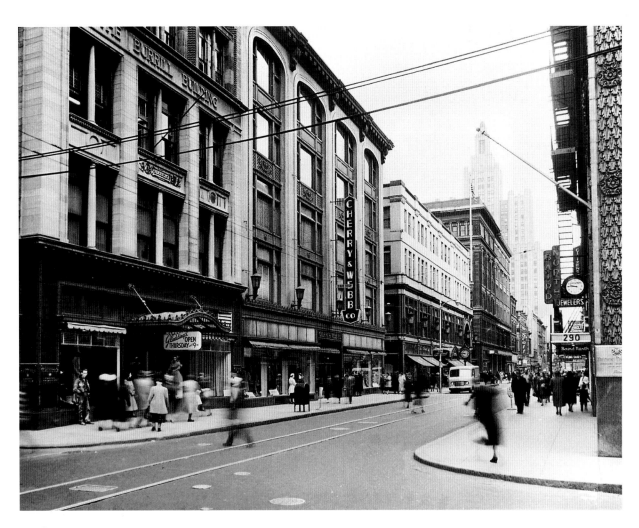

Fig. 36
Department stores on Westminster Street in downtown
Providence, which competed with the Tirocchi dressmaking shop
for clients; ca. 1951. Courtesy Rhode Island Historical Society,
Providence (photograph by Allan B. McCoy).

SUSAN PORTER BENSON
Associate Professor of History
University of Connecticut, Storrs

Clients and Craftswomen:

The Pursuit of Elegance

Two very different groups of women frequented the A. & L. Tirocchi dressmaking shop at 514 Broadway: the mostly Italian working-class immigrants and immigrant daughters who did the sewing and the wealthy Yankee women of the Providence elite who bought and wore the products of their hands. From one point of view, a vast gulf measured by differences in economic position, nativity, residence, religion, and language yawned between them. At the same time, they shared a small patch of common ground in a world increasingly given over to the impersonal transactions of mass production and mass consumption. Tirocchi seamstresses and clients alike had deep roots in a more old-fashioned world, one in which custom production and reuse of material goods testified to a more individualized and frugal sensibility. That world was certainly not egalitarian, but it was one in which a humble apprentice earning three dollars a week and the wife of a powerful industrialist shared certain values. Each could find satisfaction in fine workmanship and in the thrifty remodeling of an old but still serviceable garment.

The Tirocchi shop flourished during a transitional period in the manufacture and consumption of women's clothing. If the sisters had been plying their trade a century earlier in Providence, their business would have been typical of makers and purveyors of women's clothing. In early nineteenth-century America, women generally acquired their apparel in one of three ways: they made it themselves; they bought it second-hand; or they had it custom-made by seamstresses like Anna and Laura Tirocchi. Most well-to-do women relied primarily on custom dressmaking. During the first half of the nineteenth century, ready-made women's clothing was limited to cloaks and corsets, items that could be made in relatively standard ways. Underwear had joined this array by the 1870s.[1] Ready-made dresses, suits, skirts, and waists (blouses) were widely available by the turn of the century, but most were too crude and unfashionable for the tastes of the Tirocchi clientele. By the eve of World War I, however, manufacturers were offering women a combination of fashion and quality in off-the-rack garments. Ironically, it was just at this point in the development of the larger dressmaking world that the Tirocchi sisters established their business. They were clearly going against the tide of change, as the market for custom-made clothes was declining in importance. It is a testimony to the sewing skills, artistic sense, and business acumen of the sisters, especially Anna, that the enterprise flourished in an increasingly hostile economic context.

A new awareness of fashion, emerging in the 1920s, fueled the expansion of the ready-made women's clothing industry and had a mixed effect on custom dressmaking. Elite Americans had long been aware of the trends emanating from Paris and other fashion centers, but after World War I, haute couture received extensive coverage in the mass media as well as in high-end publications like *Vogue*. Custom dressmakers stood ready to provide wealthy women with wardrobes that would distinguish them from the legions who bought ever more fashionable clothes off the rack. At the same time, though, retail advertising and the fashion press urged upper-class ladies to change their costumes more often and to build larger and more varied wardrobes of garments suitable for every conceivable occasion. The higher price of custom-made apparel forced even wealthy women to choose between distinctive smaller wardrobes of custom-made frocks and larger wardrobes that mixed ready-made with custom-tailored garments.

Changes in retailing as well as manufacturing and fashion were also undercutting the position of the custom dressmaker. Department stores [fig. 36] and small specialty shops catered to the wealthy by offering high-quality and high-fashion clothing in lavish settings that echoed the homes and clubs to which these women were accustomed. Department stores such as the Shepard Company and the Outlet Company in downtown Providence produced the illusion of democracy by opening their stores to shoppers who were "just looking," by charging fixed prices rather than bargaining with customers, and by offering a broad range of clothing and household goods in price-segregated departments. In fact, however, all shoppers were emphatically not seen as equal by the merchants who ran these enormous stores. They sought most eagerly the same customers who frequented the Tirocchi establishment: those with substantial disposable income that allowed them to purchase more lavish wardrobes than the working-class majority, who could only afford an occasional extravagance. For their wealthiest customers, department stores reserved luxurious accommodations on the premises and offered a wide range of special services. Small department stores – for example, Gladding's in downtown Providence – and specialty shops offering similar high-end merchandise competed for elite customers' dollars. More frankly exclusive than large department stores, these businesses also used lavish décor and personal service to attract wealthy clients who would return again and again. Although both types of stores primarily sold ready-made clothing, they offered alteration services and some custom tailoring to meet the demands of well-to-do clients.[2]

Shops such as A. & L. Tirocchi faced stiff competition. The new ways of making and selling apparel offered an approximation of the exclusivity, fashion, and precise fit that had long been the dressmaker's stock-in-trade. To a large extent, Anna and Laura fought fire with fire, albeit with their own special flair. The Tirocchi sisters moved from a downtown office building to a substantial mansion on fashionable Broadway and fitted it out as luxuriously as their most pretentious competitors. Dr. Louis J. Cella, Jr., son of Laura Tirocchi, remembered that the first-floor parlor, which customers passed on their way to the showroom in the second-floor billiard room, featured an elaborate round three-person Victorian seat centered under an imposing chandelier. In the billiard room, customers could choose their fabrics from artfully draped arrays. Although the Broadway mansion housed both manufacturing and sales, the spaces devoted to making the garments were hidden away on the third floor. Stuart Blumin pointed to this separation between the venues of consumption and production as a mark of developing middle-class life in the nineteenth century, an economic and social experience limited to a minority of the population until World War II.[3] As shopping became more of a mass experience conducted in a very public setting, the Tirocchis offered personal attention and privacy. Tirocchi service was extremely individualized. Each garment could be made from a customer's fabric of choice and tailored to her figure and specifications. Although a customer might be just as warmly received and well known at an exclusive ready-to-wear shop, it was only at 514 Broadway that her exact dimensions were embodied in two sets of measurements on a dress form, one for her torso and another for her arm. A woman went to the Tirocchis not to be dazzled by the huge array of goods and spectacular, brightly-lit displays that characterized the downtown shopping district, nor to rendezvous with friends as they might at the Shepard Company's tearoom. The wealthy client sought out the Tirocchis for an experience of quiet elegance, heavily insulated from the public world of commerce.

Anna and Laura Tirocchi took a second leaf from the ready-made retailers' book in the mid-1920s, when they began to stock some ready-made items and to order high-end ready-made dresses for their customers, so that entire ensembles from underwear to hats and purses could be purchased at their shop. It is a maxim of retailing that the more one can sell to each customer, the higher the profits. The Tirocchi sisters offered their customers fine underwear imported from Italy and France, accessories, and table and bed linens. As seamstress and Tirocchi niece Emily Valcarenghi Martinelli put it: "Well, they used to sell everything and anything. When a customer wanted it, she had it." Another technique for competing with larger retailers was the use of "robes": pieces of beaded and/or embroidered cloth bearing the general outline of a gown, ready to be cut and fashioned into custom-tailored dresses. The Tirocchis ordered their "robes" from New York manufacturers/importers. Because much of the handwork had been done outside the shop, dresses made from "robes" were less expensive than comparable garments made entirely on the shop's premises. An extensive stock of "robes" was found in the Tirocchi workshop when its contents were inventoried in 1990–92 by RISD curators. These embellished dress pieces were especially well suited to the unconstructed chemise style of dress that became popular during the 1920s. The establishment also offered specialty services such as washing and restoring fine lace.[4]

The Tirocchi shop flourished despite its competitors. Anna, especially, was a canny businesswoman, but more crucial to the shop's appeal was the sisters' artistic and technical skill. They designed and supervised the construction of clothing that pleased and flattered their customers, and they were craftswomen of the first rank, probably the equal of any plying their trade in Europe or America. Ruth Trowbridge Smith remembered that when she wore her Tirocchi-made going-away suit on her honeymoon in Paris, people "thought it was the snappiest – where was it made they wanted to know."[5] Both the dressmakers and their customers valued this type of work, but they also rejected planned obsolescence, which became increasingly pervasive in the United States as the twentieth century progressed. They saw custom-made garments as long-term investments rather than throwaways. The fine apparel constructed by the Tirocchis was repeatedly retailored to fit changing fashions, social needs, and body shapes. Many wealthy clients shared the old-fashioned, thrifty mentality of Emily Valcarenghi Martinelli, who asked rhetorically, "Why throw anything away?" Mrs. Richard LeBaron Bowen typified this attitude when she purchased four new custom-tailored outfits in a single year, but also had four older ones made over.

Other aspects of their lives also predisposed Anna's clients to patronize the Tirocchi shop. As a group, their activities included a variety of social events, each occasion requiring its appropriate dress [fig. 37]. They demanded clothing that was not just suitable, but also attractive, fashionable, and new. Very few such customers held paying jobs, devoting themselves instead to the unpaid work that was a mark of their social class: home management, entertaining, and activity in clubs and social-service

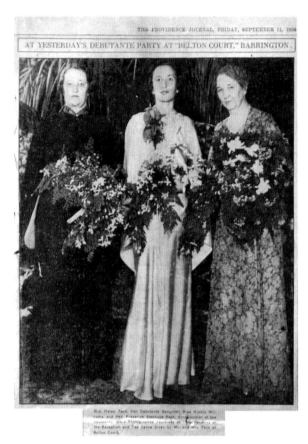

Fig. 37
Three generations of Tirocchi clients: (left to right) Helen Peck Williams, her daughter Marcia Williams, and her mother Mary Burlingame Peck (Mrs. Frederick Stanhope Peck) at Marcia's "coming-out" party in 1930 (reproduced by permission of the *Providence Journal*); Tirocchi Archive.

organizations. Among the shop's few wage-earning clients were Alice P. Brownell, an assistant court clerk, and sisters Anna and Mary Daley, who were nurses. It is not at all surprising that Brownell appears in the Tirocchi record books only for $15 worth of alterations in 1921, but it is notable that the Daley sisters together spent nearly $400 in the early 1920s for three custom-made garments and one "make-over." These expenditures probably made them the best-dressed nurses in the city, but perhaps they were not typical nurses. In 1919, Mary (and most likely her sister as well) traveled to Europe, and by 1923, she was writing to Anna Tirocchi from fashionable Brookline, Massachusetts, where she lived with her manufacturer husband.[6]

The overwhelming majority of Tirocchi clients spent money that they had inherited or their husbands had earned. The spouses of Providence customers were prominent lawyers (Harvey A. Baker); physicians (Martin S. Budlong); bankers (Michael F. Dooley); brokers (Frank D. Lisle, Pardon Miller); insurance executives (Harold J. Gross, William E. Maynard, James F. Phetteplace); and executives in the state's industrial concerns: textiles (Richard LeBaron Bowen, Arthur D. Champlin, Henry A. DuVillard, E. Fielding Jones, David S. Seaman, Edward R. Trowbridge), jewelry (William P. Chapin, Jr; Ashbel T. Wall, Sr.), precision tools (Paul Churchill DeWolf), and office equipment (Thomas Arnold Briggs and Frank D. Simmons). Some were involved in the expansion of the thriving city. Benjamin Harris was a construction engineer, Stephen Harris a real estate agent, and William M. Harris a prominent lumber dealer. Byron S. Watson was a supplier of wholesale boots and shoes. Others were engaged in less obviously remunerative but genteel occupations, such as Howard Chapin, librarian of the Rhode Island Historical Society, or sculptor E. Edwin Codman. Many husbands had broad interests bridging the manufacturing and financial sectors, such as Samuel Mowry Nicholson, who was president of American Screw Company and Nicholson File Company and chaired the Board of Directors of the Industrial Trust Company; and Frederick Stanhope Peck, who was involved in textile manufacture, coal and oil supply, and stock and bond dealing, as well as Republican party politics. Mrs. Walter (Ivy) Callender, married to the president of a major downtown Providence clothing store (Callender, McAuslan and Troup), spent nearly $1500 with the Tirocchis in 1930, instead of wearing the ready-mades available in her husband's store.

One of the puzzles of this project has been to discover why certain members of the Rhode Island and nearby Connecticut and Fall River elites came to the Tirocchi shop. Clients shared a variety of characteristics in addition to their wealth. They belonged to many of the same organizations and many lived in some proximity to one another. Of one hundred Providence clients whose addresses were found for the period 1916 to 1920, ninety lived on Providence's East Side, mostly on streets where large single-family houses of a certain grandeur set the standard [see fig. 3, p. 13; figs. 8–9, p. 19]. Of those ninety, moreover, sixty-four lived in the sector bounded by Olney Street, Hope Street, Stimson Avenue, Governor Street, Williams Street, and Benefit Street in the East Side's stately, aristocratic core, built primarily in the eighteenth and nineteenth centuries. Some clients were very close neighbors: Ivy Callender and Ella Jones lived next door to each other at 196 and 198 Hope Street; Florence Elgar and Elizabeth Smith resided across the street from each other at 169 and 170 Brown Street. At least five Tirocchi clients each were to be found on Brown, Lloyd, Bowen, Waterman, and George Streets, and six lived at the Minden, a residential hotel at 123 Waterman Street [fig. 38]. All but one of the remaining twenty-six East Side clients lived east of Hope Street and north of Waterman Street, an area with somewhat newer but still substantial homes built in the early twentieth century. This group of clients was more widely dispersed than those in the core East Side area. Of the ten Providence clients who did not live on the East Side, nine resided on the West Side, within a radius of about a mile and a half of the Tirocchi shop. The surviving client record books show no clear change over time in the residential patterns of the clientele [see p. 74].

The Tirocchis' Providence customers were further linked by their shared leisure and civic activities. Out of a sample of eighty-five women (roughly one fourth of the clients), fifty were listed in the 1932 edition of *The Blue Book for Providence and Nearby Cities*, in effect a social register for the city. *The Blue Book* asked those named therein to report club membership. The Women's Republican Club of Rhode Island received more mentions (thirty) than any other single organization named by either clients or their husbands. It is not surprising that these women and their families would cast their lot with the Republican Party, which dominated state politics until the Great Depression and, with some Democratic defectors, kept a brake on regulatory and protective legislation in the state. It is notable, however, that the Women's Republican Club attracted even more members than exclusive social organizations such as the Agawam Hunt Club [fig. 39], in

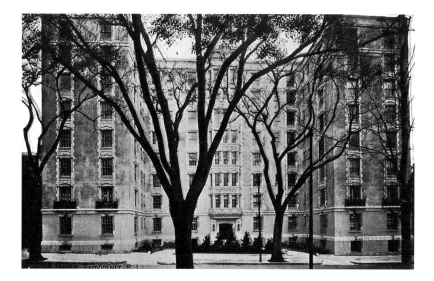

Fig. 38
The Minden, Waterman and Brook Streets, a residential hotel on Providence's East Side where a number of customers lived; ca. 1910. Courtesy Rhode Island Historical Society, Providence (photograph by Charles H. Seddon Publisher).

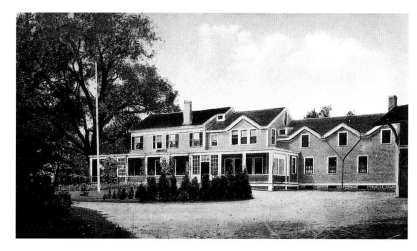

Fig. 39
The Agawam Hunt Club in East Providence (across the Seekonk River from Providence's East Side), most popular of the social clubs to which Tirocchi clients belonged; ca. 1900. Courtesy Rhode Island Historical Society, Providence (photograph by Rhode Island News Company).

which twenty-seven women reported membership. In general, though, the Tirocchi clients and their husbands reported the largest number of memberships (125) in elite social clubs that included the Agawam Hunt, the Rhode Island Country Club, and the East Side Skating Club. Organizations devoted to intellectual and artistic pursuits, still within an exclusive social context, were the second most popular category. Clients and their husbands reported 101 memberships in such groups as the Rhode Island Historical Society, the Providence Athenaeum [figs. 40–41], the Providence Art Club [figs. 42–43], and the Handicraft Club. Exclusive

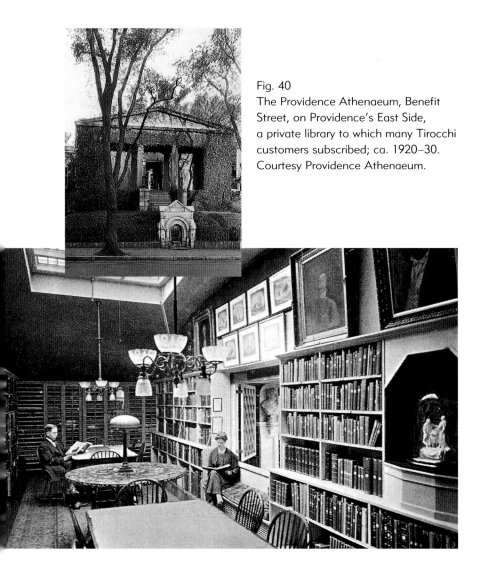

Fig. 40
The Providence Athenaeum, Benefit Street, on Providence's East Side, a private library to which many Tirocchi customers subscribed; ca. 1920–30. Courtesy Providence Athenaeum.

Fig. 41
Reading room in the Providence Athenaeum; ca. 1920–30. Courtesy Providence Athenaeum.

men's clubs, such as the Turk's Head Club, the Hope Club [fig. 44], and the Squantum Association [fig. 45], counted fifty-nine customers' husbands among their members. Thirty-two belonged to organizations for those of early American lineage, among them the National Society of Colonial Dames and the Society of Colonial Wars.[7]

As a group, the Tirocchi customers and their husbands were focused on the local rather than the national scene. Only three customers reported membership in national organizations or organizations outside Rhode Island, all of which were either affiliated with the Republican Party or were similar to the in-state clubs to which they belonged. Clients' husbands also were locally focused. A handful belonged to national groups celebrating family lineage or to clubs in other states similar to the yacht clubs and city clubs that they frequented in Rhode Island.

The most glaring omission in the list of Providence customers' club memberships is the absence of women's reform organizations devoted to "social housekeeping" in the early twentieth century. Even the relatively staid but still feminist American Association of University Women, although it did attract other women listed in *The Blue Book*, did not number a single Tirocchi client in its ranks. *The Blue Book* did not list memberships in organizations more active in social reform, but a search of such organizations' records reveals that Tirocchi customers took part only in the most conservative and timid of them. Twenty-nine of the women in the sample of eighty-five were affiliated in some way with the Irrepressible Society. Founded in 1863, the Irrepressible Society brought women together to sew first for Union soldiers, then later for former slaves; but after the Civil War its attention shifted to "the general charitable work of the city." The Irrepressible members distributed coal and food to the city's poor, as well as garments they either sewed themselves or paid poor women to sew [fig. 46]. As charity work became more professionalized and rationalized, the Irrepressibles gradually de-emphasized volunteer participation, turned much of the casework over to professionals, and focused more narrowly on aiding the disabled rather than the larger universe of the poor. By the 1920s, its focus was almost

Fig. 42
The Providence Art Club (on the downtown edge of the East Side), an organization with many Tirocchi customers among its membership; ca. 1920–30. Courtesy Providence Art Club.

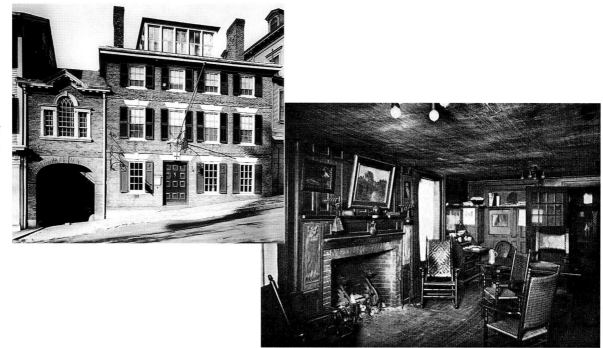

Fig. 43
Interior view of the Providence Art Club; ca. 1920–30. Courtesy Providence Art Club.

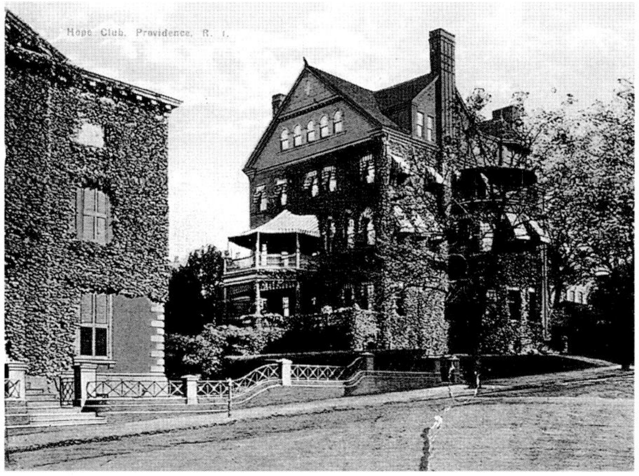

Fig. 44
The Hope Club, Benevolent Street, on Providence's East Side, a men's city club numbering husbands of Tirocchi customers among its members, ca. 1920–30: a corner of the home of Tirocchi client Mrs. Jack (Harriet Sprague Watson) Lewis at 2 Benevolent Street appears on the left side of the photograph and may be seen to almost equal the size of the Hope Club. Courtesy Hope Club, Providence.

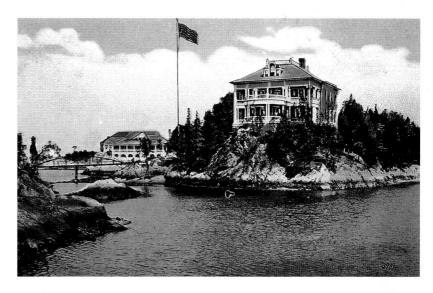

Fig. 45
The Squantum Association in East Providence (across the Seekonk River from Providence's East Side), a social resort frequented by Tirocchi customers and their families. Courtesy Squantum Association, East Providence.

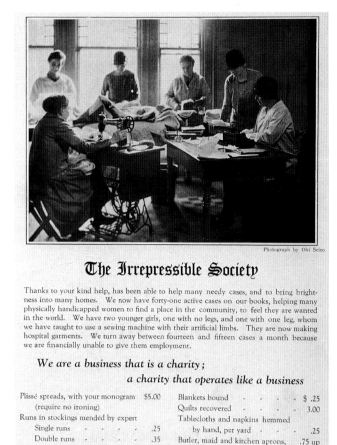

Photograph by Oki Seizo

The Irrepressible Society

Thanks to your kind help, has been able to help many needy cases, and to bring brightness into many homes. We now have forty-one active cases on our books, helping many physically handicapped women to find a place in the community, to feel they are wanted in the world. We have two younger girls, one with no legs, and one with one leg, whom we have taught to use a sewing machine with their artificial limbs. They are now making hospital garments. We turn away between fourteen and fifteen cases a month because we are financially unable to give them employment.

We are a business that is a charity;

a charity that operates like a business

Plissé spreads, with your monogram $5.00	Blankets bound	- - -	$ .25
(require no ironing)	Quilts recovered	- - -	3.00
Runs in stockings mended by expert	Tablecloths and napkins hemmed		
Single runs - - - - .25	by hand, per yard	- -	.25
Double runs - - - - .35	Butler, maid and kitchen aprons,		.75 up

We make anything. See our attractive articles on sale at

THE JUNIOR LEAGUE SHOP

Fig. 46
Page from the Junior League's 1928 program for *Oh Boy,*
a theatrical presentation/fundraiser: the Irrepressible Society
was a group that attracted many Tirocchi customers to its
approach to aiding the poor (reproduced by permission of the
Junior League of Providence). Tirocchi Archive.

exclusively on running a store to sell poor women's sewing products. Most of the Tirocchi clients were minimally involved with the Irrepressible Society as subscribers, a status which required only a dollar's annual contribution. By 1926, the organization had been absorbed into the Junior League, and Junior League programs for the late 1920s indicate that Tirocchi customers sewed clothing for sale in the Junior League shop.[8]

Eight customers in the sample were affiliated with the Women's City Missionary Society (founded in 1867), which continued the tradition of friendly visits to the poor in their homes into the 1930s, long after it had become an obsolete tactic in the fight against poverty. Two clients were prominent in the Ladies' Aid Association of the Homeopathic Hospital of Rhode Island: Mary Burlingame Peck, one of the Tirocchis' most faithful customers, and Mary Colt Gross, who wore Tirocchi clothes throughout the 1920s and 30s [figs. 47–48]. In short, Providence customers tended to engage social problems through long-standing organizations rooted in a tradition that was linked to small-scale, meliorist relief of individuals' poverty or to conventional charity work, rather than to the building of a regulatory welfare state that would undertake systemic reform.[9]

Despite the fact that Tirocchi customers tended to live in the same neighborhood and to belong to the same conservative social and charitable organizations, the fact remains that most members of those clubs and most residents of those neighborhoods did not frequent the Tirocchi shop. All of the factors that led women to patronize the Tirocchis will never be known, but kinship and close friendship certainly played a powerful role. In the firm's address books, especially those for the 1930s, many entries include such notations as "Mrs. Brayton's friend," "Peck's sister-in-law," "Mrs. Horton's daughter," and "Mrs. Booth her mother." Presumably, many customers and the connections among them were so well known to the Tirocchi sisters that such notations were unnecessary, and the recorded connections were but a small fraction of the total number of family relationships. This interpretation is supported by the fact that these notations most

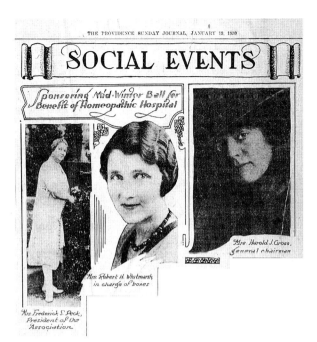

SOCIAL EVENTS

Sponsoring Mid-Winter Ball for
Benefit of Homeopathic Hospital

Mrs. Harold J. Gross,
general chairman

Mrs. Robert H. Whitmarsh,
in charge of boxes

Mrs. Frederick S. Peck,
President of the
Association

Fig. 47
Mrs. Frederick S. (Mary Burlingame) Peck (left)
and Mrs. Harold J. (Mary Colt) Gross (right)
planned the Annual Ball of the Ladies' Aid
Association of the Homeopathic Hospital of
Rhode Island; 1930 (reproduced by permission
of the *Providence Journal*). Tirocchi Archive.

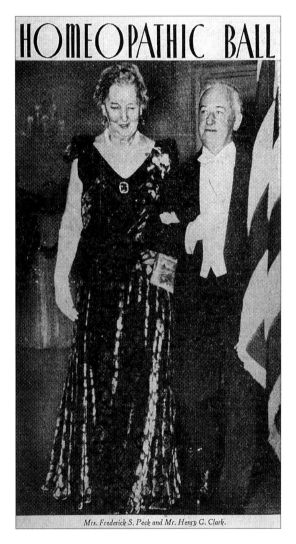

HOMEOPATHIC BALL

Mrs. Frederick S. Peck and Mr. Henry G. Clark.

Fig. 48
Mrs. Frederick S. (Mary Burlingame) Peck enjoying
the Homeopathic Hospital Ball, which she had
helped to organize; 1930 (reproduced by permission
of the *Providence Journal*). Tirocchi Archive.

often referred to out-of-town clients, identifying
those whose ties might not have been so well known
as those of local customers.

A close look at the largest cluster of out-of-town
clients – those from Fall River, Massachusetts (about
seventeen miles to the east of Providence) – rein-
forces the importance of kin ties among the Tirocchi
clientele. Twelve Fall River women bought clothing from the Tirocchis. Of these, nine were close kin:
two mother-daughter pairs, a mother and her two
daughters, and a mother-in-law and her daughter-
in-law. Clearly, clothes shopping was an activity with
intergenerational appeal. Of the three women not
linked by kinship, one lived across the street from
the mother in one of the mother-daughter pairs.
Once again, however, kin connections were part of
a larger web of class-based links. If anything, these
women were part of an even tighter economic elite
than their Providence counterparts. Seven of eleven
husbands whose occupations were found held powerful positions in the city's textile industry; one of
the seven also led two of Fall River's largest banks.
The other four husbands were a physician, a leading
coal dealer, a newspaper publisher, and a retired
admiral. What remains murky, however tightly

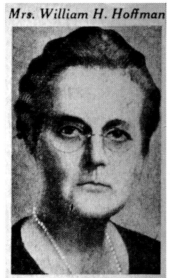

Mrs. William H. Hoffman

RHODE ISLAND Girl Scout organizer who died yesterday after a long illness.

Fig. 49
Mrs. William H. (Mira) Hoffman; 1940 (reproduced by permission of the *Providence Journal*). Tirocchi Archive.

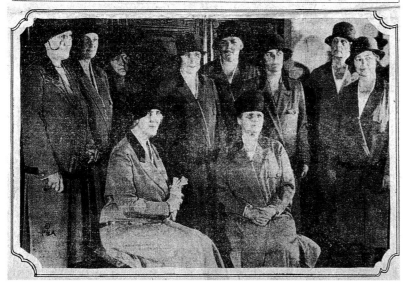

National Executives of Girl Scouts at New York Exhibition

They opened the showing of antiques loaned from some of the finest collections, now on at the American Art Galleries in New York City and the $3,900,000 drive for a five-year development program of this organization. Photo taken at the American Galleries shows, left to right, back row, Mrs. Louis Myers, Mrs. A. O. Choate, Miss Elizabeth Gunther, Mrs. Nicholas Brady, Mrs. Jane D. Rippin, National Director; Mrs. Walter Rothchild, Mrs. Frederick Edey, Mrs. Arthur Hartt. Front row, Mrs. Herbert Hoover, and Mrs. William H. Hoffman, President of the organization.

Fig. 50
Mrs. William H. (Mira) Hoffman (bottom right) and other Girl Scout executives with Mrs. Herbert Hoover (bottom left), as noted in the *Providence Evening Bulletin* (September 28, 1929): Mira Hoffman dedicated much of her life to Girl Scouting in Rhode Island, as well as to local organizations in her hometown of Barrington, Rhode Island (reproduced by permission of the *Providence Journal*). Tirocchi Archive.

linked the Fall River women may have been, is what brought them first to the Tirocchi shop. One connection may have been Adelaide Danforth of Providence, who began to frequent the shop in 1916 and who was an aunt of Dorothy Newton and a friend of Charlotte Robinson, two of the Fall River clients.[10]

Seven of the Fall River women's civic activities have left traces in the historical record. All of these belonged to the Women's Union, six were members of the Fall River Women's Club, and two were members of the Junior League. The Women's Union served the city's wage-earning women in a manner similar to a big-city YWCA, operating a residence, a store at which women's products were sold, and a center for social and educational activities. Three Tirocchi customers sat on the boards of local institutions – two served the hospital, one the children's home. The Fall River women were more engaged with the city's civic and welfare activities than their Providence counterparts, perhaps because Fall River was a smaller, single-industry city, while Providence was more populous and economically diversified.[11]

The possibility that customers in smaller towns were more involved in social-welfare activities is further supported by the long and distinguished career of Mira Hoffman of Barrington, Rhode Island [fig. 49]. In some respects, she fit the profile of the typical customer, residing with her husband William H. Hoffman on fashionable Rumstick Point in Barrington and belonging to such organizations as the Women's Republican Club, the Agawam Hunt Club, the Rhode Island Country Club, and the Society of Colonial Dames. She was far more active, however, both nationally and locally than most of those who wore Tirocchi clothes. A founder of Girl Scouting in Rhode Island, she was the state Commissioner of Girl Scouts from 1923 to 1926 and the national president of the Girl Scouts from 1926 to 1928 [fig. 50]. On the state level, she sat on the Rhode Island Board of Education from 1921 to 1932 and worked with the Rhode Island Infantile Paralysis Association. At the same time, this energetic woman was deeply involved in Barrington "social housekeeping." She founded the Maple Avenue Community House Association, a kind of settlement house for Italian immigrants, as well as the Barrington District Nurses' Association. She was also a trustee of the St. Andrew's Industrial School for Boys.[12]

Another way to examine the composition of the Tirocchi clientele is to ask who was not represented among the customers. Although Anna and Laura Tirocchi were themselves Italian immigrants and lived near other Italian immigrants, Italian names appear only once in the client books. In 1927, the Tirocchi sisters made a wedding gown and dress for Rochele Vervena's marriage to Ferdinando Tortolani. Her mother [fig. 70, p. 89] and father lived on Cushing Street, and the newlyweds took up residence on South Angell Street – both fashionable East Side streets where the Tirocchi clientele were clustered. Mariano Vervena, the Italian vice-consul in Providence, shared class and cultural connections (he was president of the Columbus Exchange Trust Company and a member of the Providence Art Club, among others) with other Tirocchi customers' husbands and was almost certainly perceived as socially distinct from the Italian immigrants who populated the West Side of the city, a predominantly working-class group engaged in unskilled labor, factory work, or skilled crafts such as stonecutting, barbering, or baking.[13]

That few Providence Italians wore Tirocchi clothing was neither an accident nor a function of poverty. Many wealthy Italians, such as the members of the Aurora Club, could easily have afforded the prices charged at 514 Broadway. Primrose Tirocchi pointed out that Anna had begun her career in Rome as an apprentice to a dressmaker with an aristocratic clientele and that Anna "aimed for the same thing when she came to this country." In the United States, Anna targeted wealthy old-stock clients – the American equivalent of the aristocrats to whom her Roman employer catered – rather than the newly rich. Primrose noted that "she would turn Italians down. Not that she was prejudiced; it's just their attitude and what they expected. Anna said she was just going to handle who appreciates what I'm [sic] doing." Anna Tirocchi's reliance on the patronage of the established elite was not evidence of social climbing, for she appears to have kept her social life separate from that of her clients. She never, according to former worker Mary Rosa Traverso, mingled with her clients either in their homes or at her vacation retreat in Narragansett, a summer resort popular with well to to Rhode Islanders. Anna Tirocchi used the power that her artistry, skill, and sense of style brought her to choose the class of people for whom she would work. The husband of seamstress Mary Riccitelli Basilico, who worked for Anna throughout the early 1930s, remembered that Anna turned away Italian clients even during the worst years of the Depression, and Traverso emphasized that it was word of mouth more than advertising (Anna advertised only in the Junior League programs) that brought clients to the shop door.

Letters in the Tirocchi Archive offer a unique picture of relations between the Tirocchi shop and its customers. Most were written by clients, but a few are copies of letters written by Anna. They reveal relationships that range from the hostile and occasionally threatening through the businesslike and matter-of-fact to the friendly and even affectionate. The obvious caveat in using these letters as research materials is that most of them come from clients who lived or were traveling outside of Providence. They give us only the rarest glimpses of the more frequent dressmaker-client contacts over the telephone or in the house on Broadway. Such shortcomings aside, this correspondence constitutes the finest and fullest collection of letters to a single dressmaker in the United States. Wendy Gamber, author of the definitive study of custom dressmaking, used letters found in a search of clients' papers and was unable to construct the broad picture of one establishment that the Tirocchi Archive offers.[14]

The letters show that the relationships between the Tirocchi sisters and their clients were fraught with potential for sharp conflict and bitter recriminations, but also were graced with mutual satisfaction and deep gratification. Some reveal what appears to have been a genuine friendship between Anna and a client. Vacationing in Florida in 1940, Mira Hoffman sent Anna a gift; Anna's chatty thank-you letter bespeaks real feeling between the two, although not without a hint of flattery on Anna's part when she ended, "Please give us the pleasure to see you look twenty years younger when you return to Providence." Satisfied customers' letters reflected the pleasure they took in their Tirocchi clothing: Mrs. E. G. Butler wrote, "I know that you will be interested to know that my two gowns arrived safely on Monday and I was delighted to receive them. I have not yet tried them on but doubt not that they will be alright. Thank you so much for sending them."[15]

Clients were especially generous in their praise when the clothing was for a special occasion such as a wedding, and their letters indicate that when things went well between dressmaker and client, it could be gratifying to both. Alice Trowbridge wrote in the warmest terms to the Tirocchi sisters after her daughter Ruth's wedding: "I take great pleasure in sending you the enclosed check and wish you both to know that Mr. Trowbridge and I both appreciate the attention you showed us and the pleasure you evidently took in your work for our daughter, and we feel that your charges are very fair indeed." The Trowbridge wedding was not the only one for which Anna extended herself. Fall River bride Dorothy Newton thanked Anna for her gift of velvet for her wedding slippers. Weddings apparently created the ideal conditions for mutual satisfaction: elaborate clothing enhanced the pleasure of the occasion for the bride and her family at the same time that it gave the Tirocchi sisters an opportunity to showcase their talents.[16]

Satisfied customers praised the sisters' work, but with more attention to their friends' reactions to the clothes than to the dressmakers' skill and artistry. Scholars who have explored the history of female beauty in the United States have repeatedly noted the tendency to encourage women to judge themselves by the way others see them, and the letters in the Tirocchi Archive corroborate this point. When Charlotte Robinson Luther wore a new Tirocchi dress to a luncheon, "everybody thought it was lovely." Luther did not offer her own opinion of the dress, or comment on its style or construction, but only her reflection in others' eyes. On another occasion she wrote from New York, "Having a nice

time and my friends like my clothes very much – guess I look better than most people." Elizabeth Phetteplace noted that a dress and coat ensemble had "been much admired"; Lucy Wall referred to a dress as a "great hit" and "a great sensation." The clothes crafted by the Tirocchi sisters clearly played a prominent role in the social lives of these wealthy women, enhancing their ability to perform as expected of their class and gender. Rarely, though, did customers explicitly attribute the credit for their appearance to their dressmakers. Mrs. Wall was unusual in doing so when, in the letter cited above, she referred to the acclaim for her dress as "a good compliment for you" and wrote that her friends thought it had come from Paris, a comment sure to warm Anna's heart. Even so, Wall undercut the praise by using the possessive in telling her friends, "Our Anna made it for me," reducing Anna's status from skilled artist and autonomous businesswoman to servant.[17]

Indeed, the relationship between the Tirocchis and their customers had more than a whiff of the servant and mistress relationship about it, although wealthy women's dealings with their servants are rarely simple and straightforward. Despite the servant's subordination to the mistress, the cliché that "no man is a hero to his valet" would doubly apply to servants and their mistresses. Wall's use of the possessive may have put Anna in her place, but Anna's skills made her customers as dependent upon her as she was on them. Even one of the Tirocchis' most quarrelsome clients bowed to Anna's judgment when she wrote, "I don't know what I want – I guess I would be happy with either you decide as being best for me so will leave it to you to do what you think will be the best and prettiest and most appropriate for me." Mrs. E. G. Butler assured Anna that "I would be guided by your judgment." Out-of-town customers were particularly reliant upon the Tirocchi sisters to make decisions for them, but it is easy to imagine customers who visited 514 Broadway asking the same questions about the suitability of color, fabric, and cut as they looked at fabric samples in the billiard room. Emily Valcarenghi Martinelli recalled exactly this sort of scene: "They would say,

'Anna, what do you think? I'm going to this wedding.' Or 'I'm going to this so-and-so and whatever. What do you think I should wear?'"[18]

Even though Anna and Laura and their workers had tailoring skills and artistic insight that their clients may have lacked, these were women's skills and hence demystified, if not devalued. Most elite women did some sewing during their lives and had some understanding of the construction of clothing. In contrast, most elite men were not likely to share or understand the skills of an electrician, a plumber, or a shoemaker. Even though the shop's customers appreciated the Tirocchis' craft, their letters reveal that they often thought they knew both style and construction better than their dressmakers. Elizabeth Phetteplace was not entirely pleased with her "much admired" dress, wishing that "the rhinestone clasp was a little [better] and perhaps a trifle bigger." In fact, the most common theme of the surviving letters is complaint about style, cut, color, or construction.

Mood and personality shaped the customers' remarks: the relationships between clients and dressmakers were intensely personal and unconstrained by bureaucratic or formal procedures. Some women stated their complaints in a matter-of-fact, descriptive way that suggested a desire to get things right rather than to assert a class prerogative. Mrs. E. G. Butler complained mildly – "I am sorry to tell you that I am not quite satisfied with the front of my new gown" – and then wrote ten days later to thank Anna for the changes that she had made. Elizabeth A. Seaman made clear her appreciation for a dress that hadn't come out quite right when she wrote, "Will you give me more room at the bottom of the skirt – I love the dress, but wasn't able to take long enough steps." Often the complaints combine the general and the specific. One woman began an angry letter from Washington, D.C., by asserting that a dress sent to her was "impossible for me to wear as it is" and then went on to criticize the cut, the color, and fit in very concrete terms. Other customers moved beyond anger over specific features to attacks on the Tirocchis' skills. One can only imagine how the proud Anna would have reacted

to a client's allegation that "neither dress was carefully finished"; or to another's that a waist was "a failure" with flaws so obvious that "I can't understand why you could not have seen [them]"; or to a third's threat that "If it is possible to make it *fit*…, I will be glad to have it otherwise I will have to get one somewhere else." The outbursts of anger testify that customers identified so intensely with the most minor details of their clothes that they saw errors as personal insults.[19]

Clients repeatedly demanded the Tirocchis' time and attention in ways that recalled mistresses' unbounded claims on their servants' time. They failed to recognize that the dressmakers were businesswomen with demanding schedules. A Fall River woman wrote on Friday, March 2, 1923, to announce that she would be in Providence on the following Monday for a fitting, clearly assuming that she could be accommodated, and breezily announced that "I have decided to have my clothes made this month instead of April." A Providence client wrote to say that she would appear for a fitting at a certain time on the following day, and another customer wrote a long letter peremptorily demanding two fittings in one day. The latter obviously thought nothing of requiring the shop to drop other work in order to turn its primary attention to fitting, sewing, and fitting her again. A Connecticut woman wheedled instead of demanding: "Can you not arrange it that way? and *would it be possible* for you to have *both* my dresses ready?…I know you are just as busy as can be but perhaps some one who lives nearer would be willing to wait." Customers often complained childishly that someone else had gotten preferential treatment from Anna and Laura.[20]

The Tirocchi customers were covetous of the sisters' time and attention and unhappy when they felt they weren't getting enough of it. Another Fall River client scolded, "Now if you cannot promise me that time let me know immediately and I will look elsewhere. As I have a house to get furnished as well as a dress and wedding to look after." The issues of time and attention could provoke a genteel guerrilla war: when this woman paid a surprise visit to the Tirocchi workshop, she complained that she was told that Anna was "gone and I could not find out when you return." Not to be outdone, she left postage for Anna's reply with the boy – possibly Louis J. Cella, Jr. – who answered the door. A frequent customer perennially complained that Anna was neglecting her clothing, and, after being told one time too many that a fitting was to be delayed, she wrote, "I cant [*sic*] understand why I am constantly put off," and demanded a fitting at the scheduled time because she needed the dress for a luncheon engagement. Customers had a double standard about time. They made unilateral demands on the dressmakers' time, wreaking havoc with their work schedules, but they insisted that the dressmakers respect their own social schedules, thus inverting the business-oriented attitude of the day that time was money and should be valued according to its market rate. Customers' time, an unpaid commodity, took precedence because of the clients' social position. The time of the Tirocchi sisters and their employees, although compensated by wages, was devalued because of their class, painfully

recalling the testimony of domestic servants who had no quarrel with the work they did, but resented bitterly that they were on call around the clock at their employers' whim.[21]

Despite customers' determination to exact deference and coddling from the Tirocchis, in the end the relationship was still a commercial one, and the bills had to be paid. Those bills were substantial, whether compared to the cost of ready-made clothes or to the incomes of the working-class majority. Mrs. H. A. (Margaret) DuVillard ran up an account of $668.50 at the Tirocchi establishment in 1921, about sixty percent of what a male factory worker earned in that year, and the Tirocchis' work for Dorothy Newton's June 1923 wedding came to $1797, a sum substantially higher than most Rhode Island working-class families then lived on for a year. Some customers felt they were getting good value for their money. At least twice, they wrote to request bills for work done. DuVillard made a clumsy joke of asking, "Where is my bill? I have never had to ask for it before – you must be on easy street and maybe are going to make me a present of clothes etc." This sort of joking inversion of the relative financial positions and power of client and dressmaker was apparently part of the verbal byplay of the relationship. Primrose Tirocchi recalled clients – whom she called "ladies" – saying to Anna, "You know, Anna, you have a better house than I do" [fig. 51]. The luxury and beauty of the establishment at 514 Broadway may indeed have galled some of the customers, who perhaps felt that Anna and Laura were putting on airs inappropriate to their social position. Another source of resentment may have been Anna's obvious success and prosperity as an astute businesswoman. Customers uncomfortable with their own financial dependence on male kin may well have resented Anna's independence and resolute adherence to high standards of work.[22]

Money, not surprisingly, became a source of conflict between dressmakers and customers. The blame was clearly two-sided. The Tirocchis ran a custom business where the price for each garment was set individually, and that price reflected not just the Tirocchis' costs but also negotiations between dressmaker and client and the dressmakers' estima-

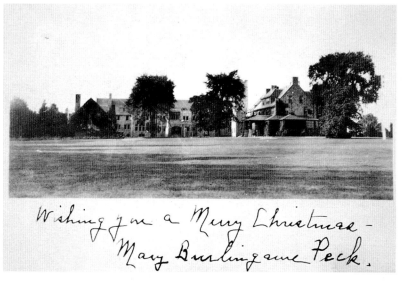

Fig. 51
Holiday card from Mrs. Frederick S. (Mary Burlingame) Peck, made from a photograph of her home on Rumstick Point in Barrington, Rhode Island: it suggests the level of comfort in which most Tirocchi customers lived. Tirocchi Archive.

tion of what the market would bear. A given style of dress would cost less if the customer chose a cheaper fabric, but cost more with every additional bit of work she requested. In the larger commercial culture, fixed prices were the rule, but in the Tirocchi workshop the older practice of mutual agreement on price still prevailed. Customers pushed the sisters to give them firm prices, but then often asked for extras, expecting that the price would remain the same. What might begin as an agreeable discussion of price could end in acrimony. After a visit to 514 Broadway in May 1922, Charlotte Robinson Luther wrote Anna that she would not be able to afford the two dresses they had talked about, saying, "I don't b[l]ame you for going up on your price but I can not this year pay as much." She also took the trouble to list the clothes she had had from the sisters and their prices. When her bill arrived in early August, however, things turned sour. There had been many problems with the garments, alterations were required, and the bill was much higher than Luther had anticipated. She placed the blame squarely on Anna: "The waist of the crepe dress was always a failure so much so that I never wore it but a few times and when I did my friends remarked they wonder if I knew how badly it looked on me that I feel that you were only rectifying your own mistakes." Fortunately, Luther and Tirocchi had a long history of good relations that survived this dispute. Her letter closed: "If I am not doing the correct thing let me know and I wont [sic] bother you again." After Charlotte Luther's death, Anna Tirocchi wrote to Luther's executor that she would "miss her very much, not only for the business part, but for her personality" and remembered her as someone who "always paid her bills very very promptly."[23]

Relations with some other clients reflected more intense conflict. A Newport customer apparently had convinced the Tirocchi sisters to give her preferential prices, which remained a secret between them. The customer characterized the agreement as one between businesswomen and negotiated her prices relentlessly, but she showed a casual attitude toward her side of the bargain when she once "forgot" to give Anna a check while at the shop and on another occasion sent a check "which I though[t] I put in the letter I wrote you a few days ago." When she received a bill, she paid only what she had expected the prices to be, offered to negotiate about the charges above that level, and treated Anna to a long recital of her logistic and financial difficulties, clearly perceiving herself as different from the ordinary Tirocchi customer when she asserted, "I cannot afford what some of your customers can."[24]

Whether peacefully resolved or a source of bitterness, disputes over prices were an integral part of the custom trade, as dressmakers and clients each argued their version of the moral economy of clothing prices. These disagreements were compounded by two other customer practices that financially hobbled the Tirocchi business. First, customers often delayed payment. A quick look at the client account books makes clear why Anna so warmly praised Charlotte Luther's promptness. While most customers paid their bills within two weeks and many sent checks by return mail, some – often those with substantial balances – delayed far longer. A bill for $678 sent on October 6, 1916, for example, was not paid until the following February. Clients' letters give the story behind some of these delays and reveal that certain persons were more considerate than others. Cornelia Ely asked to have a bill sent at once, promising that "I will send or bring check so you can have it before you go abroad." More peremptory was Mrs. E. A. Loomis, who wrote from her Maine vacation home that she had found errors in her bill and would not pay until she returned to Providence in early September. Even during the prosperous 1910s and 1920s, customers wrote to delay payment because they had not received dividends or other expected income, and sent partial payment or postdated checks. At least one customer ran up bills amounting to $4,000 during the 1930s and had serious, protracted difficulty in paying them, to the point that Anna Tirocchi charged her twelve percent interest on the balance. The only dunning letters from Anna date from the 1930s. To one customer she wrote in exasperation, "It is not the time to joke any longer, as people need their money, and I must have mine so that I can pay my bills."[25]

The Tirocchis' business calculations were also disrupted by customers' cancellations of orders. It is not always possible to know if work had already begun on the garments, but sometimes this was clearly the case. Some customers reneged with good reason, such as serious illness or mourning. When Ella Fielding-Jones lost two close relatives, she revoked her order for two evening dresses and expressed concern that "I am not inconveniencing you too much." Others canceled because of disputes about other garments. Most simply canceled because they had changed their minds. A Fall River woman baldly stated, "I don't need [the dress]. I would rather have it new sometime in the winter." Such incidents increased the overhead of a business that was already very expensive to run and made it all the more difficult for the sisters to hold to quoted prices when extra work was required. As is always the case in retailing, the customer was both the key to success and the source of ruinous problems.[26]

The historical record tells much less about the lives of the women who sewed in the Tirocchis' shop. Only one letter survives from a worker, Sofia Johnson,[27] but it is undated and her name does not appear in any of the surviving employee time books. The time books are very sketchy, usually listing only seamstresses' first names and weekly earnings and sometimes the number of hours worked. A few interviews have helped to fill in the outlines of their world, but far less documentation exists for the workers' experience than for the lives of the customers. A happy coincidence allows for the construction of a relatively complete picture of the hours and wages of Tirocchi workers in late 1920 and for a comparison with a larger group of Rhode Island wage-earning women. One of the most complete Tirocchi employee time books covers the period from April 1919 to January 1921. During the last three months of 1920, the Women's Bureau of the U.S. Department of Labor investigated the wages and hours of Rhode Island women in other branches of manufacturing (chiefly rubber, jewelry, metals, and paper-box factories), as well as in stores and laundries.

The women in the Tirocchi shop worked far longer hours than those surveyed by the Women's Bureau. Tirocchi employees were ten times more likely than the latter to work fifty-four hours a week, then the legal maximum in the state. "General mercantile," the Women's Bureau category with the longest hours worked, required only about twenty-five percent of its female employees to work fifty-four hours, while more than forty percent of the Tirocchi employees' weeks were that long. As in many occupations, overtime at night and on weekends was common. This would have been the case particularly when the shop had to respond to customer-imposed deadlines or when big projects like weddings were underway. The time books never record over fifty-four hours a week for a given worker or any Sunday work, but Sofia Johnson's letter reports that she worked three hours on a Sunday. Like many employers of the time, the Tirocchis may have required their employees to work unpaid overtime, or they may have paid overtime off the books, allowed employees compensatory time off, or given them gifts to compensate them for overtime.[28]

The Tirocchi workers did escape one practice pervasive in Rhode Island: they were not required to take work home. Wage-earners in the clothing, textiles, jewelry, and artificial flower industries were frequently expected to complete unfinished work at home, making their residences into adjuncts of the factories. Anna and Laura Tirocchi prohibited this practice, but more out of concern for the fine fabrics than for the workers. Emily Valcarenghi Martinelli explained, "You couldn't take that material out of the house! Because if you ever put it on a table and it was dirty, it would spoil, or something would happen. No, no! She never sent nothing out."[29]

Although Tirocchi workers avoided the abysmal pay rates associated with work taken home, their longer hours did not earn them fatter pay packets than those surveyed by the Women's Bureau. None of the Tirocchi seamstresses earned $20 or more per week, but nearly a third of the female employees in the Women's Bureau survey did. Nearly two-thirds of the Tirocchi workers earned less than $12 per week, while the Women's Bureau recorded only fifteen percent with such lean pay envelopes.

Tirocchi employees more closely matched the Women's Bureau statistics in the middle pay ranges, where just under forty percent of the former and over fifty percent of the latter earned between $12 and $19.99 per week. The Tirocchi median weekly wage of $9 was just over half of that found for all workers by the Women's Bureau, and only three-quarters that of the lowest-paid group (five-and-dime-store employees). The Women's Bureau tabulated its data in a way that makes broad comparisons of hourly wage rates difficult, but it is possible to compare Tirocchi workers to those women who worked fifty-four-hour weeks. The median hourly rate for those surveyed by the Women's Bureau was well over one-and-a-half times the rate for Tirocchi employees.[30]

Post-World War I inflation exerted upward pressure on wages during October, November, and December 1920, the three months under consideration, and many of the Tirocchi workers achieved handsome raises. Between April 1919 and October 1920, Theresa Marianetti's weekly rate increased from $9 to $15, Rosina Pecora's from $10 to $19, and Veronica's from $9.50 to $21.60. Impressive gains by any standards, these increases far outstripped the rate of inflation, estimated by the Women's Bureau to be at most twenty-six percent between December 1918 and December 1920. Most raises came just after the New Year or in the weeks following the summer break, but they appear to have been negotiated individually rather than offered across the board. In the fall of 1919, for example, four out of nine workers received a raise one week, two the next week, and one each in the two following weeks: thus eight of the nine women received raises within a four-week period. Whether the healthy raises recognized the seamstresses' skill or resulted from favoritism, they do show the Tirocchi sisters' efforts to retain their skilled workers at a time when wages in general were on the rise.[31]

This overall picture suggests that workers did not gravitate toward the Tirocchi workshop because of favorable hours and pay: they could clearly have done better in both respects in a variety of other jobs. The time books offer tantalizing glimpses of the attractions of work at 514 Broadway and of the

ways it may have fit into women's lives beyond the job. Medians and averages homogenize the work force, but the time books reveal notable differences among the seamstresses and suggest some of the small dramas of daily life in the Tirocchi workshop. One of the most obvious divisions was the length of time women had spent working for the Tirocchi sisters. Just as the customers generally fit the prevailing pattern for women of their class, ethnicity, and race in that few were employed for pay, the workers generally fit what was by the 1910s a dominant pattern for women of the white immigrant working class. Mostly born in the United States, these immigrant daughters typically held jobs after leaving school and before either marrying, becoming pregnant, or having their first child. Mary Riccitelli Basilico appeared in the employee books off and on between 1921 and 1933, but her husband Panfilo Basilico remembered that she left the Tirocchis' employ when she became pregnant immediately after their marriage in 1936. Mary Rosa Traverso noted that "once they got married, they didn't go back. The husbands didn't want them to." As we shall see, however, women's wage-earning didn't necessarily end after marriage, although its visibility decreased.[32]

Because of the episodic quality of the employee books, it is difficult to know with certainty how long women worked for the Tirocchi sisters, and of course they may well have labored for other employers before or after they sewed at 514 Broadway. The data, however, suggests that of the thirty-nine women who could be traced in public records through the 1920s and 1930s, seven may be placed in a "career" category because they appear in the employee books over at least a ten-year span. To these might be added an eighth (Anna Del Matto) who probably worked that long. By contrast, twenty-two seamstresses appear to have been employed by the Tirocchis for three years or less. The result was a segmented work force with a relatively stable long-term component and a larger, more transient group of short-termers. This is precisely the pattern of labor that many late-twentieth-century corporations intentionally created, but in the case of the Tirocchi shop it is not clear whether the sisters desired such a distribution or whether it evolved because of the goals and desires of the workers themselves.

The needle trades have been and remain seasonal, both in the U.S. and Europe. The Tirocchi shop was no exception, closing each year during the 1920s for six to eight weeks in late summer, and for an additional few weeks in February and March during the mid-to-late 1930s. The 1919–21 time book shows some of the complexities of seamstresses' comings and goings. Theresa Marianetti began her summer break a month or two before the others in both 1919 and 1920. Perhaps she had schoolchildren who required her care. If so, the Tirocchi sisters valued her enough to allow her flexibility, for she returned to 514 Broadway in the fall of each year and received a pay increase of sixty-seven percent during these two years. (Theresa was an in-law of Salvatore Tirocchi's daughter Elvira Tirocchi Marianetti and also of Salvatore's granddaughter Louisa.) Some other work-force changes also seemed to have been seasonal in nature, with many employees disappearing during the summer break and many new workers appearing in the fall. In 1919, for example, five workers did not return at the end of the break, and five new ones took their places; but there were constant arrivals and departures. Seven weeks was the longest period in this time book during which the labor force remained the same.

Some women seem to have entered and left the Tirocchi work force in pairs or groups. Five women – Laura (definitely not Laura Tirocchi), Veronica, Margaret Volta, Marie, and Margaret C. – all left Tirocchi employ at the end of the week of January 17, 1920. Laura, Veronica, and Margaret Volta had been sewing for the Tirocchis at least since the first entry in that book, which was for the week of April 19, 1919, and they worked steadily until mid-January 1920. Laura returned only for two two-week stints in the late spring and early summer of 1920. Veronica and Margaret Volta returned to 514 Broadway within a week of each other in October 1920 and left forever within a week of each other in December. Judging by their pay rates, Veronica was a more skilled and/or experienced worker than Margaret Volta. Perhaps they worked as a team. Marie and Margaret C. began working

for the Tirocchis at the end of the summer 1919 break and worked steadily until mid-January 1920. Because their names are so common, it is difficult to trace their subsequent history. Were all five laid off in the post-Christmas business lull? Were they friends who quit in some act of solidarity? Were they on the losing end of a workplace dispute?[33]

The five women were almost certainly not laid off for lack of work. Their total weekly salary rates added up to $41.50, but within the next three weeks they were replaced by seven new workers whose aggregate wages were $66.90. The Tirocchis were clearly not cutting the overall payroll or seeking to hire cheaper workers, since the average salary of the new hires was $1.25 a week more than that of the departed seamstresses. Some, but far from all, of the higher wages are attributable to the fact that post-World War I inflation had not yet run its course. More likely, the Tirocchis were trying to upgrade their work force. Three of those who departed were paid at middling rates and two at low rates; two of their replacements earned top rates, four earned middling rates, and only one a low rate. This interpretation is supported by the fact that three of the new employees – Emily Valcarenghi Martinelli, Patricia Scalera, and Ida Del Matto – became "career" workers who each spent well over ten years with the Tirocchi shop.

The eight "career" women might be considered a core group of Tirocchi employees, an interpretation strengthened by the testimony of oral history. In addition to their longevity at the Tirocchi firm, Anna and Ida del Matto, Mary Riccitelli Basilico, Patricia Scalera, Emily Valcarenghi Martinelli, Grace Venagro, Theresa Marianetti, and Rosina Pecora were all Italian, and all of those who are known to have married wedded Italian men. In this, they were distinct from the short-term employees. The latter were still predominantly Italian (nineteen), but eleven did not have Italian last names. Two each had Irish and Jewish last names, one French, and five were of uncertain but clearly non-Italian ethnicity, while the eleventh was born in the Azores. This ethnic pattern fits into the larger picture for young wage-earning women in the United States at the time. Although workplaces often had a dominant ethnic character, hiring and job-seeking practices were imperfect segregation devices. As a result, workers usually encountered people of different ethnicities, religions, and cultural backgrounds on the job. Despite the heterogeneity of the early Tirocchi work force, its predominant character was Italian and became more so over time. By the late 1930s, all were Italian. Even more telling is the fact that Italian women were listed in the time books by first name or, more rarely, by first and last names, but women with obviously non-Italian last names – Larkin, Morey, and Remus – were referred to as "Mrs."

As the longest-term workers, this group of eight Italian women formed the core of the labor force. They were the best paid and presumably the most skilled seamstresses in a group with varying degrees of experience and ability. Skill differences were reflected in widely varying pay scales. The Tirocchi workers during those last three months of 1920 fell into three categories. Six women at the top of the pay scale earned from twenty-eight to forty cents an hour. Four in the middle range earned about seventeen cents an hour, and three at the bottom earned from nine to eleven cents per hour. This stratification persisted through the 1920s and well into the 1930s, but the differences between the highest and lowest paid narrowed sharply. In 1919–20, the lowest-paid worker earned about eleven percent of what the highest-paid earned. In 1926 the ratio was fourteen percent, and it grew to forty-two percent in 1934 and to seventy-four percent in 1937–38. The narrower spread in wages was probably linked to the decline in custom work, which required much low-skilled work such as basting.

Some women came to the shop without a great deal of sewing experience and started at the bottom of the ladder. Emily Valcarenghi Martinelli, who herself was to become one of the career workers, remembered this hierarchy. When she began working at the Tirocchi workshop in 1920, she looked up to four of the other career workers: Anna and Ida del Matto, Grace Venagro, and Mary Riccitelli Basilico. As Martinelli put it: "They were the oldest girls that would do all the best. We would sew too, but they would do the better work." Mary

Rosa Traverso recalled starting in 1934 as an unpaid "apprentice" who basted the clothing together and overcast the seams inside the garments to finish them. By this time, however, the ancient system of apprenticeship had decayed, and Traverso's "apprenticeship" was more of a dead-end entry-level position than one that guaranteed her a mastery of the entire range of the craft. By the time she left, after three years, she had learned little more than her initial tasks of basting and overcasting. In this respect, Traverso's history was typical of young and inexperienced women: she worked briefly and learned some limited skills, but not an entire craft.

Tirocchi associates interviewed for this project repeatedly stated that the shop was like a family: in Emily Valcarenghi Martinelli's words, "Even better than family because we never argued." Given that the majority were short-term workers, however, it was probably a very hierarchical family with the career workers at top. By the time Mary Riccitelli married Panfilo Basilico, he recalled that she had attained the position of head sewer. Primrose Tirocchi remembered that one of the Del Matto sisters performed as the model. Other career workers very likely had their own distinct roles. Martinelli noted that relationships among the workers were so close that even though they were not blood kin, "We were all related when we lived there. And we didn't have to be related because we were one family. We always stuck together. We stuck up for one another like nobody's business." Anna del Matto was godmother to Martinelli's children. According to Italian custom, this made Anna and Emily kin. The notions of family held by the Tirocchi workers were sharply at variance with those held by the customers. Family for the clients referred to blood kin, the connections embodied in such lineage organizations as the Daughters of the American Revolution that were so popular among them. For the workers, family went beyond blood and incorporated relationships based on godparenting, neighborhood, and working together.

The connections within the shop were reinforced in the outside world. Mary Riccitelli Basilico's husband Panfilo told interviewers that his wife obtained her job when "somebody took her in there

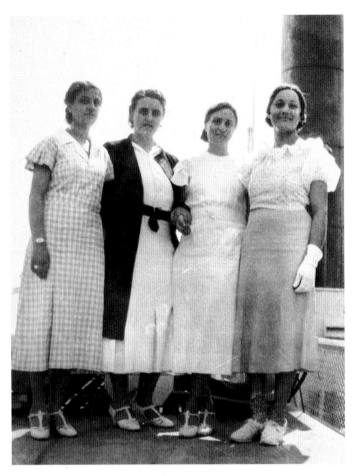

Fig. 52
Tirocchi employees on holiday in Narragansett, where Anna's
summer home was located: (left to right) Mary Rosa [not
Traverso], Gwendolyn, Mary Riccitelli, Miss DeLuca; ca. 1930.
Private collection.

the workers were expected to clean the house; then Anna Tirocchi went to her retreat in Narragansett, to which the workers were invited for a week [fig. 52]. Employer-sponsored leisure became increasingly popular during the period between the World Wars, and both factories and department stores organized such excursions. In the case of large companies, this practice was designed to promote workers' loyalty to the firm and to make them feel like part of a contrived, industrial "family," as well as to encourage efficiency. In the case of the Tirocchi shop, it grew more organically out of the close relationships among workers and employers.[34]

The "family" had a strong head. As Martinelli remembered, "We listened to Mrs. Tirocchi [meaning Anna, although it was Laura who was married]. She had the whole say, and we would listen to her." Anna's artistry translated into perfectionism in her management of the workshop. Mary Riccitelli's husband, Panfilo Basilico, recalled his wife telling him that "Madame [Anna] – she was very strict. The rules were very strict. You had to be – to do everything perfect. You couldn't do anything... even on the outside, anything wrong. You had to be a perfect person and you got to be exact in your work." When Basilico began to court Riccitelli, Anna summoned him to the shop, and only after interrogating him did she give Mary her approval to go out with him. By all accounts, the workers admired Anna enormously for her skills, her manner, and her intelligence. Mary Rosa Traverso, who never rose beyond the lowest rank of the shop hierarchy, reminisced that it was "wonderful to work for her. It really was." Emily Valcarenghi Martinelli described the way in which she taught and corrected the seamstresses: "She used to get you in a nice way. She never scolded anybody. No, she never scolded." Disputes among the employees were, she remembered, always settled by Anna. Basilico spoke admiringly of Anna, praising "her intelligence and her drive," and Martinelli referred to her as "the brains" and "an artist in her way."

This "family" was also to some extent ethnically exclusive. Traverso recalled that they conversed in Italian among themselves, although they all spoke English. Communicating in Italian would

– that's the only way you got in." Grace Venagro brought her downstairs neighbor, Mary Rosa Traverso, into the Tirocchi shop. Neighborhood contacts probably contributed widely to staffing the shop. All of the employees whose addresses could be ascertained resided on the West Side of Providence, in sharp contrast to the customers, who nearly all lived on the East Side. The largest and most concentrated group of worker residences (nine) was located in Federal Hill, then the center of Italian settlement in Providence, and a similar number were scattered more widely in the Silver Lake and Olneyville areas.

Tirocchi employees even vacationed together. When the shop closed down during the summer, have been a way to marginalize the non-Italian short-term workers and to draw the Italian short-term or low-ranking employees into the career workers' circle, as apparently happened with Traverso. The shared ethnicity of the owners, the career workers, and the majority of the short-term workers gave them a bond that went beyond other communal experiences of the shop.

The familial nature of the Tirocchi establishment was reinforced by its small size. At its largest, during the 1920s, the median number of seamstresses in any given week was fourteen, a group large enough to have its cliques and divisions, but also small enough to have a common experience. At a time when more and more wage earners were laboring in large establishments – the sites investigated by the Women's Bureau averaged 404 workers, and even the jewelry factories averaged 100 – these women continued to work in a small shop where they knew one another and their employers well. Ready-made clothing outsold custom-made garments at the Tirocchi establishment from 1924 on, but the shift did not have a dramatic effect on the size of the work force. In 1926, the median weekly roster was still fourteen, and it fell only to twelve in 1928. Even the Depression had a delayed effect on the sewing room at 514 Broadway. The work force remained at around ten until early 1933, and only then did it sharply contract, to a median of five per week after the 1933 summer break and to three per week in 1937–38. The seamstresses' experience went against the historical trend toward larger and larger workplaces, but it was shared with Italian immigrant men, about two in every five of whom worked in a similar setting. Even as late as 1940, over a fifth of self-employed Italian craftsmen had daughters who were also employed in the crafts.[35]

The women sewed at two tables pulled close to the windows. Conversation would have been easy since most of the work was done by hand, although at least by the 1930s there were both sewing and hemstitching machines in the shop. The workers ate together either in a small dining room near their third-floor workroom or, in good weather, out on a porch. Some were provided with lunches by the Tirocchis, and some brought their own food. They took turns making coffee. Occasionally, Martinelli remembered, "the girls used to go out and take a walk." The most vivid description of life in the sewing room came from Mary Riccitelli Basilico's husband. Panfilo recalled that when he came home from his work in an East Side bakery, he passed by 514 Broadway. After he and Mary had begun courting, the sewing women would drop their work and come to the windows to shout greetings to him, using his nickname of "Bombi." Like young women throughout the country, the seamstresses incorporated the talk and rituals of courtship into their work lives.

The workshop was clearly separate from the customers' territory on the second floor of the house, but the needlewomen themselves were not entirely isolated from the clientele. All of those interviewed named some of the customers, were well aware of their social positions, and knew a few details about their families and their personalities. Presumably, the customers were as much the subject of third-floor gossip as the workers' romances. The seamstresses knew enough about the customers' visits to indicate that they were sometimes in the room when clients had fittings or viewed fabrics. Dr. Louis J. Cella, Jr., recalled that "when the little girls were working they would use all the premises during the day." The sewing women also made deliveries. Emily Valcarenghi Martinelli remembered "go[ing] out nights" with Anna del Matto to deliver dresses. Martinelli also recalled that she, Anna and Ida del Matto, and Mary Riccitelli Basilico ("We were the smallest ones") would help dress brides for their weddings.

The seamstresses could easily have become resentful because of the obvious economic gulf between themselves and the clients, but this seems not to have been the case. While a few customers were notorious for their high-handed behavior, such as the one who "just wanted to show her power…because of her husband's power," the workers did not tar them all with the same brush. Basilico remembered his wife's judgment that some clients "were nice and some of them were cranky old ladies," but that she had no hostility toward them as a group. The interviews indicate

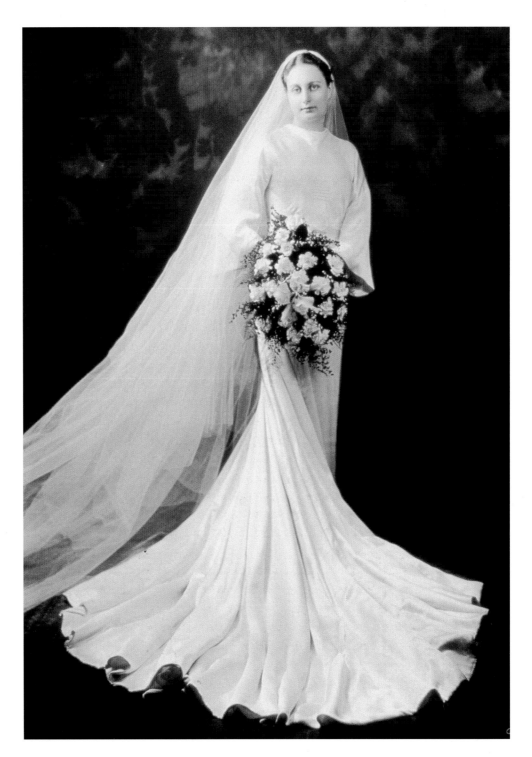

Fig. 53
Seamstress Mary Riccitelli in her wedding gown, made for her by her
colleagues at the Tirocchi shop for her marriage to Panfilo Basilico; 1931.
Tirocchi Archive (photograph by Bachrach).

that Tirocchi seamstresses took enormous pride in their skills, in creating beautiful clothing, and in working in a fine mansion. Emily Valcarenghi Martinelli, while telling interviewers about restoring a customer's piece of fine lace, sighed, "That was a place to work. So beautiful." Even more importantly, and in sharp contrast to most workers who made luxury goods, Tirocchi seamstresses were able to share in what they made. Each worker who married received as a gift from Anna and Laura a wedding gown that was the equal of any created for the paying customers [fig. 53]. Making these gowns, of course, would have been another practice that bonded the workers together.

The skills and experience gained in the Tirocchi shop served many of the workers well after they left 514 Broadway. The later occupations of thirteen of them are known: eleven remained in the needle trades, all in small-shop settings. Lino Picolo married a tailor in 1929, the same year that she worked for the Tirocchi sisters. In all likelihood, she would have plied her craft alongside him in his shop. Anna del Matto, who never married, went on to sew for Topal-Carlson and Jean's Inc. At these exclusive Providence shops, she would have altered ready-to-wear garments rather than making custom clothing, but she would have been sewing on quality garments as well as serving a clientele very like that of the Tirocchis. Mary Rosa Traverso became a free-lance seamstress after leaving A. & L. Tirocchi, but then worked for Mrs. Bernstein, a downtown Providence dressmaker, for about twelve years. Sometime before 1935, Patricia Scalera opened her own custom dress shop on a side street not far from the Tirocchis; apparently the Tirocchis did not regard this move with disfavor, because Dr. Louis J. Cella, Jr., reported that she was "of great assistance" in taking on some of the Tirocchi clients after the shop at 514 Broadway closed.[36]

Sewing was not just the center of the workers' wage-earning lives, but an important part of their family and social lives as well. Mary Riccitelli Basilico, her husband reported, "went on sewing… because she loved it, she loved to create, she loved… making things." She had, he recalled, the same ability as Anna Tirocchi to design apparel without patterns and made beautiful clothes for their daughter. Mary Rosa Traverso also sewed "tailor-made" garments for her daughter and continued to make wedding gowns, having somewhere picked up the art of beading, one of the skills she had not learned in the Tirocchi workshop. Emily Valcarenghi Martinelli spoke lovingly of the finely finished snowsuits she made for her daughters. Even so, the evidence of written documents and interviews undoubtedly captures only a small part of the role that sewing played in the lives of these women. Mary Riccitelli Basilico continued to make wedding gowns in her home, assisted by Mary Rosa Traverso and Grace Venagro during the evenings, and Panfilo Basilico would drive the two home afterwards. This activity is not recorded in the 1935 census report, which lists Mary Basilico as neither working at a gainful occupation nor seeking work. Even more telling is the fact that Panfilo Basilico mentioned Mary's continued dedication to sewing, but neither its collective nor money-making functions. Like much of the workers' lives, their sewing remains partly invisible in the historical record, but there is enough evidence to conclude with certainty that their skills were an enduring source of support, pride, and community. Mary Rosa Traverso reported that the career workers with whom she remained friendly were close "until they all died." One may indeed wonder if these seamstresses did not garner more satisfaction from their work than the clients experienced in wearing the fine apparel constructed at 514 Broadway.

Tirocchi Clients Resident on the East Side, Providence

Arranged by street address to show proximity to each other

56 Alumni Avenue	Mrs. David S. (Elizabeth A.) Seaman
63 Angell Street	Mrs. Charles Fletcher
170 Angell Street	Mrs. Michael F. (Ellen F.) Dooley
500 Angell Street*	Mrs. Theodora Colt Barrows
545 Angell Street	Mrs. Elizabeth Colt Anthony
60 South Angell Street	Mrs. Thomas A. (Esther) Briggs
30 Barnes Street	Mrs. James F. (Elizabeth) Phetteplace
74 Benefit Street	Mrs. Mariano (Catherine S.) Vervena
2 Benevolent Street	Mrs. John B. (Edith M.) Lewis
20 Benevolent Street	Mrs. Byron S. (Isabel) Watson
	Miss Annie P. S. Watson
	Miss Betty Watson
112 Benevolent Street	Mrs. Charles M. (Ruth Trowbridge) Smith III
110 Bowen Street	Mrs. Charles Dexter (Alice Evelyn Cooke) Owen
187 Bowen Street	Mrs. Richard LeBaron Bowen
215 Bowen Street	Mrs. Edward A. (Phoebe or Phebe D.) Loomis
251 Bowen Street	Mrs. Stephen C. (Mary L.) Harris
252 Bowen Street	Mrs. Harvey A. (Marrion B.) Baker
442 Brook Street	Mrs. Benjamin P. (Mona E.) Harris
27 Brown Street	Mrs. Barnes (Elizabeth) Newberry
83 (93?) Brown Street	Mrs. Howard M. (Hope C. B.) Chapin
109 Brown Street	Mrs. Pardon (Edna) Miller
111 Brown Street	Mrs. Stuart (Martha L.) Aldrich
111 Brown Street	Mrs. Wallace W. (Louise Aldrich) Hoge
117 Brown Street	Mrs. Charles S. (Elizabeth) Smith
169 Brown Street	Mrs. James (Florence Mc K.) Elgar
170 Brown Street	Mrs. Charles S. (Elizabeth) Smith
173 Brown Street	Mrs. Charles M. (Ruth Trowbridge) Smith III
180 (136?) Brown Street	Mrs. Arthur D. (Harriett) Champlin
16 Cabot Street	Mrs. Benjamin P. (Mona E.) Harris
26 Cooke Street	Mrs. Charles H. (Anne Kilvert) Merriman
61 (65?) Cooke Street	Mrs. Erling C. (Helen B.) Ostby
47 Doyle Avenue	Mrs. David S. (Elizabeth A.) Seaman
714 Doyle Avenue	Mrs. David S. (Elizabeth A.) Seaman

25 Freeman Parkway	Mrs. Paul Churchill (Olive B.) De Wolf
59 George Street	Mrs. Pardon (Edna) Miller
67 George Street	Mrs. Ashbel T. (Lucy) Wall, Sr.
71 George Street	Mrs. Samuel Mowry (Mary Coe) Nicholson
173 George Street	Mrs. Henry A. (Margaret D.) DuVillard
129 Hope Street	Mrs. John B. (Edith M.) Lewis
196 Hope Street	Mrs. Walter (Ivy L.) Callender
198 Hope Street	Miss Ilene Jones
63 John Street	Mrs. Edgar (Isabel Brown) Brunschwig
91 Keene Street	Mrs. Theodora Colt Barrows
195 Laurel Avenue	Mrs. Elizabeth Colt Anthony
295 Laurel Avenue	Mrs. Charles M. (Ruth Trowbridge) Smith III
81 Lloyd Avenue	Mrs. Edgar (Isabel Brown) Brunschwig
102 Lloyd Avenue	Mrs. Frank D. (Mary E.) Simmons
168 Lloyd Avenue	Mrs. William E. (Harriet B.) Maynard
555 Lloyd Avenue	Mrs. Harold J. (Mary Colt) Gross
1 Magee Street	Mrs. William (Adelaide) Ely
59 Manning Street	Mrs. Frank D. (Helen S.) Lisle
60 Manning Street	Mrs. Bruce E. (Helen A.) Merriman
144 Meeting Street	Mrs. Edward R. Trowbridge
156 Meeting Street	Mrs. Arthur D. (Harriett) Champlin
26 Olive Street	Mrs. David S. (Elizabeth A.) Seaman
43 Orchard Avenue	Mrs. Harold J. (Mary Colt) Gross
67 Prospect Street	Mrs. Frank D. (Mary E.) Simmons
353 Slater Avenue	Mrs. E. Edwin (Janet) Codman
123 Waterman Street†	Mrs. Edgar (Isabel Brown) Brunschwig
	Mrs. James F. (Elizabeth) Phetteplace
320 Wayland Avenue	Mrs. William P. Chapin, Jr.
349 Wayland Avenue	Mrs. Harold J. (Mary Colt) Gross
10 Young Orchard Avenue	Mrs. Charles M. (Ruth Trowbridge) Smith III
	Mrs. Edward R. Trowbridge

*Wayland Manor
†The Minden

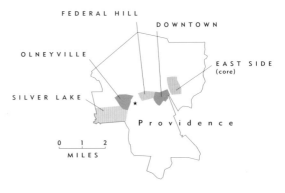

★ 514 Broadway

Many thanks to Edward Benson, Katherine Benson, and Sharon Hartman Strom for their very helpful comments on an earlier version of this essay.

The interviews referred to and quoted in this essay are to be found in the A. & L. Tirocchi Archive, Museum of Art, Rhode Island School of Design, Providence. Such references have not been footnoted. All letters sent or received by Anna or Laura Tirocchi are understood to be found in the Tirocchi Archive. See "Note on the A. & L. Tirocchi Archive, Collection, and Catalogue," p. 23.

1. Claudia B. Kidwell and Margaret C. Christman, *Suiting Everyone: The Democratization of Clothing in America.* Washington, D.C.: 1974, pp. 135–37.

2. See Susan Porter Benson, *Counter Cultures: Saleswomen, Managers, and Customers in American Department Stores.* Urbana: 1986.

3. Stuart Blumin, *The Emergence of the Middle Class: Social Experience in the American City, 1760–1900.* Cambridge (England) and New York: 1989, pp. 83–107.

4. Anna Tirocchi to Ivory Flakes Soap, June 3, 1940, and June 4, 1940.

5. Cf. pp. 38–39 in this volume.

6. Biographical information on clients and descriptions of their purchases may be found in the Tirocchi Archive client data base. See also Mary D. Doherty to Miss T., May 1923; and *Street List of Residents over Twenty Years of Age in the Town of Brookline, 1923.* Brookline (Massachusetts): 1923. The latter reference was kindly supplied by Anne Clark of the Brookline Public Library.

7. John S. Gilkeson, Jr., *Middle-Class Providence, 1820–1940.* Princeton: 1986, pp. 204–10, 318–20. In addition to those mentioned in the text, "general social organizations" include the Jacobs Hill Hunt, Warwick Country Club, Dunes Club, Wannamoisett Country Club, and the Providence Plantations Club; intellectual/artistic organizations include the Providence Athenaeum, the Needlework Guild, Rhode Island School of Design and its museum, The Players, and the University Glee Club; other elite men's clubs are the Economic Club of Providence and the University Club; and lineage societies include the Society of Mayflower Descendants, Sons of the American Revolution, and Daughters of the American Revolution.

8. Kathryn Manson Tomasek, "Irrepressible Women, Work, and Benevolence in Providence, Rhode Island, 1860–1936," paper presented at the conference "Rhode Island Reconsidered," John Nicholas Brown Center, Brown University, November 15, 1997; see also *Sixty-Third Report of Irrepressible Society for the Year Ending April 30, 1926.* Providence: 1926.

9. *Providence Journal* (January 19, 1930); Tirocchi Archive.

10. Dorothy Newton to Anna Tirocchi, n.d., 1923; Mrs. Charles B. Luther [Charlotte Robinson Luther] to Anna Tirocchi, n.d.

11. "Women's Union at 100 changes with times," "Union has changed with the times," and "Over the years many groups have been aided by the Union," *Fall River Herald* (June 18, 1987); *Fall River Women's Union: A Brief History Celebrating the Hundredth Anniversary of Incorporation, 1887–1987.* 1987, n.p. Janelle Tanous Lyons of the Fall River Historical Society generously supplied these references.

12. Obituary of Mrs. W. H. [Mira] Hoffman, n.d. (1940); Tirocchi Archive.

13. Judith E. Smith, *Family Connections: A History of Italian and Jewish Immigrant Lives in Providence, Rhode Island 1900–1940.* Albany: 1985, pp. 35–44.

14. Wendy Gamber, *The Female Economy: The Millinery and Dressmaking Trades, 1860–1930.* Urbana: 1997. A related problem in using the letters in the Tirocchi Archive is that there is no way to know what proportion of the incoming correspondence was saved or of the outgoing correspondence copied. Over half (52%) of the letters date from 1919 to 1923, but even these appear not to be all the letters received in these years, since those from 1919 are almost all dated September through December and those from 1923 are almost all dated from March through July. Another fifth of the letters (19.7%) are undated. The most one can say is that the best selection of the letters comes from the four years after the end of World War I, an era of inflation followed by a sharp deflation, during which the dollars of the wealthy went even further than usual.

15. Anna Tirocchi to Mrs. Hoffman, March 20, 1940; and Mrs. E. G. Butler to My dear Madam, November 1919. Because it is often not clear to which of the sisters a letter was directed, they are herein identified by salutation. "Madam" or "Madame," however, was the common form of address to Anna Tirocchi.

16. Alice E. Trowbridge to Anna and Laura [Tirocchi], November 1, 1922; Dorothy Newton to Anna [Tirocchi], May 6, 1923.

17. Mrs. Luther to Anna [Tirocchi], June 1923. Mrs. Luther to Anna [Tirocchi], Tuesday. Elizabeth Phetteplace to Anna [Tirocchi], n.d. Lucy L. Wall, no salutation, n.d.

18. J. S. Bateman to Anna [Tirocchi], November 1919. Mrs. E. G. Butler to Madame Tirocchi, November 6, 1919.

19. Mrs. E. G. Butler to Madam Tirocchi, December 9, 1919, and December 19, 1919. Elizabeth A. Seaman to Madame, n.d. Mrs. A. D. Champlin to Anna [Tirocchi], 1918? Mrs. M. A. Davis to A & L. Tirocchi, 1920. Mrs. Luther to Anna [Tirocchi], January 1920. E. A. Loomis to Anna [Tirocchi], May 10, 1920.

20. Dorothy Newton to Anna [Tirocchi], March 2, 1923. A. N. Brown to Miss Tirocchi, July 1, 1923. Adelaide W. Danforth to Miss Anna [Tirocchi], April 15, 1923. Mrs. E. G. Butler to Madam Tirocchi, November 13, 1919. Mrs. Charles B. Luther to Anna [Tirocchi], n.d.: Lucy L. Wall to Anna [Tirocchi], November 22, 1919.

21. Mrs. Mary O. P. Rounseville to Madame Dirocchi [*sic*], n.d. Mrs. Charles B. Luther to Anna [Tirocchi], n.d.; see also

Mrs. Charles B. Luther to Anna [Tirocchi], January 1920. David M. Katzman, *Seven Days a Week: Women and Domestic Service in Industrializing America*. Urbana: 1981, pp. 110–15.

22. U.S. Department of Labor, Bureau of Labor Statistics, *Handbook of Labor Statistics 1975 – Reference Edition*. Washington, D.C.: 1975, p. 254, table 102. This table gives the average weekly salary for a nonsupervisory manufacturing employee as $21.94. I multiplied this by 50 to get a yearly figure, but this is almost certainly too high, because so many workers at that time were unable to secure a full year's work. See weddings folder; Tirocchi Archive. Mrs. O. H. Williams to Misses Tirocchi, September 26, 1919; Alice E. Trowbridge to Anna and Laura [Tirocchi], November 1, 1922. Margaret D. DuVillard to Anna [Tirocchi], July 12, 1940.

23. Charlotte Luther to Anna [Tirocchi], May 1922, two letters. Lottie Luther to Anna [Tirocchi], August 2, 1922. Anna L. Tirocchi to Richard Hawes, January 14, 1932. For another example of a price dispute amicably resolved, see Mary Burlingame Peck to Anna [Tirocchi], July 26 and August 1, 1939.

24. J. S. Bateman to Anna [Tirocchi], November 1919; Jennie L. Bateman to Anna Tirocchi, 1923. Jennie L. Bateman to Madam Tirocchi, October 1920.

25. Cornelia L. W. Ely to Anna [Tirocchi], July 3, 1923. E. A. Loomis to Anna and Laura Tirocchi, n.d. See, for example, Nina A. Williamson to Mrs. Tirocchi, 1916; Florence Beresford to Anna [Tirocchi], November 20, 1919; E. A. Loomis to Anna [Tirocchi], 1922. Mary Colt Gross, 1934; Mrs. Harold J. Gross to Miss Tirocchi, June 11, 1934; Anna Tirocchi to Mrs. Gross, July 10, 1934; Mary Colt Gross to Miss Tirocchi, January 29, 1940. Anna Tirocchi to Mrs. T. C. Barrows, September 20, 1932.

26. M. B. Baker to Anna Tirocchi, November 19, 1919; Florence P. Maxwell to Anna [Tirocchi], November 7, 1922; Lucien L. Butler to Madame Tirocchi, November 18, 1922; Bessie H. Sweet to Miss Tirocchi, December 3, 1922. Ella Fielding-Jones to Anna [Tirocchi], January 25, 1915. Mrs. A. D. Champlin to Anna and Laura Tirocchi, 1918. Hetty Newton to Anna Tirocchi, n.d.; see also Abbie H. R. Stearns to Anna and Laura Tirocchi, December 2, 1919; Bessie H. Sweet, October 11, 1922; Marion R. Vonsiatsky to Anna [Tirocchi], January 18, 1937; Mary Burlingame Peck to Anna [Tirocchi], July 26, 1939; Mary E. Gardner to Madame Tirocchi, n.d.

27. Sofia Johnson to miss Tirochi [*sic*], n.d.

28. This conclusion is based on a comparison of data in table I in the U.S. Department of Labor, Women's Bureau, *Women in Rhode Island Industries*. Washington, D.C.: 1922, p. 61, which gives the number of hours worked in one unspecified weekly pay period, and the weekly hours of each woman listed in the Tirocchi time book during October, November, and December 1920, excluding Anna and Laura (who always reported themselves as working fifty-four hours) and Christmas week (the last week of the year). The latter tabulation included 109 woman-weeks of work at the Tirocchi shop. Corroborating evidence for hours at the Tirocchi shop may be found in the letter from Sofia Johnson to miss Tirochi [*sic*], n.d.; and in the Emily Valcarenghi Martinelli and Mary Rosa Traverso interviews in the Tirocchi Archive.

29. U.S. Department of Labor, Women's Bureau, *Industrial Homework in Rhode Island*, Bulletin 131. Washington, D.C.: 1935; U.S. Department of Labor, Children's Bureau, *Industrial Homework of Children: A Study Made in Providence, Pawtucket, and Central Falls, Rhode Island*, Bulletin 100. Washington, D.C.: 1922; Susan Porter Benson, "Women, Work, and Family: Industrial Homework in Rhode Island," in Eileen Boris and Cynthia R. Daniels, eds., *Homework: Historical and Contemporary Perspectives on Paid Labor at Home*. Urbana: 1989, pp. 53–74.

30.

	Tirocchi	Women's Bureau
under $7	33%	2.8%
under $10	56.8%	7.7%
under $12	63.3%	15.4%
$10–$19.99	45.7%	60.2%
$12–$19.99	39.3%	52.5%
$20+	0%	32.1%

Tirocchi data calculated from the time records for all weeks in October, November, and December 1920, omitting the pay rates for Anna and Laura Tirocchi. For Women's Bureau data, see *op. cit.*, 1922, p. 64, table IV. The Tirocchi median wage was $9; the Women's Bureau median for all industries was $16.85 and for 5-and-10-cent stores, $11.90. See *ibid.*, p. 27.

31. *Ibid.*, p. 25.

32. Kathy Peiss, *Cheap Amusements: Working Women and Leisure in Turn-of-the-Century New York*. Philadelphia: 1986, pp. 38–41.

33. It first seemed possible that Margaret C. was the same as Margherita, who appeared in the time book at the end of January 1920, a week after Margaret's last appearance. Margherita worked until early fall of 1920 and disappeared from the record just before Margaret reappeared. A promising hypothesis, however, fell by the wayside when the time book showed both at work the week of December 12, 1920.

34. National Industrial Conference Board, *What Employers Are Doing for Employees: A Survey of Voluntary Activities for Improvement of Working Conditions in American Business Concerns*. New York: 1936, pp. 44–45.

35. U.S. Department of Labor, Women's Bureau, *op. cit.*, 1922, p. 4. Smith, *op. cit.*, pp. 37, 69.

36. See data base of Tirocchi workers; Tirocchi Archive.

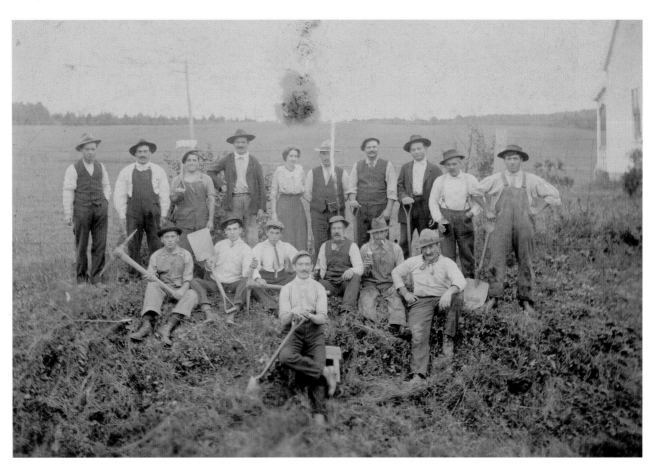

Fig. 54
Laura Tirocchi and her brother Frank, the
padrone (back row, fifth and sixth from left),
with the laborers who were building the Bangor
and Aroostook Railroad in Canada; 1909.
Private collection.

JOHN W. BRIGGS
Associate Professor, Education and History
Syracuse University

Strategies for Success:

The Tirocchis, Immigration, and the Italian American Experience

ranches of the Tirocchi family began to assemble in Providence in the early years of the twentieth century. They joined over four million Italians and other Southern and Eastern Europeans who entered the United States during the forty years prior to World War I. In waves of heavy and sustained immigration, these people came to America in search of employment within a rapidly expanding urban industrial economy [fig.54]. Like so many of them, the Tirocchis came from a small rural village. Their hometown of Guarcino lies south of Rome in the province of Frosinone among the foothills of the mountainous center of the Italian peninsula [fig. 55]. At the time of their emigration, the nearest railroad was about ten miles away in the provincial capital. Later, a spur line was constructed to the town [fig. 56]. As late as 1930, the local hotel offered twenty beds to the tourists who used Guarcino as a base from which to climb the seven-thousand-foot Monte Viglio. Guarcino today remains a small, remote community with a population of approximately eighteen hundred inhabitants.[1]

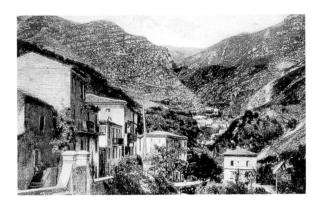

Fig. 55
Guarcino, Italy, home to the progenitors
of the Tirocchi families living in Providence;
ca. 1938. Tirocchi Archive.

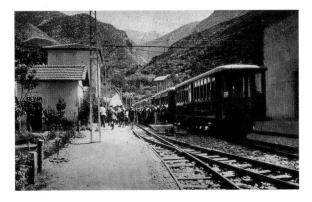

Fig. 56
View of Guarcino showing the railroad
spur line; ca. 1938. Tirocchi Archive.

The Tirocchi families, like most immigrants, came from the middle ranges of the working classes and not from the most impoverished segments of the home society. The very poor, in addition to lacking resources to finance emigration, were also generally disheartened and did not possess the psychological capital necessary to embark on such a wrenching experience. The wealthy and professional classes seldom left their homeland. The former had no need to pursue greater opportunities, and the latter, if they did leave, found that their European training seldom qualified them for practice in the United States, thus immigrant professionals usually experienced significant loss of status. Even in times of severe hardship, emigration was a selective process. Far more people stayed behind than relocated. Those, such as Anna Tirocchi and her family, who chose to risk all in search of opportunity, were a special subset of the larger population. Their skills and personal characteristics would be put to good use in the United States.[2] As Anna's niece Primrose Tirocchi put it, their family came "to get ahead."

Eugenio Tirocchi and Maria Rossi Tirocchi, progenitors to nearly all of the family members in Providence, were listed as "*contadini*" – "peasants" or "farmers" in the rural Italian status classification system – in the Stato Civile records for Guarcino. Three of their sons, Nazzareno, Giuseppe, and Tito, as well as their daughters-in-law, were likewise recorded as "*contadini*." The category of "*contadini*" did not preclude other undertakings beyond an individual's primary economic activity. Two of Tito's sons indicated that their family worked as teamsters transporting paper from a factory in Guarcino to Rome by mule and wagon. Only the father of Maria Rossi was listed as "*possidente*," suggesting that he had substantial holdings in land or other agricultural capital (see the Tirocchi genealogy on pp. 98–99 for an outline of the family relationships).[3]

The birth, death, and marriage records for fifty other Tirocchis in Guarcino suggest that they were all from modest social and economic backgrounds. Twenty were listed as "*contadini*." An equal number were identified as "*pastori*" ("shepherds"). Four women were listed as "*pecorare*" ("sheep herders"),

and an equal number merited "*donne di casa*" or "*cassalinge*," which usually suggested a somewhat higher status. There were only three references to "*possidenti*." Other families in Guarcino with whom the Tirocchis were associated either by marriage or business included the Del Signores [fig. 57], De Meis, and Furias. All but one Del Signore listing were "*muratori*" or "*falegnami*": "masons" or "carpenters." The largest number of De Meis entries were "*possidenti*," but there were also "*contadini*," two "*falegnami*," and one "*cavaliere*" ("gentleman"). Furia listings were almost all "*contadini*." The lowest occupational classification, "*braccianti*" ("day laborers"), was not used by the community clerk to label any of the numerous persons considered above.[4]

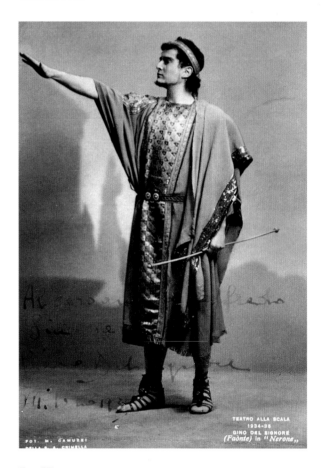

Fig. 57
Opera singer Gino Del Signore in costume at La Scala, Milan; 1934–35: Anna and Laura Tirocchi's brother Frank married Gino's cousin Maria. Gino remained in Italy and prospered with an international career in the theater. Private collection (photograph by M. Camuzzi).

In a classic chain migration, three branches of the Tirocchi family had settled by 1910 in the southwest corner of Providence at its border with Cranston and Johnston, an area referred to then and now as the Silver Lake district (see map, p. 97). Silver Lake would remain the locale for many of the future business enterprises initiated by the family. This Italian community, while not the largest in the Providence area, had been a center of settlement for immigrants since the late nineteenth century. There were five areas of Italian settlement in Providence before World War I. Federal Hill was the largest. In addition to Silver Lake, there also were enclaves in the North End, Eagle Park, and South Providence. Early arrivals, often from northern Italy, worked in agriculture, and a number eventually owned and operated their own farms. Through the years, Providence newspapers published generally complimentary accounts of this community.[5]

Salvatore Tirocchi, son of Eugenio and Maria and brother to Nazzareno, Giuseppe, and Tito, was one of the first family members to come to the United States. He and two of his older sons, Luigi and Gerardo, entered the U.S. in 1902. It is unclear when they arrived in Providence, but this was probably by 1907, when Salvatore's wife Luisa and their younger children joined him. In 1908, Salvatore was listed as residing at 18 Alto Avenue in the *Providence City Directory*. According to the 1910 federal census, he lived with his wife and children at 50 What Cheer Avenue. In that year, Salvatore was operating a cement-block manufacturing enterprise, while three of his older boys (Gerardo, Giuseppe, and Augusto) worked as laborers for a railroad and Luigi was employed by the City of Providence. The only daughter, Elvira, was a spinner in a worsted mill, and the youngest son, Giovanni, attended school. While the parents are listed as speaking Italian, all of the children spoke English and, like their father, were literate.[6] Between 1910 and 1920, Salvatore with five of his six sons – Luigi, Gerardo, Giuseppe, Augusto, and Giovanni – developed the Rhode Island Improved Cement Works Company and the Rhode Island Laundry Company. By 1920, Salvatore was managing the Tirocchi Brothers Motor Trucking, which offered local and long-distance hauling.

After Salvatore's death in 1925, his son Luigi assumed presidency of the family enterprises. Other brothers filled the vice-president, secretary, and treasurer positions. After World War II, the brothers added a real estate firm to the list.

A second branch of the family – children of Salvatore's brother Tito Tirocchi – first appeared in the 1906 *Providence City Directory*, where one of Tito's sons was recorded as a laborer boarding at 25 Hillhurst Street. Tito's daughter Maria and his son Giuseppe arrived in 1907. The 1910 census placed Maria and her husband Francesco Furia at 489 Union Avenue with their ten-month-old daughter Armelinda. Francesco had immigrated in 1906 and was working as a street laborer for the City of Providence. Maria's brother Giuseppe boarded with the family and was also a street laborer. In 1914, Tito's sons Eugenio and Mario were boarding at 140 Prudence Avenue. Two years later the Furias moved to 144 Prudence Avenue, which became their longtime family home. Tito left Italy for Providence late in life to be near his children after the death of his wife. Like Salvatore and his sons, male members of Tito's family were first employed as laborers; and like their uncle and cousins, they soon turned to business ventures. By 1921, Eugenio and his brother Giuseppe were respectively vice president and secretary/general manager of Ideal Concrete Products Company, Inc., on Hartford Avenue. Within a few years Giuseppe was functioning as president and general manager, while his wife Assunta served as secretary for the business. Eugenio moved on to cement contracting. Giuseppe then established J. Tirocchi Construction, which his grandchildren continue to operate as AA Construction in Johnston. The Hartford Avenue property was the location for a number of businesses, including a tire-retreading plant and a miniature golf course. Through the late 1920s and early 1930s, Tito's son Angelo worked as a laborer and janitor. In 1935, he opened an auto service station at 314 Hartford Avenue, which he continued to operate after World War II. Tito's youngest son, Mario, listed himself as a contractor and builder in 1925 and branched out with the Tirocchi Cement Block Company. In the latter years of the 1920s, he established the Rhode Island

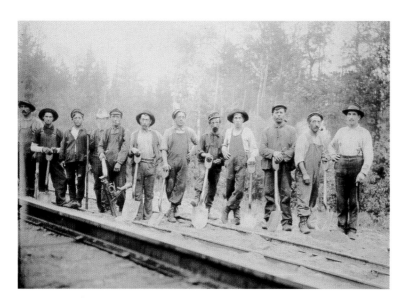

Fig. 58
Frank Tirocchi (far right) and his crew at work on the
Bangor and Aroostook Railroad in Canada; 1909.
Private collection.

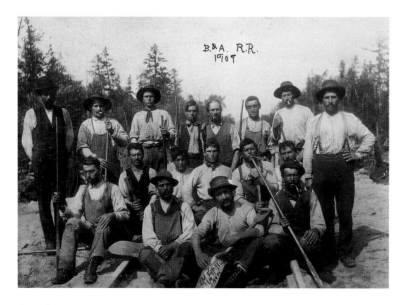

Fig. 59
Padrone Frank Tirocchi (far right) and his group of
laborers with their tools; 1909. Private collection.

Column Company, then moved into the auto-service
sector in 1932 with the Huntington Avenue Filling
Station. After the Second World War, he opened a
tire-retreading company. Later, he would operate a
milk delivery business, an auto service station, and
another tire-retreading business.

Anna, Laura, Eugenia, and Frank Tirocchi
represent the third, but not necessarily the latest,
branch of the family to settle in Providence. Anna
and Laura came to the United States in 1905. Anna,
Eugenia, and Frank were the children of Nazzareno
and Rosa Fraticalli Tirocchi, and Laura was their
half-sister, the daughter of Rosa's second husband,
Giuseppe Tirocchi (the deceased Nazzareno's
brother). Family oral tradition holds that Anna and
Laura first worked in New York before arriving in
Providence. By 1910, they were boarding with their
sister Eugenia and her second husband Luigi
Valcarenghi at a store-and-apartment block at 324
Pocasset Avenue in Providence, about two blocks
from their uncle Salvatore and their cousins in uncle
Tito's family. Eugenia and Luigi Valcarenghi had
entered the United States in 1907 and most likely
settled in Providence soon thereafter. Their son
William was born in Rhode Island in 1908 or early
1909. By 1910, Luigi was working as a house painter
and owned the block on Pocasset Avenue with the
help of a mortgage. Frank Tirocchi, brother to Anna
and Eugenia and half-brother to Laura, also immigrated in 1905, but does not appear in the *Providence
City Directory* until 1914. Frank Tirocchi spent a
part of the time between 1905 and 1914 as a labor
contractor (*padrone*) for railroad construction in
Canada [fig. 58]. A dated photograph in the Tirocchi
Archive captures him and his crew at a "B. & A.
R. R." (Bangor and Aroostoock Railroad) work site
in 1909 [fig. 59]. Laura appears in another photo
with Frank and a gang of construction workers [fig.
54, p. 78]. Railroad work and sojourns in Canada
were also a part of the early experience of other family members. Tito's sons Eugenio and Giuseppe told
their children of laying rail in the Canadian "wilder-
ness." Another son, Angelo, spent time in Maine,
where he joined the American military in 1908.
Salvatore's eldest son, Federico Achille Tirocchi,

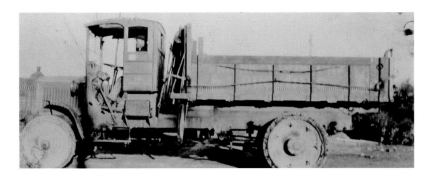

Fig. 60
Frank Tirocchi's truck; ca. 1930.
Private collection.

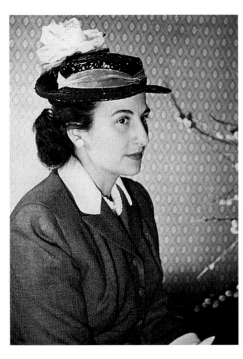

Fig. 61
Anna and Laura's niece Primrose Tirocchi (Frank
Tirocchi's daughter) modeling one of her millinery
creations; 1940. Private collection.

served as a priest in Quebec before being assigned
to build a parish for Italian and French Canadian
immigrants in the Natick section of West Warwick,
Rhode Island.[7]

In 1914, Frank and his new bride Maria Del
Signore, a woman with artisan and middle-class
family ties in Italy, set up housekeeping at 39 Bradford Street on Federal Hill following their marriage
in February. Frank was listed in the 1914 *Directory*

as a clerk at the Roma Pharmacy on Federal Hill's
Atwells Avenue, the heart of Providence's largest
Italian settlement.[8] He also worked in a machine
shop briefly before starting a trucking business and
hiring out his services to the City of Providence.
From 1928 through 1931, he ran his trucking business [fig. 60] from Anna's Broadway residence and
lived in one of her apartments on nearby Tobey
Street. His son, Frank Jr., became a dentist. His
daughter, Primrose, had a long career in fashion
and sales at the Outlet Department Store, where
she specialized in millinery. She designed hats and
had her own show downtown at the Biltmore Hotel
in the 1930s [fig. 61].

Anna and her siblings were adults at the time
of their departure from Italy. According to the 1910
federal census, Anna at thirty-five years of age was
the oldest, Eugenia was thirty, Frank was twenty-
five, and Laura twenty-two.[9] Both Anna and Laura
spoke English and were literate, according to the
census, although it is not known where they
acquired this learning. Perhaps it was during their
first years in the United States, when they worked
for others. Eugenia was literate, but spoke only
Italian. The 1920 census lists Frank as literate. Given
his labor contracting and trucking activities, it may
probably be assumed that he was proficient in his
use of English. Such facility was an essential quality
for *padroni*, who served as middlemen between
North American employers and immigrant laborers
having little or no English.

The Tirocchis found Providence a thriving
industrial city of just under a quarter of a million

inhabitants in 1910. During the previous two decades the population had increased by thirty-three percent and twenty-eight percent respectively, slowing by 1910 and increasing only around six percent for the next two decades. In 1910, Providence was the twentieth largest city in the United States. By 1950, it had slipped to forty-third and was one hundredth in 1980. At the beginning of the century its economy was built around cotton and worsted mills, rubber products, machine-tool fabrication, and jewelry and silver manufacture. A few of the Tirocchis found employment in these industries, but most turned to entrepreneurship. Salvatore's cement-block company and Anna and Laura's dress shop were the first family enterprises, followed by a grocery store, two more cement-product companies, a laundry, two trucking concerns, three gas-station/auto-service firms, two tire-retreading shops, rental properties, a miniature golf course, a dairy, a plumbing business, and a real-estate company. With the exception of the Valcarenghis and Laura and Anna, all adult members of the family's branches were in the contracting, construction, and trucking business at one time or another, and most owned gravel banks, which provided raw materials for some of their various enterprises. They also sold sand, gravel, and loam. Collectively, the family enterprises represent a vertical integration of the construction business.

The 1910 census lists Anna and Laura Tirocchi as wage-earning tailors. Family history indicates that they worked briefly for Rose Carraer-Eastman, later Madam Zarr, a prominent dressmaker patronized by wealthy East Side women. Whatever their earlier employment in Providence, they wasted little time in setting up their own business. In 1911, they opened their dress shop in the Butler Exchange [fig. 62], situated downtown in the center of Providence. They shared their Westminster Street business address with lawyers, doctors, dentists, and other professionals. Wholesalers, insurance agents, music teachers, the Republican State Committee, the Rhode Island Women's Christian Temperance Union, and the Rhode Island Sunday School Association were also among the tenants of that building. In 1913, a firm of patent attorneys and the Crown

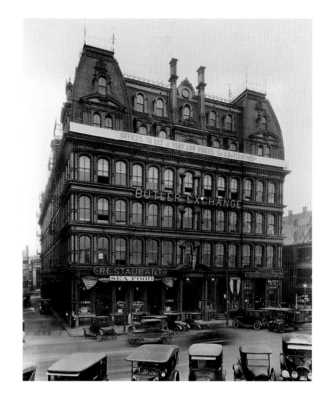

Fig. 62
The Butler Exchange, a vast emporium occupying an entire block on Westminster Street in downtown Providence, the site of the first Tirocchi shop; ca. 1915. Courtesy Rhode Island Historical Society, Providence.

Gold Mining and Milling Company of Nova Scotia flanked the Tirocchi "gown" suite on the fourth floor. The fifth and sixth floors were given over largely to music teachers.

Anna and Laura joined their brother Frank and his wife as boarders in the newlyweds' home, but the sisters' stay was short. In 1915, Laura married a young American-born physician, Louis J. Cella,[10] who had set up his practice in the Valcarenghis' building on Pocasset Avenue. Anna purchased a large mansion at 514 Broadway in a then fashionable section of the city [see frontispiece]. She and the new couple converted part of the first floor into a doctor's office and the second into a dressmaking shop, living primarily on the third floor, which also housed the workshop for the dressmaking business. As self-designated "gown makers," the Tirocchi sisters sought to distinguish themselves from others who were simply identified as "dressmakers." Moving to the stately Victorian house on Broadway [fig. 63] was a major step in this direction. While in the Butler Exchange, they had been directly across Westminster Street from twenty-five milliners and five dressmakers who had shops located in the historic Arcade [fig. 64]. Other dressmakers and tailors for ladies were scattered about the city center. Through marriage and geography the sisters were moving away from the larger Italian immigrant community and toward middle-class status.

Dressmaking as a trade in Providence had reached its peak in 1906, when 890 practitioners were listed in the *City Directory*. This was six times the number of dressmakers recorded in 1880 (146). By 1910, the number had decreased to 754. Anna thus built her successful business in the context of a declining market for custom-made women's clothing. Increasing competition from the ready-made clothing market and department-store dressmaking departments was driving a large number of independent dressmakers from the trade. During the next twenty years their numbers continued to drop rapidly, falling to 466 in 1920 and to 245 in 1930. By 1937, dressmakers in Providence numbered 144, equal to the 1880 level, a mere sixteen and a half percent of the 1906 peak.

In the face of competition, the Tirocchi sisters distinguished themselves through the prime location of their shop, their self-identification as makers of "gowns," and the employ of upwards of a dozen women in their operation. According to the family account, the sisters' vocational preparation resulted from contacts their mother had made while working as a cook in Rome, where Anna and Laura became apprenticed to a dressmaker whose customers were upper-class city dwellers. In Providence, Anna – the driving force in the enterprise – quickly demonstrated her skill at cultivating an exclusive clientele, as well as her dressmaking artistry.[11]

Dressmaking was characterized by features not common to other occupations popular with immigrants in the U.S. Producers and consumers joined together, often across class lines, to create original and highly personal products. Dressmakers found

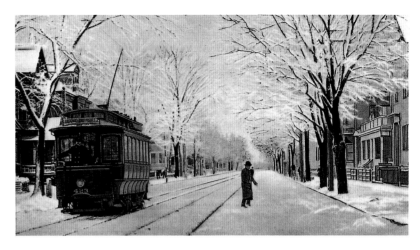

Fig. 63
Scene of a trolley on Broadway, showing the residential character of the street at that time; ca. 1910. Courtesy Rhode Island Historical Society, Providence.

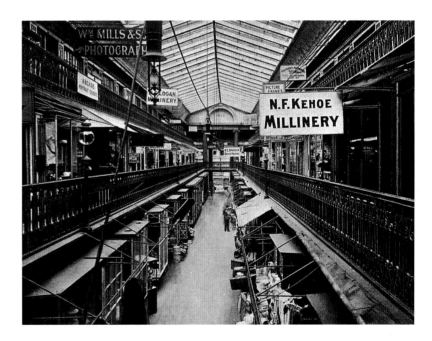

Fig. 64
The Arcade, downtown Providence (built in 1810); ca. 1910. Courtesy Rhode Island Historical Society, Providence (photograph by the Metropolitan News Company).

that social distance from their clients presented challenges to their free assertion of creativity and taste. Upper-class clients did not necessarily feel comfortable relying on their social inferiors in so intimate an area as fashion and also may have experienced some discomfort in exposing their bodies and tastes to tradeswomen. Dressmakers often sought to camouflage or reduce perceived class differences by adopting and projecting characteristics that reinforced their status and authority as artists and experts, thus clouding their working-class and immigrant origins. One of the most common strategies was to assert personal ties to the centers of high fashion, especially Paris. Claims of frequent trips to international style centers and the appropriation of the title "Madam" or "Madame" were used to distinguish a "gown maker" from her more common

sister artisans who did not enjoy upper-class patronage. Anna employed both of these tactics. She decorated the mansion on Broadway with fine European antiques and other furnishings. Her shop stationary in the 1920s was headed by a blue band highlighting the words "Di Renaissance," which suggested the European connection she sought to establish, and she did nothing to undermine the family's idea that while in Rome she had been employed by a dressmaker to the queen of Italy. Her full-page advertisement in the program for the 1928 Junior League presentation of the musical comedy *Oh Boy* [figs. 65–66] proclaimed "Exclusive Importations of Sportswear Coats and Suits" and included the following announcement: "Madam Tirocchi is now abroad attending the opening and selecting models and merchandise from different

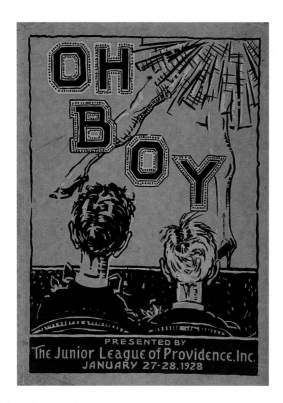

Fig. 65
Program cover of 1928 for *Oh Boy*: the Junior League of Providence held a theatrical performance each year to raise funds for its enterprises. Anna and Laura Tirocchi actively targeted the Junior League. They do not appear to have advertised in any publication other than the Junior League programs (reproduced by permission). Private collection.

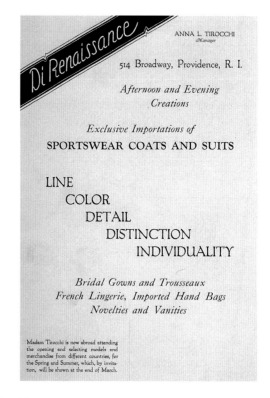

Fig. 66
Advertisement for the Tirocchi shop, then called "Di Renaissance": it appeared on p. 71 of the 1928 program for the musical-comedy production *Oh Boy* (reproduced by permission). Private collection.

countries, for the Spring and Summer, which, by invitation, will be shown at the end of March."[12]

Although frequent travel to Paris and New York is often mentioned with regard to Anna, there is no real documentation to verify annual "buying trips." Shop accounts and other written material in the Tirocchi Archive does indicate that she went to Europe on business in 1924, 1926–27, 1931, and 1938. While Anna listed customs duties as an expense only in her 1926 tax calculations, there are substantial customs declarations in the Tirocchi Archive for merchandise purchased in Paris in both 1924 and 1926. In early 1927, as she continued the journey begun in 1926, Anna bought some merchandise in Florence. While attempting to recover her health during an extended European trip in 1938, she visited Nice, where she saw no dresses that she wanted and was put off by the prices and the prospect of paying customs on any imports. Anna's employee and niece Emily Valcarenghi Martinelli, other workers, and family members have mentioned frequent trips abroad, but extant evidence remains only for the four noted above. The easy acceptance of regular sojourns in European fashion capitals in the accounts of various dressmakers is not especially puzzling, as the self-aggrandizement of both client and provider was served by the general acceptance of claims of a dressmaker's close and regular connection to the centers of haute couture. Historian Lois Banner explores the role of dressmakers "as a power in the land" promoting standards of fashion and beauty in the United States: "…the most successful had…also mastered the relationship between salesperson and client and were effectively able to manipulate their patrons by a subtle mixture of flattery and imperiousness." These phrases perfectly encapsulate much of the surviving description of Anna as an artist-businesswoman.[13]

Accounts of Anna as an employer indicate she was respected, but was not particularly generous in her pay rates. Following the classic pattern for proprietors of successful shops, she hired young women or girls as "apprentices" and paid them low wages, a practice justified by the theory that the girls were learning a valuable trade. While in high school, Louisa Furia D'Amore, the daughter of Anna's

cousin Maria and the granddaughter of Tito Tirocchi, worked briefly in the shop at her mother's urging, but Louisa recalled being frustrated by the slow pace at which Anna taught her the trade. While Anna kept her close by and exposed her to the business by allowing her to be present when clients were being served, she was not allowed to talk or report to others about what transpired. Louisa's duties consisted largely of picking up pins and sewing hooks on the insides of garments. She eventually left the shop to work in a handkerchief factory. Mary Rosa Traverso recalled that she herself began working in the shop at age sixteen but eventually moved on because she did not make much money. After leaving Anna's employ, Traverso worked twelve years for Mrs. Bernstein, who had a downtown shop in the Lapham Building on Westminster Street. On one occasion at least, Anna may have flouted child-labor and school-attendance laws when attempting to hire young girls.[14]

Anna paid more substantial wages to her most skilled workers. She is remembered as an exacting supervisor who insisted on high quality work from her employees. Both Louisa Furia D'Amore and Dr. Louis J. Cella, Jr., recalled her directing the third-floor workers by calling instructions down the hall from her room on days when she was too ill to leave her bed. Anna took an interest in the lives of her employees, advising them on the choice of a husband and providing trousseaus for some. Panfilo Basilico recalls being summoned to meet with Madam Tirocchi and to receive her approval before marrying one of the shop workers, Mary Riccitelli. Anna also provided a week's vacation at her summer retreat at Narragansett Pier for her "shop girls." They stayed in an apartment over the garage and had their meals in a log cabin attached to the main house. Beatrice Cella, Laura's daughter, anticipated their arrival for their week of vacation [figs. 67–69], for "then the fun begins. We play tennis every day and have a fine time." "There [sic] doing all the cooking so I think it will be our holiday instead of theirs."[15]

Something of Anna's personality and self-confidence is reflected in a letter she sent to E. L. DuPont de Nemours in 1939, following her return

Fig. 67
Tirocchi family members at the shore: (center) Louisa Furia D'Amore, (left) Evelyn Tirocchi, (right) Concetta Tirocchi (Evelyn and Concetta were daughters-in-law of Giuseppe and Assunta Tirocchi); ca. 1940. Private collection.

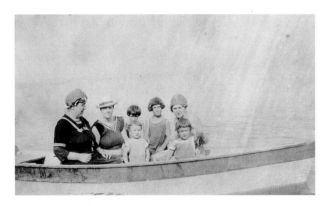

Fig. 68
Narragansett, Rhode Island, where Anna Tirocchi owned a summer home: pictured are some of the seamstresses from the Tirocchi shop on holiday; ca. 1930. Private collection.

Fig. 69
Tirocchi family members on vacation: (left to right) Anna Tirocchi, Laura Tirocchi Cella, and Maria del Signore Tirocchi with their children, Beatrice Cella, Louis J. Cella, Jr., Primrose Tirocchi, and Frank Tirocchi, Jr.; ca. 1918. Private collection.

from an extended stay in Europe, during which she visited Italian and French factories. She suggested mixing rayon with milk and soya beans to produce an elastic thread for stockings. Anna thought they might be called "MILK TRADE STOCKINGS by DUPONT."[16] She sent the letter by registered mail. Vincenzo (Jimmy) Tirocchi recalled occasionally chauffeuring Anna around town when he was a youth. On one trip she insisted that he double park in front of the Columbus Exchange Trust Company so that she could go in and "show him how to do business." With Jimmy in tow she marched into the manager's office and proceeded to aggressively negotiate a much reduced interest rate for a loan she was seeking.

Anna's two physical disabilities also may have contributed to the aura that impressed and somewhat intimidated her workers. She had some sort of problem with one leg and one arm and used these maladies to her advantage on occasion. An Internal Revenue Service auditor reported that her disabilities justified the expenses she claimed on her tax return and that although there were irregularities, she should be assessed no further tax. Bus drivers also adjusted the Broadway route and schedule to accommodate her "limited mobility."[17]

A certain exclusivity was most likely important for attracting and retaining upper-class customers. Anna's choice to seek an elite clientele probably also contributed to her self-imposed isolation from the larger Italian community in Providence. At a time when Italians suffered from substantial prejudice in the United States, Anna's rejection of Italian customers assured her upper-class clients that they would not have to contemplate sharing their dressmaker with socially inferior women, much less encountering them in person as fellow customers.[18] The young Italian American women who worked in the shop generally occupied the third-floor workroom and did not interact often with the clients who came for fittings or to transact other business. Anna's Italian workers did not always receive respect from the shop's patrons. Her niece and employee Emily Valcarenghi Martinelli recalls the often abrupt or indifferent treatment she received as a young girl while delivering dresses to clients.

"They'd just about open the door and they'd chop your little hand off if you didn't get over there and take it out."

Anna's isolation from the local Italian community extended beyond her choice of clients. Other than her family and the women hired to work in her shop, she seems to have had only limited and rather formal contact with her fellow countryfolk in Providence. Her Italian American social interactions were with persons prominent at the state level in Rhode Island, such as lawyer Antonio Capotosto, who became a State Supreme Court judge, and Mariano Vervena, the president of Columbus Exchange Trust Company and Italian vice-consul for Rhode Island. Mrs. Vervena [fig. 70] is the only Italian customer listed in the Tirocchi client books: the Columbus Exchange Trust Company was an important source for Anna's business capital. As Mariano's wife, she was at the top of the social ranking of Italians in the state. The Vervenas were among the handful of Italians who merited mention in press accounts of the wedding of Anna's sister Laura. Included, also, was Capotosto, then an Assistant State Attorney General, who was best man to Louis J. Cella. According to Primrose Tirocchi, Anna's shop made the dress for the wedding of Judge Capotosto's daughter, although the transaction does not appear in the shop records. Primrose also reported that Anna rejected business from Italian women whose husbands had become prosperous in the United States because they lacked the background to appreciate her artistry and status. Perhaps as fellow immigrants they were more aware of Anna's humble origins and less inclined than her upper-class American clients to accept or be manipulated by her strategies for status enhancement.[19]

Anna did not have many native-born American customers of middling status; however, Isabel Brown (later Mrs. Edgar Brunschwig), personal secretary to one of Anna's most prominent clients – Mrs. Stuart (Martha L.) Aldrich – was one of the few. The close relationship that developed between Anna and Isabel is an exception that suggests the impact of social status in the business. The personal and friendly communications between the two women contrast sharply with the more formal

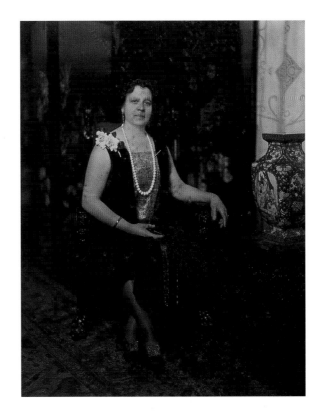

Fig. 70
Mrs. Mariano Vervena, the only Italian client listed in the records of the Tirocchi shop. Private collection.

business-style correspondence of Anna's elite customers. Anna was able to impress middle-class Americans with her cosmopolitanism. A real-estate agent from Narragansett, Mrs. S. A. Walsh, after a meeting with Anna, wrote: "It was a pleasure to listen to one who had really seen so much of the world and was big enough to take it in and be able to give others some idea of it all."[20]

In 1915, the *Providence City Directory* did not record any Italians in the neighborhood of Anna's new residence and shop at 514 Broadway, nor on the streets that intersected it. Directly to the west of it was Saint Mary's, a large, prosperous Irish Catholic parish. It was at this time that the household established a pattern of regularly attending services at the conveniently placed Saint Mary's, while still holding major family religious events at Holy Ghost on Federal Hill, the nearest Italian parish church. They also sent the children in their care to Saint Mary's for schooling. Frank's daughter Primrose

Tirocchi graduated from St. Mary's, but when it came to her religious instruction and First Communion, her mother insisted that those Catholic essentials take place at Holy Ghost, where proper Italian traditions would be honored. Primrose recalled that her mother objected to the Irish methods for designating godparents at St. Mary's.

Although Saint Mary's often received larger donations from Anna, her Christmas list included the priests at both parishes. Records of Anna's charitable contributions date from the early years on Broadway. If anything, they suggest an even further remove from the local Italian community. She donated to general charities in the Providence area, such as the Girl Scouts, Red Cross, Easter Seal Campaign, Catholic Charities, Rhode Island Hospital Fund, and the Society for the Prevention of Cruelty to Children. In some cases it seems likely that these were in part business-related, as her clients solicited them. Anna's gifts to the Girl Scouts and the Homeopathic Hospital supported favorite charities of two of her most important clients. When she gave to Italian causes, they were not local but national campaigns directed toward Italy, such as the Italian World War Veterans in the United States, a fund for families of war victims in Italy. She made donations to various religious orders and charities in Italy, as well as contributing substantially to the

reconstruction of the church in Guarcino. There is no indication that she supported local feast-day celebrations or other Italian American community activities in Rhode Island.[21]

Laura's choice of husband also suggests the Tirocchi sisters' distancing of themselves from the large southern Italian working-class population of Providence and a rise to middle-class status. Louis J. Cella [fig. 71] was one of the younger children in a large family. His parents emigrated from northern Italy in the nineteenth century: his mother entered the U. S. in 1879 and gained her citizenship in 1886. Louis had graduated from Rhode Island College of Pharmacy and University of Vermont Medical School before obtaining his Rhode Island license to practice medicine in 1915. At that time, he had two unmarried sisters and a brother living with his mother in Providence. Nina, the older sister, was a dressmaker for a department store, ironically, an institution that would eventually doom the dressmaking trade. Nina and sister Ida soon moved to California, where they purchased property and wrote optimistically to Louis about the prospects for real estate investment in the Los Angeles area. Dr. Cella was active in Providence Republican politics, served in China as a medical missionary, received an honor from the Italian government, but tellingly was not active in local Italian American social organizations. There is no evidence, for example, that he was physician to any mutual-benefit societies, as was common practice for Italian American doctors. He was awarded a brief entry in Ubaldo Pesaturo's 1936 compendium of prominent individuals in Rhode Island Italian communities, but no Cellas or Tirocchis were listed in the 1940 edition.[22]

As her dressmaking business prospered, Anna accumulated a number of real-estate holdings. Realtors solicited her, which suggests that she was known as a prospective investor in commercial properties. The purchase of the Broadway mansion was followed by the acquisition of an existing duplex on nearby Bainbridge Avenue and a lot fronting on Tobey Street, where Anna had a duplex and garage built in 1917. Soon thereafter, she and Dr. Cella together bought a set of leaseholds at 97–99 and 101–09 North Main Street, at the foot of the East

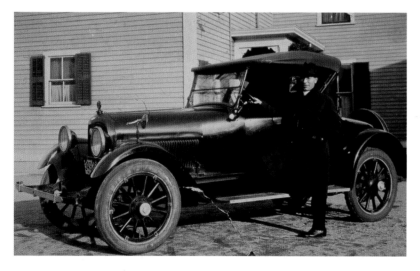

Fig. 71
Laura's husband Dr. Louis J. Cella beside his car; ca. 1930.
Private collection.

Side's College Hill just a short distance from Market Square [figs. 72–73]. These were substantial properties that included an auto-repair garage, a diner/restaurant, and a multistory commercial block. Scattered records seem to indicate that Anna managed the financial side of this joint holding for herself and Dr. Cella. She paid the taxes and rent due to the City of Providence on the lots, arranged for insurance, and kept accounts of tenant rents and capital costs.[23]

In subsequent years, Anna acquired a vacation home at Narragansett Pier, which also produced rental income for her, and a property in Cranston on which stood an auto service station. In the 1930s, as the dress business declined, rents from these holdings produced a larger proportion of her income. She also lent money to others. In 1922, the Columbus Exchange Trust Company collected payments on a mortgage held by Anna and credited them to her collateral loan with the bank. Over a decade later, she called in a mortgage from Giuseppe Scungio of Simmonsville, Rhode Island, in order to meet her own mortgage commitments. Anna had investments in Italy as well. She purchased Italian bonds and lent money to businessmen Agnello De Meis and Giovanni Castagnacci of Guarcino. The Castagnacci family manufactured felt as well as hats of straw and wool there. These Italian investments proved problematic. She had difficulty obtaining repayment of the loans, and the bonds became worthless after World War II.[24]

It is not easy to reconstruct an exact account of Anna's finances. The shop records indicate that Anna maintained personal funds not included in the shop records, from which she occasionally made loans to the business. She also regularly borrowed sums from her family and two banks to even out the shop's cash flow. Anna's sister Eugenia made several substantial loans, and her brother Frank advanced the business $1,000 [$9,500 in 1999 dollars] on at least one occasion. In addition to family sources, Anna secured her business financing and mortgages from the Columbus Exchange Trust Company and the Union Trust. In 1931, Anna borrowed $3,345 [$32,500] for A. & L. Tirocchi. Two years later she notes further loans amounting to $2,425 [$28,800].

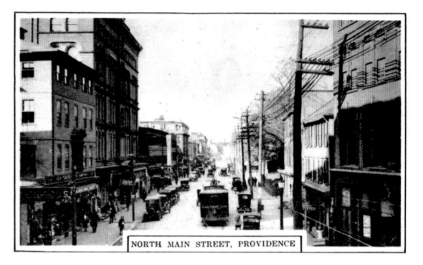

Fig. 72
North Main Street, Providence (looking north): Anna Tirocchi and Dr. Louis J. Cella owned the property at Nos. 101–09 (building at extreme right); ca. 1910. Courtesy State of Rhode Island, Archives, Providence.

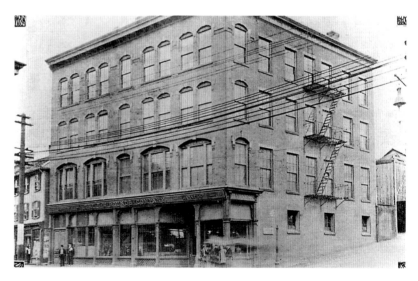

Fig. 73
The property owned by Anna Tirocchi and Dr. Louis J. Cella at 101–09 North Main Street, showing the auto repair garage at the rear (sometime after the photograph was taken, but before they bought the property in 1923, a one-story restaurant was added to the side of the building at right in the photograph); ca. 1890. Courtesy Rhode Island Historical Society, Providence.

Tirocchi Shop Income and Expenses: Various Years*

	1923	1926	1928	1932	1933	1934	1935	1937	1943
INCOME									
FROM CLIENTS	$18,760	$14,990	$12,265	$18,431	$13,440	$11,400	$7,304	$3,898	$528
RENT	2,076	3,862	4,517					3,414	2,997
DIVIDEND/INTEREST	300	360	300						356
TOTAL INCOME	$21,136	$19,212	$17,082	$18,431	$13,440	$11,400	$7,304	$7,312	$3,881
EXPENSES									
LABOR/WAGES	$7,097	$12,500	$8,291	$4,559	$2,743	$3,220	$2,570	$674	
MATERIALS/SUPPLIES	8,489	145	3,356	2,203	1,014		777	416	
MERCHANDISE FOR RESALE		22,000	33,685	7,828	7,391	4,644	3,120	2,031	402
TELEPHONE/TELEGRAPH	95		175	112		82	73	103	111
UTILITIES	545			606	576		159	894	612
POSTAGE/FREIGHT/BOXES	21		424	125	165	75	77	144	
INTEREST	1,320	1,710	1,440	2,081					674
TAXES	874	1,364	1,630					1,696	1,897
DEPRECIATION	1,099	2,305	2,325						
ADVERTISING	26			9	9	22		5	
CHARITY	50	95		91	85		38	158	144
INSURANCE				279	154		96	582	564
REPAIRS/MISC.	797	1,625	1,137	777	201		874		1,064
TRAVEL			510	100					
CUSTOMS DUTIES		632							
BAD DEBTS	696								
TOTAL EXPENSES	$21,109	$42,376	$52,973	$18,770	$12,338	$8,043	$7,784	$6,703	$5,441
NET INCOME	$27	$(23,164)	$(35,891)	$(339)	$1,102	$3,357	$(480)	$609	$(1,560)

*The data in this table are derived from informal work sheets used in the preparation
of Anna's federal income-tax returns; Tirocchi Archive.

Drafts of income-tax statements in the 1920s, when the shop's gross sales were as high as $18,000 [$174,353] and rents and dividends would add nearly $5,000 [$42,322] more income, indicate that after expenses were subtracted, the bottom line was not large. She had ongoing interest payments on mortgages and business loans, as well as substantial incurred costs for merchandise and materials for the shop. The Broadway, Tobey, and Bainbridge properties were often mortgaged, and there was a heavy loan against the Park Avenue gas station in Cranston. Anna also may have taken out loans against the Narragansett house. Assuming the interest on her loans to have averaged six percent, her reported annual interest payments indicate that she was carrying debts that varied between $22,000 and $34,683 [$213,097 and $369,510]. As the effects of the Depression and the changing nature of the women's clothing industry eroded her business in the 1930s, she tried unsuccessfully to sell her vacation property, although she wrote to her real estate agent that she "never liked a home so well" and regretted that her current poor health prevented her from enjoying the cottage and the Narragansett community.[25]

The table at left summarizes the data Anna used in completing some of her federal income tax returns. Several generalizations may be drawn. She did not keep systematic accounts and financial records that would allow her readily to summarize and monitor the performance of her various business activities. Erratic reporting of certain categories of expenses suggests that she concentrated on the assembly of sufficient "expenses" to eliminate any tax liability, rather than the production of a full accounting of her business and properties.[26] The sporadic notation of rental income probably results from her use of substantial depreciation figures to produce paper losses from her real-estate operations. The figures for the 1920s are those of rents received before any deductions. The absence of rents listed during the 1930s may have resulted from offsetting deductions that also went unreported. In 1943, she tallied $2,997 [$29,786] in rental income. Collections for December of that year produced $487. Annualized, these figures produce the yearly sum of $5,844 [$58,081], a number close to the amount

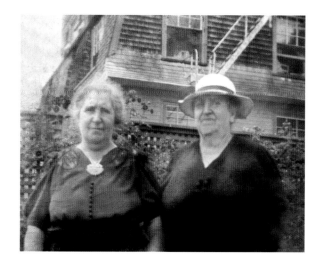

Fig. 74
Anna Tirocchi (right) and her sister Eugenia Tirocchi Valcarenghi in Providence; ca. 1930. Private collection.

of annual rents appearing on an undated calculation in the records for that time period. Unnoted deductions for depreciation, real estate taxes, and maintenance may account for the lower reported figure.

Anna's dressmaking business began a precipitous decline after 1932. Prior to that, her labor and materials expenses came close to offsetting the shop income. She also accrued sizable expenditures for "goods for resale," which resulted in large operating deficits. While she continued to purchase merchandise after 1932, a part of the shop's income in later years appears to have come from the sale of the extensive inventory, much of it purchased in the 1920s.

The inventory of Anna's estate, assembled after her death in 1947, valued the North Main Street leaseholds at $46,500 and Industrial Trust Company common stock at $1,140, yielding a total of $47,640 [$395,073]. Worthless assets included gold bonds of the defunct Philippine Railroad Company, 300 shares in the closed Columbus Exchange Trust Company, and $1,600 (the face value) in Kingdom of Italy gold bonds. There is no mention of the other real estate or any value placed on the business. This may indicate that there was no remaining value in the real estate after the mortgages were paid off. Anna also left $3,000 [$24,894] in life insurance, which was distributed among her sisters, Laura and Eugenia [fig. 74], and her brother Frank's children.

After expenses, the remainder of the estate was placed in trust for the support of Laura. Laura's daughter Beatrice was the executrix and inherited the residual upon the death of her mother.[27]

In parlaying her dressmaking skill into a substantial business, and by virtue of her selective social contacts, Anna exemplified the qualities of middle-class immigrants in the United States. This group is representative of a very small portion of immigrant women. Their experiences have been less well studied than the lives of their working-class sisters in the early twentieth century. From the beginning, Anna's situation deviated from the common pattern. Her successful dressmaking business catered to the American-born upper and upper-middle classes. Few other immigrant businesses relied exclusively on nonimmigrant customers. Caterers, barbers, tailors, gardeners, contractors, and the like might eventually enjoy the patronage of the broader American community, but they usually began by serving their fellow immigrants. Her sister Eugenia's grocery store represents this more common form of entrepreneurship. Such businesses typically found their niche by serving the ethnic tastes of fellow immigrants. In 1909, the *Providence Sunday Journal* published a description of an Italian grocery in the Silver Lake enclave, comparing it to an old-fashioned country store.

> There is an almost infinite variety of products not found anywhere else. The ceilings and walls present an interesting study for the student of domestic sciences. Long strings of silver-shelled garlic hang side by side with large, flat Italian hams, queer balls of meat minced with spices and pressed tightly into bags; bright peppers that look like trimmings for a christmas [sic] tree, festoons of dark sausage and bunches of things that have the appearance of earthen bottles of a wax in color [sic], the outside shell being of the consistency of granite, but really a fine brand of cheese. On the counters and shelves are great loaves of bread, vegetables, a variety of canned goods and packages of olive oil. In the center of the room is a pyramid of long boxes of macaroni.[28]

This account is very close to Primrose Tirocchi's description of her aunt Eugenia's store.

Perhaps the most important feature of Anna's life and career was her continued status as a single woman, which varied from the typical experience. Married immigrant women contributed to their families' financial well-being in a variety of ways. Some, like Anna's sister Eugenia Valcarenghi, operated groceries or other family businesses with their husbands. In Eugenia's case, the extraordinary entrepreneurial spirit displayed by many of the Tirocchis and the fact that she ran the business alone for many years after her husband's untimely death suggest that she may have been the moving force behind the grocery all along. Eugenia's husband, moreover, had continued in Providence to pursue his former Italian employment as a house painter. In some years, Luigi is listed in the *Providence City Directories* as a grocer; in others, he is designated a painter or decorator. Eugenia also regularly took in boarders, a common means by which immigrant women contributed to their family income without working outside the home, and rented storefront space in her building to other businesses. Primrose Tirocchi remembered both her aunts Eugenia and Anna as powerful personalities in the family. Another Tirocchi woman who played an important role in a family business was Assunta, the wife of Tito's son Giuseppe, who for years merited a separate entry in the *Providence City Directory* as secretary for her husband's Ideal Concrete Products Company. Often, immigrant women supplemented the family income through labor accomplished at home. Mary Riccitelli worked in the Tirocchi shop for years, becoming one of its most skilled seamstresses. After her marriage to Panfilo Basilico, she left 514 Broadway but contributed to her new family as many Italian women did, by sewing at home.[29]

In remaining unmarried, Anna avoided any possibility of having to share authority or defer to a husband. The patriarchal family governance often attributed to Italian culture did not touch her. With Dr. Cella, her American-born brother-in-law, Anna invested in several commercial properties, and his practice was located at 514 Broadway. Anna managed the business aspects associated with their properties, such as paying taxes and arranging insurance. When it came to the shared expenses of the Broadway businesses (Dr. Cella's medical practice and the dress shop), Anna paid the bills and Louis reimbursed her for his share. On occasion he would deal with the shop's bookkeeper "so as not to disturb Miss Tirocchi."[30] The assumption that women generally should be subject to male authority was, of course, not limited to Italians. In 1920, the census enumerator first recorded the Broadway house as Anna's property, but then crossed out the entry and made Dr. Cella the household "head," giving him ownership of the property. Anna was designated as the "sister-in-law" in her own home.

Taken together, the Tirocchis illustrate a number of themes common to the immigrant experience of the time; yet, paradoxically, they also go beyond it as well. They migrated in search of greater economic opportunity, and the family displayed unusual spirit, talent, and business acumen. The men established businesses in construction and service industries, common areas for immigrant entrepreneurship, and the women sometimes played important roles in these endeavors, as well as earning money through work done at home. Anna represents an exception to the common experience for women and for immigrants in general. She remained single, independent, and the proprietor of a business that put her in intimate contact with upper- and upper-middle-class Americans. She and Laura cultivated a middle-class life, limiting their contacts with the larger Italian working class in Providence to members of their own family. Personal inclinations as well as business strategies undoubtedly prompted this social mobility. Anna made a number of trips back to Italy; but, if the surviving correspondence is any indication, she focused her attention on middle-class members of the family while there, the Del Signores and the priests Andrea and Ignazio Tirocchi, members of an Italian Franciscan religious order. Kin such as Salvatore's eldest son Federico Achille Tirocchi, pastor of the Roman Catholic parish of the Sacred Heart in the Natick section of West Warwick, Rhode Island, also maintained close ties with Anna [fig. 75].[31]

Family solidarity was a major asset in the Tirocchi successes in Providence. Anna entertained the families of her brother, sisters, and cousins at her

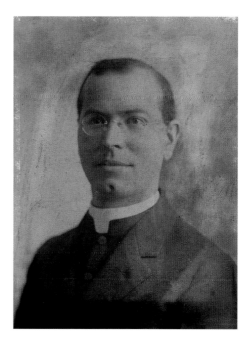

Fig. 75
Father Federico Achille Tirocchi, a Roman Catholic priest and son of Salvatore Tirocchi: Father Tirocchi served the Church in Canada and later in Natick, an area in West Warwick, Rhode Island. Private collection.

Narragansett Pier home. Surviving cousins fondly recalled vacations there, as well as the silver dollars Anna distributed to the Tirocchi children. Mention has been made of the important loans family members made to Anna's business. Anna also contributed to the economic health of other family members. Frank's trucking business was the beneficiary of a number of sums from Anna over the years. She also paid off a mortgage he and Maria had contracted in 1917. Dr. Cella continued to maintain his office in Eugenia's Pocasset business block for a brief time after his marriage to Laura, and he relied on his brother-in-law Frank as agent in the management of his farm. Anna managed some financial tasks for her Uncle Tito in both Providence and Italy. She received a number of nephews and nieces into the Broadway house for periods of time and supported their schooling at the neighboring St. Mary's Parish School. She also supported their further education and professional aspirations. Laura's daughter Beatrice received the bulk of these contributions. Beatrice's brother, Dr. Louis J. Cella, Jr., believes that Anna vetoed Laura's desire that her daughter Beatrice become a nun. Certainly Anna played a prominent role in Beatrice's education, paying for music lessons, supporting a correspondence course, and assuming the cost of her college tuition. Anna also took an interest in the education of male members of the younger generation of Tirocchis. She wrote to a cousin once removed, Carlo C. Tirocchi, while he was in military service, telling him that she had opened a savings account for him and was sure that he, like Angelo, another of the younger generation of Tirocchis under her wing, would have enough money to finish high school, college, and "get a nice profession." Carlo died while in the military, and Anna took responsibility for reporting the unhappy event in the Rhode Island records.[32]

Family support was central to the flourishing of other Tirocchi undertakings as well. Anthony

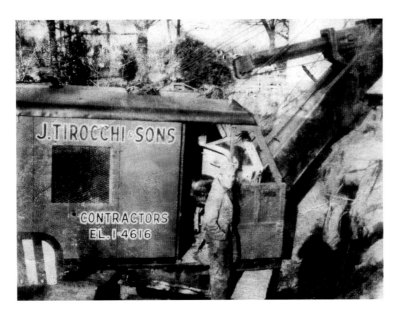

Fig. 76
Eugene Tirocchi (son of Giuseppe and Assunta Tirocchi and grandson of Tito Tirocchi) with a power excavating shovel; ca. 1950–60. Private collection.

Tirocchi observed that the family "came together and went apart" as they established businesses and made their way in Providence. They competed in the gravel, construction, and cement business, as well as in trucking. Mario Tirocchi entered the tire retreading business after seeing his sister Maria Tirocchi Furia's family open the Hartford Tire Company on the Hartford Avenue family property. His brother, Giuseppe, negotiated the political arrangements necessitated by wartime economic controls. Between the two firms, they serviced all the major tire retailers in the Providence area. Most of the male second-generation Tirocchis worked for their uncles' businesses, as well as for their fathers. Mario was a bachelor and something of a character. He managed to get the women of the family to wash and sterilize the bottles for his milk business. They complained that they worked at a nasty job while he was out driving around in the milk truck. His nephews recall that he managed to get them to do all the heavy work, while he traveled from job to job, supervising the work of others. When Salvatore's sons sold the Rhode Island Laundry, it went to their cousins, the grandchildren of Tito. As Tito's family acquired more heavy-duty construction equipment, including the first crane in Rhode Island, they shared it with the various Tirocchi businesses [fig. 76].

In the end, Anna Tirocchi, for all her independence and business initiative, was constrained by the traditions that shaped her early life. At a time when the women's clothing industry was undergoing revolutionary change, she persisted in an earlier artisan mode, relying on her fashion skills, artistic taste, and strong personality to resist the tide for some time. When she looked beyond dressmaking for investment opportunities, she chose the well trodden path of real estate. Like her sister dressmakers and milliners, she remained apart from the new industrial and commercial order.

The Tirocchis' Providence

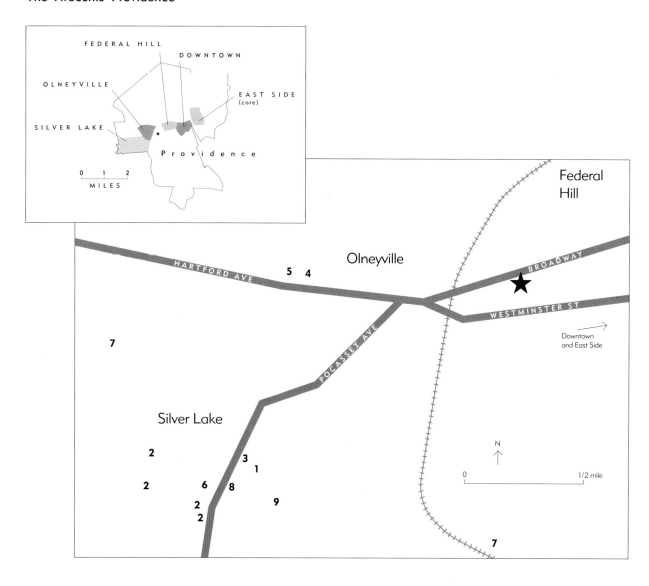

KEY TO MAP

★ Anna Tirocchi and Laura Tirocchi Cella's family home and business, A. & L. Tirocchi,
  and Dr. Louis J. Cella's medical office. 514 Broadway.

1 Salvatore Tirocchi's first residence in Providence. 50 What Cheer Avenue.

2 Salvatore Tirocchi's family home and businesses, including Tirocchi Brothers Trucking Company, Rhode Island Laundry, Rhode Island Improved
  Cement Company. 836 Plainfield Street, 131 Farmington Avenue, 136 Silver Lake Avenue, 371 Dyer Avenue, and 80 Eliza Street.

3 Eugenio Tirocchi's first residence in Providence (the first Tirocchi listed in Providence records). 25 Hillhurst Avenue.

4 Giuseppe and Eugenio Tirocchi's family homes and businesses, including Ideal Concrete Products, Hartford Tire Company,
  and a miniature golf course. 266–72 Hartford Avenue.

5 Angelo Tirocchi's auto service station. 314 Hartford Avenue.

6 Maria Tirocchi Furia and Francesco Furia's home and business. 144 Prudence Avenue.

7 Mario Tirocchi's home and businesses, including his auto service station and various other ventures. 540 Huntington Avenue, 105 Sunset Avenue.

8 Eugenia Tirocchi Valcarenghi's business block with family home, grocery, and rentals. 322–24 Pocasset Avenue.

9 Frank Tirocchi's family home and business. 71 Alto Street.

Tirocchi Family Genealogy

EUGENIO TIROCCHI* AND MARIA ROSSI*
(Guarcino, Italy)

Nazzareno Tirocchi* and Rosa Fraticalli*①
(Guarcino, Italy)

1. Anna Tirocchi†
No issue

2. Eugenia Tirocchi† and ? Federici*①   and Luigi Valcarenghi†②
Ida Federici [Tirocchi]†

Emily Valcarenghi [Martinelli]
William Valcarenghi
Rosa Valcarenghi
Georgina Valcarenghi
Henry Valcarenghi

3. Frank Tirocchi† and Maria Del Signore
Primrose Tirocchi
Frank Tirocchi, Jr.

Giuseppe Tirocchi* and Rosa Fraticalli Tirocchi*②
(Guarcino, Italy)

1. Laura Tirocchi† and Louis J. Cella
Beatrice Cella (no issue)
Louis J. Cella, Jr. (father of L. J. Cella III and Edward Cella)

① First marriage
② Second marriage
[ ] Married name, if known
* Never left Italy
† Born in Italy and came to the U.S.

Tito Tirocchi† and Luisa Iacobelli*
(Guarcino, Italy – Providence, RI) and (Guarcino, Italy)

1. **Eugenio Tirocchi**† and Maria Verdecchia
   Laura Tirocchi
   Tito Tirocchi
   Dora Tirocchi
   Josephine Tirocchi
   Joseph Tirocchi

2. **Angelo Tirocchi**† and Anna Ludovici
   Angelo Tirocchi
   Louise Tirocchi
   Joseph Tirocchi
   Mary Tirocchi
   Jenny Tirocchi
   Selma Tirocchi
   Tresa Tirocchi

3. **Guiseppe Tirocchi**† and Assunta Moriconi
   Vincenzo (Jimmy) Tirocchi
   Valentino Tirocchi
   Eugene Tirocchi
   Giuseppe Tirocchi
   Louis Tirocchi
   Carlo Tirocchi
   Anthony Tirocchi (father of Lisa)

4. **Maria Tirocchi**† and Francesco Furia†
   Luigi Furia
   Vincenzo Furia
   Louisa Furia [D'Amore]
   Armelinda Furia

5. **Mario Tirocchi**†
   No issue

Salvatore Tirocchi† and Luisa Guadrana†
(Guarcino, Italy – Providence, RI)

1. **Fr. Federico Achille Tirocchi**†
   No issue

2. **Elvira Tirocchi**† and Cesare Marianetti
   ?

3. **Luigi Tirocchi**† and Antonia Renzi
   Valerimina Tirocchi
   Louis Tirocchi
   Elvira Tirocchi
   Achille Tirocchi
   Salvatore Tirocchi
   Anna Tirocchi
   Elizabeth Tirocchi

4. **Gerardo Tirocchi**† and Luisa ?
   ?

5. **Giuseppe Tirocchi**† and Anna ?
   Elvira Tirocchi
   Louisa Tirocchi [Marianetti]
   Vincenza Tirocchi

6. **Augusto Tirocchi**† and Ida Federici
   Gloria Tirocchi
   Mary Tirocchi
   Frederick Tirocchi

7. **Giovanni Tirocchi**† and Concetta DeSimone
   John Tirocchi
   Dolores Tirocchi
   Gerald Tirocchi
   Louise Tirocchi
   Marie Tirocchi

The interviews referred to and quoted in this essay are to be found in the A. & L. Tirocchi Archive, Museum of Art, Rhode Island School of Design, Providence (hereafter referred to as Tirocchi Archive). Such references have not been footnoted. All letters sent or received by Anna or Laura Tirocchi are understood to be found in the Tirocchi Archive. See "Note on the A. & L. Tirocchi Archive, Collection, and Catalogue," p. 23.

Additional interviews were conducted by the author and are not included in the Tirocchi Archive. References to and quotations from the author's interviews are not footnoted. The following paragraph includes all such material and stands in place of footnoting.

Members of the Tirocchi family provided information and guidance that contributed substantially to this author's research and to this essay. The author is especially indebted to Anthony Tirocchi and his daughter Lisa, Vincenzo (Jimmy) Tirocchi, Louisa Furia D'Amore, and Joseph Tirocchi, who spent two evenings talking with me about their family history (April 10 and 12, 2000). Anthony and Lisa generously shared their extensive genealogical research, which was invaluable in my reconstruction of the Tirocchi family in Providence. Primrose Tirocchi graciously provided information and family photographs in an interview with the author (May 18, 1999) and subsequent telephone conversations.

1. Karl Baedeker, *Southern Italy and Sicily, with Excursions to Malta, Sardinia, Tunis, and Corfu: Handbook for Travellers.* Leipzig, London, New York: 1930, p. 15. The 1909 Baedeker guide *Central Italy and Rome: Handbook for Travellers* indicates that there was no rail connection with Guarcino. Http://www.eurolink.it/ciociaria/c_guarc.htm and http://www.rtmol.stt.it/ciociaria/citta/guarcino.html provide online information on contemporary Guarcino.

2. An expanded statement of this argument is found in John W. Briggs, *An Italian Passage, Immigrants to Three American Cities, 1890–1930.* New Haven: 1978; see especially the introduction and chap. 1.

3. Municipio di Guarcino, Ufficio dello Stato Civilie, *Registro – Atti di Morti*, 1879, no. 29; 1882, no. 72; 1893, nos. 10, 14, 23; and Municipio di Guarcino, Ufficio dello Stato Civile, *Registro – Atti di Nascita*, 1891, no. 22; also, the author's interviews with Tirocchi family members. Microfilm copies are available through the genealogy service of the Church of Jesus Christ of the Latter Day Saints.

4. The summary that lists other Tirocchis and associated families is the result of a search of records in the Archivio di Stato, Frosinone, Italia: Municipio di Guarcino, Ufficio dello Stato Civile, *Atti di Nascita*, 1889, 1891; *Atti di Matrimoni*, 1876–77, 1882, 1885, 1895; *Atti di Morti*, 1877, 1879–80, 1882–83, 1885, 1893, 1895; *Registro delle Publicazione di Matrimonio*, 1876–78, 1881, 1883, 1885, 1887, 1890–91, 1898.

5. "Chain migration" refers to a pattern of supported migration wherein the earliest migrants encourage and sponsor subsequent migration by other family members and close associates. Chain migrations usually result in a concentration of family members in one city of immigration, as pioneer migrants persuade and assist brothers, sisters, cousins, parents, etc., to join them in their adopted country. St. Bartholomew Parish on Laurel Hill Avenue in the Silver Lake community still acknowledges Guarcino as one of two Italian communes that provided its early parishioners. See the history of the parish Holy Name Society at http://www.rc.net/providence/stbartholomew/holyname.html

Also see "Italian Farmers," *Providence Sunday Journal* (October 18, 1891), p. 16; "The Italians of Silver Lake," *Providence Sunday Journal* (June 29, 1902), p. 18; and "Where Thrift and Enterprise Convert Rocky Wastes Into Fertile Acres," *Providence Sunday Journal* (June 6, 1915), sect. 5, p. 3. I am indebted to Father Robert W. Hayman of Providence College for bringing these references to my attention and allowing me to work from his clippings.

6. U.S. Bureau of the Census, *Thirteenth Census of the United States: 1910 Population.*

7. A later census lists Anna and Laura as entering the country in 1907, but this may indicate the year they arrived in Providence. The author has relied on the 1910 census, since the enumerator carefully recorded different dates of migration for different individual members of the families. In the photographs, Frank's status as boss is indicated by his hands. He holds a cigarette in one, and in the other grasps a piece of paper. The workers typically hold shovels, picks, crow bars, or other tools in such photographs. It would be interesting to know if Frank Tirocchi's stint as a labor contractor in Canada was connected to Father Federico Achille Tirocchi's mission there.

8. Among Maria's relatives, Gino Del Signore had a successful career in the Italian opera [see fig. 57]. His father Gino was a merchant in Rome. Vincenzo Del Signore operated a building and road construction business in Guarcino. Other Del Signores listed in the Guarcino Stato Civile records were either masons or carpenters.

Primrose Tirocchi reported that her father managed a drug store on Atwells Avenue for Anna at this time. Primrose possesses a mortar and pestle from that shop, and chairs from the ice cream parlor in the store ended up in the third-floor workroom at 514 Broadway. No written records from this enterprise survive in the Tirocchi Archive. The author's account of Tirocchi enterprises is constructed from *Providence City Directories*, state and federal manuscripts, and family interviews.

9. Other evidence indicates that Eugenia was most likely thirty-one or thirty-two years of age and Laura might have been nineteen or twenty years old in 1910. It is not unusual to find ages reported in censuses to be "averaged" down or occasionally up.

10. Dr. Cella's mother's maiden name was Garibaldi, and the family claimed a connection to the Italian hero.

11. While Laura Tirocchi was at Anna's side throughout the history of the dressmaking shop, the evidence indicates that Anna

was the prime mover at each stage of the business and the architect of her financial and professional life. This essay thus makes Anna the center of its story. Wendy Gamber, *The Female Economy, The Millinery and Dressmaking Trades, 1860–1930*, part II. Urbana: 1997, documents the rise of department stores and their effect on independent dressmakers and milliners. See also Lois W. Banner, *American Beauty*. New York: 1983, chap. 2, for the rise of the ready-to-wear clothing industry and the success of department stores in attracting upper-class women. See Pat Trautman, "Personal Clothiers: A Demographic Study of Dressmakers, Seamstresses and Tailors, 1880–1920," *Dress*, vol. 5 (1979), pp. 74–95, for a general description of the waxing and waning of the custom-clothing industry.

12. *Oh Boy, presented by the Junior League of Providence, Inc.* (January 27–28, 1928), p. 77. Madam Zarr also purchased a full-page advertisement at the cost of $50 [or about $467 in 1999 dollars]. Throughout this essay the author has included conversions of monetary figures into 1999 dollars and enclosed the present-day figures within brackets. Data since 1975 are from the annual *Statistical Abstracts of the United States*. Prior to 1975, they are based on the Consumer Price Index from *Historical Statistics of the United States* (USGPO, 1975). The calculations were made with a program created by S. Morgan Friedman and available at http://www.westegg.com/inflation.

13. There are only a few references in the shop records to U.S. Customs payments that suggest substantial imports. On April 2, 1924, Anna paid a $5 customs bill for "increased duties" following her European trip that year. The 25,326 francs worth of goods that she declared in Paris convert to about $4600 [$43,768 in 1999 dollars]. The duty for her imports in 1926, after she received a refund for overpayments, still approached $600 [$5500 in 1999 dollars]. On each of these trips she also purchased household furnishings and antiques: see the itemized customs declarations for March 10, 1924, and August 11, 1926, among the travel documents in the shop records; and Iqina Catelani to "Gentilissma Signora" [Anna], Firenze, April 25, 1924. Also see correspondence and itemized bill from the firm G. Gandola, "Trine-Ricami" [lace-embroidery], Firenze, to Anna Tirocchi, February 14, 16, and 19, 1927, in the Italian-language Tirocchi correspondence. Anna Tirocchi to Mrs. Martella, Anna's bookkeeper, n.d., in which Anna discusses a variety of business matters, including her income tax, the renting of her vacation home at Narragansett Pier, insurance policies, and the high utility bills resulting from too many hot baths, an issue she had also raised with Dr. Cella. Apparently, her niece Emily Valcarenghi Martinelli was managing the shop in her absence. Anna worried that Emily might be buying too much merchandise and advised that she return dresses that proved unsalable. Anna recommends not purchasing from one supplier, Colli, who had refused to take back unsold goods in the past. Gamber, *op.cit.*, explores the social-class dynamics of these trades in chap. 4 and *passim*. Mary Molloy, the daughter of an Irish immigrant, built a customer base in St. Paul, Minnesota, by 1900 that resembles Anna's. Molloy's business closed the year after Anna and Laura opened their establishment at the Butler Exchange. Accounts of Molloy's career include references to her French connections, including trips to Paris at least annually to keep up on the latest in fashion. Judith Jerde, "Mary Molloy: St. Paul's Extraordinary Dressmaker," *Minnesota History*, vol. 47, no. 3 (Fall 1980), pp. 93–99. Another Twin Cities modiste, Madame Rose Boyd, also was believed to make trips to Paris twice a year "to view the latest fashions"; see Julieanne Trautmann, "'Sizing up' the client, Minneapolis dressmaker Madame Rose Boyd," MA thesis, University of Minnesota, October 1997, pp. 2, 37, 159, 167. Banner, *op. cit.*, p. 29.

14. Shop records include age certificates for Mary Barone, who was fourteen years and five months old on September 29, 1919; and Francesca Caito, age fourteen years and three months on January 27, 1922. Lucy Restivo began working at age fourteen years and three months: Lucy's mother "made her work." The Tirocchi Archive includes a note from a truant officer: "To whom it may concern – It is impossible for any child to secure an Employment Certificate until they are fourteen years old."

15. Beatrice Cella to Mother, Father, and Brother, July 19 and 24, 1935. She reported having fun on the ride down to Narragansett in her uncle's laundry truck.

16. Anna Tirocchi to E. L. DuPoint [*sic*] de Nemours, December 11, 1939.

17. Dr. Louis J. Cella, Jr., described her leg problem as "tuberculosis of the knee which caused her to walk with a stiff gait for life." Report of audit of 1929 return, February 5, 1931, found that the taxpayer was an "individual who is crippled and has to hire help to do her work being unable to do it herself." Anna's 1930 return was also audited without any additional tax levies. See the copy of the auditor's report, May 26, 1932; Tirocchi Archive.

18. Gamber, *op. cit.*, p. 195, notes that department stores often sought to attract wealthy customers with private showrooms, where their most elite clientele could enjoy "all the privacy that they would enjoy in their own chambers."

19. According to Primrose Tirocchi, Anna claimed that the wives of newly well-to-do Italians lacked the culture and taste to appreciate her artistry. Perhaps as upwardly mobile persons themselves, they would not accept Anna's claims to higher social status. In an ironic series of events, Mariano Vervena, after serving in the Italian diplomatic service for thirty years, became an American citizen in 1932. He was quoted in the *Providence Evening Bulletin* (April 25, 1932) as explaining "America is my homeland. My wife and five of my six children were born here…my business is here"; Tirocchi Archive. Less than a year later, his Columbus Exchange Trust Company failed, and he returned to Italy permanently. See obituaries in the *Providence Evening Bulletin* (July 26, 1955), *New York Herald Tribune* (July 27, 1955), and a paper in Sorrento, Italy (July 27, 1955); Tirocchi Archive. The account of Laura's wedding in the *Providence Evening Tribune* (July 2, 1915) includes a sizable list of guests with non-Italian names; Tirocchi Archive.

20. See Isabel R. Brown to My Dear Anna, October 12, 1919, and I. R. Brown to Anna, November 23, 1919. Mrs. S. A. Walsh to Anna Tirocchi, Sept. 13, 1933.

21. Due bill from Vincenzo Del Signore, October 2, 1928, for "Riparazioni alla Chiesa Parrocchiale di S. Michele Arcangelo chesi asiguesione per conto della Signa. Anna Tirocchi"; Tirocchi Archive. The charge was 11,811 lire, or about $622 [$5800 in 1999 dollars]. Anna did contribute to a fund for the repair of Holy Ghost Church, which earned her a ticket to sit in the VIP section at the rededication of the church by the Bishop. Anna's contributions are listed in the shop checkbook stubs and in her income tax returns for the 1920s; Tirocchi Archive. The Tirocchis were strongly religious. In addition to Father Federico, at least two others were members of the Franciscan order in Italy. Anna and Laura regularly gave to religious charities, while the Silver Lake Tirocchis were major supporters of St. Bartholomew's and Holy Cross, the mission parish that developed in Johnston, Rhode Island, after World War II. Angelo's son Joseph was one of at least two American-born children that the family sought to direct to the clergy. He was sent to Brothers of Charity schools in Massachusetts and Quebec.

22. The history of dressmaking in the United States is recounted in Gamber, op. cit. Much of the family information is constructed from the 1920 census manuscripts. The letters are in the Tirocchi Archive. Dr. Cella's obituary ran in the Providence Journal (January 12, 1965), p. 30; Tirocchi Archive. The account of his China service came from his son, Dr. Louis J. Cella, Jr., who recalled visiting him in China. See Ubaldo U. M. Pesaturo, Italo-Americans in Rhode Island. Providence: 1936 and 1940, pp. 106–7.

23. Members of other branches of the Tirocchi family had established the Rhode Island Cement Works Company and worked as contractors. Not surprisingly, Anna employed them in the Tobey project. She paid $50 to John Miller for plans for the house and hired the Ideal Concrete Products Company (her cousins Giuseppe and Eugenio) to pour the cellar foundations. See entries for June 20, 1917, and July 5, 1917 in the shop account books; Tirocchi Archive. Anna and Dr. Cella took possession of the Main Street building on October 3, 1923. Payment and financing of this transaction are indicated in the 1923–24 shop financial records; Tirocchi Archive. Anna's payments are recorded in the shop financial records; Tirocchi Archive. P. Russo to Anna Tirocchi, November 23, 1922. The mortgage to Harvey Becthkas was for $3500 [$31,766 in 1999 dollars]. Her note with the bank had a $2500 [$22,690] balance. For the Simmonsville mortgage, see shop financial records, February 4, 1934; Tirocchi Archive.

24. See shop financial record entries for September 28, 1927, and January 21, 1929, for interest from Italian Consolidated Bonds; Tirocchi Archive. Giovanni Castagnacci to Laura Cella, September 10, 1928, acknowledges the loan from Anna. De Meis's stationary identifies him as "Appaltatore Delle Esattorie" (contractor/agent of tax collector's offices) for Trivigliano and Torre Caietani with his office in Guarcino. In the nineteenth century, the De Meis family was most often listed as substantial landholders in the community records. After De Meis died in 1927, Anna sought to recover her investment through receipts from a tax sale of the deceased's house and garden; Affino Giggalconi to Anna, n.d. On March 26, 1929 (Anna Tirocchi to Loreta De Meis), she wrote the widow seeking

repayment of 2500 lire [$1,241 in 1999 dollars]. Anna expressed sensitivity for the widow, but sought sympathy for the costs to her health involved in earning the money in the first place. She also stressed the importance of maintaining Agnello's good name and indicated that her patience was waning, suggesting that she might be forced to legal action.

25. Anna Tirocchi to Mrs. S. A. Walsh, November 16, 1934.

26. Banner, op. cit., pp. 28–32, asserts that dressmakers typically emphasized their craft and artistry over astute business strategy.

27. Anna's will and estate settlement are filed in Providence City Probate Court, no. 48948.

28. "Federal Hill's Growing Rival Silver Lake," Providence Sunday Journal (September 19, 1909); see also the Providence Journal (October 7, 1888), p. 10; these clippings from Father Hayman's files give an indication of the important role played by groceries in Italian communities (see n. 5); Eugenia, for example, extended credit to her customers, according to Primrose Tirocchi.

29. Panfilo Basilico built a popular and successful bakery on the East Side of Providence. He spoke in his interview with high respect for and praise of Anna's ability to develop a business based on a wealthy East Side "Anglo" patronage.

30. Notes from Dr. Cella to Mrs. Mastella, 1940 (no day or month given), and December 30, 1940, in the shop financial records; Tirocchi Archive.

31. See correspondence in the Tirocchi Archive.

32. Tirocchi Archive and author's interviews: evidence of Anna's support of Frank's business is scattered throughout the shop records for the 1920s (Tirocchi Archive) in the form of insurance payments on his truck and a Ford touring car; a down payment for a Packard truck, January 13, 1921; and payments prompted by an automobile accident; as well as the paying off of a mortgage on June 25, 1923. As mentioned before, Frank ran his business from the Broadway house and lived in one of Anna's apartments in the late 1920s. Other indications of family support includes a typed note from Ida [Federici, Eugenia Tirocchi Valcarenghi's daughter by her first husband], 324 Pocasset Avenue, November 2, 1920, returning a check from Anna and explaining that what she did for Anna "was done with a free heart with no intention of being repaid." At the time, Ida was a bookkeeper. She also discusses a coat that Anna bought for her. Tito Tirocchi to My dear niece, August 13, 1925; and Anna Tirocchi to Esteemed Mister Agnello, n.d.; Anna Tirocchi to Carlo C. Tirocchi, May 8, 1940, and May 21, 1940. Also see Angelo G. Tirocchi to Anna, July 13, 1934, and November 11, 1934, reporting on his progress in the Civilian Conservation Corps and his self-education efforts; Mrs. A. Martella [for Anna Tirocchi], January 23, 1942; and Anna Tirocchi to Tony Tirocchi, May 12, 1941. State death records, November 26, 1941, no. 379.

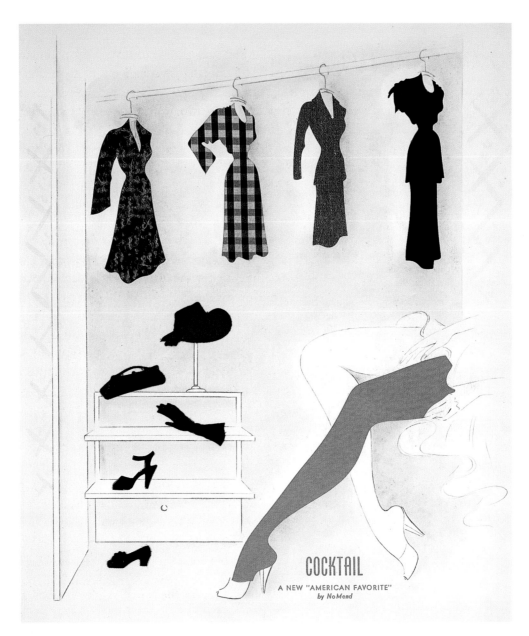

COCKTAIL

A NEW "AMERICAN FAVORITE"
by No Mend

Fig. 77
"Cocktail," one of the eight hosiery shades offered in the fashion guide
American Favorites by No-Mend Hosiery, Inc. (Fall–Winter 1941–42; see fig. 81,
p. 111). Courtesy Museum at the Fashion Institute of Technology, New York.

MADELYN SHAW
Associate Curator of Costume and Textiles
Museum of Art, Rhode Island School of Design

American Fashion:

The Tirocchi Sisters in Context

Anna and Laura Tirocchi maintained a small, personalized dress business in Providence for over thirty years. These decades saw two world wars, a global economic depression, and the transformation of the industry of which they were a small part; however, the knowledge gained through study of the surviving Tirocchi shop inventory and records is only a fragment of the story of the women's garment industry in America. Were the Tirocchis and their clients unique or typical? Was their experience of and response to the changes in their industry singular or common? To understand the Tirocchis' place in the dressmaking hierarchy of their day and the changes in the structure of their business, one must examine the wider world of American fashion.

Between 1900 and 1950, the ways in which American women of all social and economic levels thought about and acquired their clothing changed considerably. Any pretense to true high fashion in the early twentieth century required the purchase of a custom-made and custom-fitted wardrobe from Paris couturiers or from American importers and reproducers of Paris models.[1] Although Paris was generally the source of high fashion for what was considered at various times "high society," "the smart set," or "café society," it is also true for most of this period that to be well dressed in Paris required both money and social position, or money and celebrity. Women outside the small circle of wealthy frequenters of Paris couturiers did not exist for the style makers. Bettina Ballard wrote of this "small egocentric group of…chic Parisiennes…who inspired the couturiers and the modistes, the women for whom fashion was really created." She pointed out that during this time, society women "wouldn't have been considered eligible for a fashionable reputation until they were at least 35 and with their children behind them."[2] The youth cult of the post-World War II years was foreign to the elegance of haute couture. True high fashion was always the preserve of the few, but, as a later writer pointed out, "No style is fashionable until it is imitated."[3]

American fashion was seen by most critics as primarily imitative, with few original stylists. In spite of this, at all price levels American-made garments clothed the vast majority of American women. During the commercial life of the Tirocchi shop, the American garment industry learned to combine Art with Big Business. The notion that fashion and style could be made available to the majority of women, whether they were working class or leisure class, was an American original [fig. 77]. In the first decades of the twentieth century, class and social structure in the United States were much more fluid than in Europe. Social position was based not only on family and property, but also on wealth, however it was acquired, and on education: it was possible to cross boundaries. The definition of "society" began to broaden, as the aristocracy by birth and old money began to find competition from a new aristocracy of achievement, celebrity, and notoriety: the "café society" of the 1920s. While there was without doubt a leisured "Society" deserving of the capital "S" in the United States, there was also a need for stylish apparel among the countless women who worked outside the home, whether as volunteers or as wage earners.

Manufacturing, clerical, academic, administrative, and management positions blurred and broadened the definition of "middle class." Educational opportunities in women's colleges and state schools and universities were available to more and more females. College life, clerical jobs, and careers such as teaching and social work required neat, professional clothing that was not necessarily on the cutting edge of fashion. American women were active in a wide variety of social, charitable, and political clubs and organizations. For town-dwellers it was relatively easy to participate in active sports or to attend a variety of public or private entertainments. The availability of alternative jobs made domestic service an increasingly unpopular choice of livelihood. Women with fewer or no servants needed clothing that was easier to wear and maintain. Wages, although usually much lower for women than for men, were generally higher here than in Europe. Single working women typically lived at home and contributed their earnings to the family coffers, but were given back a certain amount for clothing and entertainment.[4] This large population of women of differing economic means, all of whom required clothing suitable for their various activities, had to be addressed. Many writers on fashion from this period agreed with American apparel designer and critic Elizabeth Hawes's assessment of the growth of ready-to-wear in America, even for women who could afford custom-made clothes: "A lot of women in America are just too busy to come for fittings."[5]

All of these factors contributed to the growth of the ready-to-wear clothing industry in the United States and to the role of fashion in that industry. In turn, the industry utilized mass media to encourage consumers to respond to new fashions. The choices made by consumers eventually led to the development of a recognizably American aesthetic in fashion. The goal of the industry was not merely to make cheap, serviceable clothing to cover the masses, but to make fashionable clothing available to most income levels. Custom dressmakers, like the Tirocchis, had to adapt to the needs and wants of their customers and to the competition offered by mass production, or fail.

In order for consumers to develop a fashion consciousness, there must be effective means of spreading information about fashion. How was word about new styles disseminated throughout the United States? The program of the 1940 Fashion Group Inc. presentation, *New York's Fashion Futures*, stated: "There's no Main Street anymore…She may come from a small town, but she doesn't look it. No one's a country cousin, a jay, a hick any more." The fashion press had become increasingly important in "educating Americans about style."[6] Women learned about fashion by reading magazines and newspapers, attending motion-picture and live performances, window-shopping in their local stores or on big-city visits, and – as today – in a variety of mundane ways that are difficult to assess.

The 1940 Fashion Group program lists journalistic advertisers and supporters that covered both high and volume fashion, including: *Harper's Bazaar, Vogue, Mademoiselle, Ladies' Home Journal, Woman's Day, McCall's, The New Yorker, Town and Country, Good Housekeeping, Bride's, Woman's Home Companion,* and *Collier's* magazines. Several of these titles were descendants of nineteenth-century women's magazines, which had included fashion, etiquette, needlework and other craft patterns and instructions, and home decorating advice among their contents. Access to fashion information was not new in the twentieth century, but the scale of its distribution was.

Vogue and *Harper's Bazar* were important American showcases for French haute couture. *Vogue,* from its inception in 1892 as a biweekly magazine covering society and fashion, was meant for an audience at the higher end of the social scale. Although *Vogue* included ads for American custom dressmakers such as Thurn, Jessie Franklin Turner, and Hattie Carnegie, and both retailer's and manufacturer's ads for ready-to-wear, it was not until February 1938 that *Vogue* first devoted an entire issue to American fashion.[7] The French and British editions of *Vogue,* which had their own editorial staffs and relied on local advertising revenue, may be assumed to have promoted even fewer American designers than the parent magazine. In contrast, *Harper's Bazar* devoted serious space to American couturiers fairly early on. Even before 1900, New York and Paris fashions were reported side by side. Pages of original designs by New York designers Henri Bendel, E. M. A. Steinmetz, and Hermann Patrick Tappé appeared in issues from the 1910s and 1920s [fig. 78].

Many other women's magazines devoted some proportion of their pages to fashion and so employed fashion editors, such as Helen Koues of the *Ladies' Home Journal* and Isabel DeNyse Conover of *Woman's Home Companion.* These publications gave fashion direction to middle-class women, while paying close attention to Paris couturiers and Paris trends. This particular print medium, however, was only one of many venues for spreading the fashion gospel.

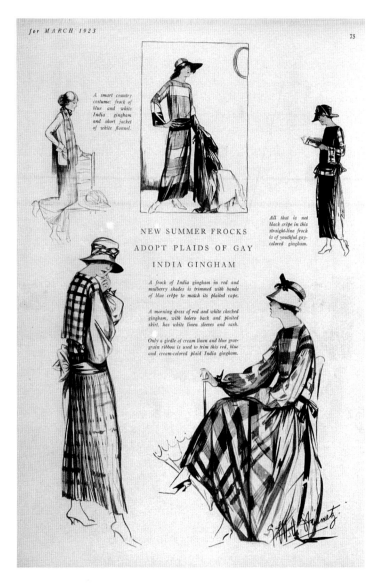

Fig. 78
Page of E. M. A. Steinmetz designs, *Harper's Bazar,* vol. LVIII, no. 3 (March 1923), p. 75: E. M. A. Steinmetz sketches of Paris fashions appeared in *Vogue* in the 1910s, and her own designs were prominently featured in *Harper's Bazar* in the 1920s (the magazine's name was changed to *Harper's Bazaar* sometime around 1930; reproduced by permission). Steinmetz was also the head designer for Stein and Blaine, a New York dress company.

Dress-pattern companies also put out magazines, such as *Vogue Pattern Quarterly*, *The Delineator*, *The Pictorial Review*, *Elite Styles*, *Le Costume Royal* (*The Royal Pattern Company*), and *The Fashionist*. *Vogue's* first patterns, from the mid-1890s, were carried in the parent magazine and were sold mail-order in one size (36″ bust) only, with each pattern cut out individually by the originator, Mrs. Rosa Payne, in her home.[8] Sized patterns had been available from other sources, however, since the 1860s. Cut-to-measure patterns copied from French couturiers (almost certainly without authorization) appeared in *Vogue* after the turn of the century. Paris models of 1911 from Francis, Paquin, Poiret, Bernard, and Bernhardt were illustrated in the May 1 issue at $1 for a coat or skirt and $2 for a suit or gown. The Royal Pattern Company included both unattributed designs and Paris couture styles among its offerings. A 1912 issue showed work by Chéruit, Drécoll, Poiret, Lanvin, Paquin, and Hallée. The company kept the imported models from which the patterns were taken on display in its New York showroom, perhaps indicating that these were actually licensed copies.[9] *McCall's Patterns* first offered licensed copies of French designs in 1927. *Vogue Patterns* published its "Paris Couture" patterns in 1931, but since the copies were unlicensed, the names of the original designers were not on the patterns. For most companies, by far the largest number of designs (then as now) were adaptations of the prevailing modes by anonymous stylists, although Butterick Pattern Company was caught making unauthorized copies of Paris models in the 1930s.[10] Except for a brief appearance by some Hollywood costume designers in Butterick's "Starred" patterns in 1933, no evidence has surfaced so far that well known American designers licensed their work to, or were copied by, pattern firms before World War II [fig. 79].[11]

These magazines may have been especially important to the home dressmaker or patron of the small dressmaking shop as aids to decisions about fabrics, trims, and accessories, as well as in the primary discussion of silhouette or style. Some publications, such as *Elite Styles*, *Le Costume Royal*, and *Le Bon Ton* were specifically aimed at professional dressmakers.[12] The Elite Styles Company even held

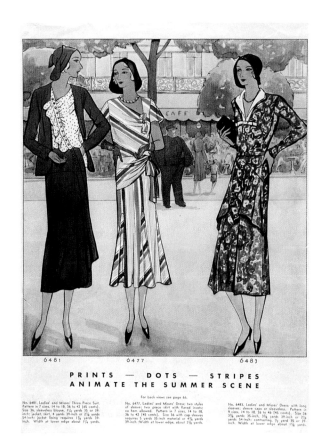

PRINTS — DOTS — STRIPES
ANIMATE THE SUMMER SCENE

Fig. 79
Models such as these dresses, which appeared in the *McCall Quarterly*, Summer 1931, p. 24, might be original designs from an anonymous staff artist or adaptations of popular Paris or New York fashions (reproduced by permission).

fashion shows at its New York headquarters to acquaint out-of-town dressmakers with the latest models. The Woman's Institute of Domestic Arts and Sciences in Scranton, Pennsylvania, published *Inspiration*, beginning in 1916, for its dressmaking students, and the *Fashion Service*, which illustrated for subscribers both Paris adaptations and patterns from American sources such as *Pictorial Review*, *Butterick*, *Ladies' Home Journal*, and *McCall's*.[13] Examples of some of the titles mentioned are found in the Tirocchi Archive.

Newspapers, of course, also had fashion information, usually in the "women's pages," which also carried reports on club activities and society doings. Sunday photogravure sections of the paper also included the latest in dress. In the 1920s and 1930s, the *Providence Sunday Journal's* fashion editor, Madeliene [*sic*] Corey, attended the Paris openings and later put together articles describing the new styles, illustrated with photos or sketches of models available locally. No Providence shops or dressmakers were mentioned in the text, although the Paris designers often were. Readers had to call or write for a list of local purveyors.[14] *Vogue*, during the same decades, also asked readers to send in for the names of shops where merchandise mentioned in features or sections such as "Seen in the Shops" or "Fashions for Limited Incomes" could be purchased.

The *Providence Journal* was not the only newspaper with a fashion editor, and some, such as Eugenia Sheppard of the *New York Herald Tribune*, wielded real power in the fashion industry. Syndicated columnists, most notably Tobé (Mrs. Tobé Coller Davis) were also extremely important in spreading a uniform fashion gospel throughout the nation. Edna Woolman Chase noted that in addition to her column, Tobé advised "more than a thousand stores on fashion trends, compiling, printing, and mailing weekly a fifty-page report telling her clients how and where to buy the clothes customers will shortly be demanding. Tobé didn't invent dirndl skirts, sweater blouses, slim pants, and years ago, Bramley dresses, but she foresaw their immense popularity and by advising the nation's stores accordingly made these clothes great fashion Fords…"[15]

Fashion critics noted that the relationship between fashion makers and fashion writers entailed a conflict of interest between journalistic integrity and advertising revenue. Designers, manufacturers, or retailers who advertised in a publication often expected favorable editorial treatment over those who bought little or no ad space, and advertising departments were often reluctant to offend an advertiser through editorial coverage of a competitor. Efforts to preserve advertising revenues often meant that local makers or retailers remained anonymous except to those few who wrote in for the information. Edna Woolman Chase detailed her efforts to keep *Vogue's* fashion features free from the tyranny of advertisers during this period. She explained to one manufacturer that in order to maintain the prestige of *Vogue*, the major attraction for advertisers,

she could not use his product: "But how do you suppose we have won that prestige?…It is because we insist on quality in the merchandise we show…You may get into *Vogue* through the advertising pages, but to come in the editorial door you must give me material we can be proud to use." This assessment of the relationship between advertising and editorial space in the magazine was not always accepted by other observers, who claimed to see a direct correlation between the amount of advertising space a company paid for and the number of times its products were featured editorially.[16]

New York was the primary American center for dissemination of fashion and style information through the publication of the bigger magazines. Most cities, however, had department stores with custom departments catering to a wealthy clientele and sections called "Budget," "Moderate," or "Better" dresses to accommodate less well-off working- and middle-class customers. Many of these stores produced mail-order catalogues of their merchandise or small in-house style magazines to distribute to customers. Chicago's Marshall Field & Company published *Fashions of the Hour* "periodically," while William Filene's & Sons Company in Boston published *Clothes* on a quarterly schedule. Store catalogues are often particularly interesting for the many different names and price levels of departments within the store. Among the Filene's departments were the French Shop (few-of-a-kind dresses), Misses' Gown Shop, Women's Inexpensive Dress Shop, Misses' Sport Shop, and the House Frocks Shop.[17] Department stores without the means to publish their own magazine could distribute a bi-monthly publication called *Modes & Manners*, which was produced with the store's name and city on the cover, but contained generic fashion and home-decorating information, including coverage of the Paris trends, and national ads [fig. 80]. Two copies exist in the RISD files, one (complete) from P. A. Bergner and Co. in Peoria, Illinois (April – May 1929) and the other (cover only) from the Jordan Marsh Company in Boston (April – May 1926).[18] Of course, mail-order catalogues from firms that had no retail outlets, such as the National Cloak and Suit Company, were also in circulation.

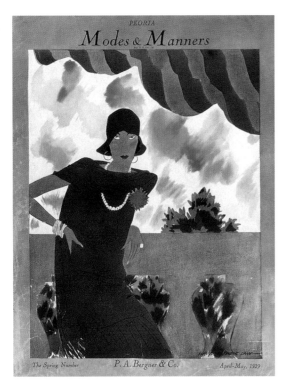

Fig. 80
Cover of *Peoria Modes & Manners* issue for April/May 1929 featuring textile designs by modernists Kem Weber and Ilonka Karasz: such magazines ensured that even in smaller urban areas, the newest fashions in dress and home furnishings were available to anyone interested in style. Museum of Art, RISD, Department of Costume and Textiles, library.

Many manufacturers of apparel, fabrics, and accessories also published style sheets or books for the trade, which illustrated how their products should be used or worn. Maurice Rentner put out "his own little fashion magazine" called *Quality Street*, for which he claimed to write most of the copy himself.[19] H. R. Mallinson & Company put out its *Blue Book of Silks* regularly. A 1921 booklet illustrated fabrics, clothing, and accessories through black-and-white photographs. The 1926 booklet that accompanied their "American National Parks" silk series included photographs of the parks, the textile designs derived from the photographs, and drawings of dress patterns from several companies to show how the fabrics might be best used.[20] According to Mallinson ads in *Harper's Bazar* in the 1920s, the booklets were available to readers by mail at a cost of ten cents. Several Haas Brothers sample books,

containing fabric samples and illustrations of garments, exist in the Tirocchi Archive. The Textile Department of The Museum at The Fashion Institute of Technology possesses several books from No-Mend Hosiery Company of the 1930s and 40s, which contain actual samples of hosiery with drawings of the season's new styles and swatches of appropriate fabrics and leathers from the textile and leather manufacturers themselves [fig. 81]. Another firm advertised that its "Holeproof Color Ensemble Book," found in hosiery departments, was an important guide for fashion-conscious consumers. E.M.A. Steinmetz illustrated the book shown in the May 1932 *Harper's Bazaar* ad. These books may also have functioned as salesmen's sample books.

Readers also saw illustrations for the new fashions in advertisements from shops and stores in the local papers and for large manufacturers, regional department stores, and bigger specialty shops in the magazines. Even general interest and business magazines such as *Fortune*, *Life*, and *Collier's* presented features on fashion designers or manufacturers, particularly in the 1930s, as interest in American designers grew and as American industries – including the fashion industries – began to prepare for the coming war in Europe.

It is also important to factor in the new, non-print medium of motion pictures, which made access to up-to-date fashions widespread. The clothing worn by stars in films could, and often did, have an impact on the style-conscious even in small towns, but the newsreels and short features shown in that era before every feature film also carried fashion information. A 1923 ad for the house of Milgrim promoted designer Sally Milgrim as fashion editor of "Selznick's Weekly Movie News."[21] In 1924, a *New York Times* article reported that Keith Theatres, a chain of movie houses, would "cooperate with retailers in showing new styles."[22]

On occasion, live fashion shows sponsored by textile and apparel manufacturers or trade organizations were held in movie theaters. A "Velvet Revue" of garments made by several ready-to-wear manufacturers from fabrics by Shelton Looms was advertised in late 1929 as a coming attraction in Loew, Stanley, and Paramount theaters throughout the

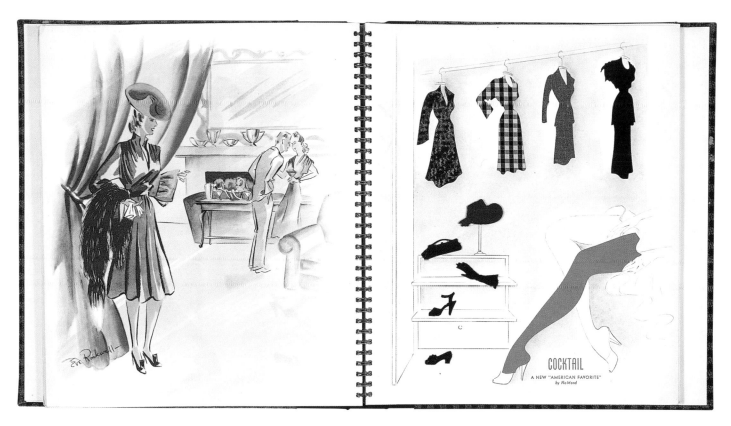

Fig. 81
"Cocktail," one of eight hosiery shades offered in the fashion guide *American Favorites* by No-Mend Hosiery, Inc. (Fall–Winter 1941–42): books such as these aided consumers by suggesting fabric and color combinations for the latest fashions and benefited manufacturers by linking their names with other high-end producers. Courtesy Museum at the Fashion Institute of Technology, New York.

country. Hotels were also common sites for live fashion shows. The Hotel Astor in New York was home to the January 1915 cooperative "fashion exposition," sponsored by the United Fashion Company of New York, and to a 1937 Velvet Guild Review featuring fashions by Helen Cookman, Walter Plunkett, and Irene, among others.[23] The *Providence Sunday Journal* of September 24, 1939, ran an ad by Fredleys, a Providence specialty shop, which invited readers to "attend a Fashion Luncheon in the Garden Restaurant of the Providence Biltmore Wednesday, September twenty seventh at twelve thirty o'clock. Mannequins will present a most brilliant collection of clothes for autumn wear." The fixed-price luncheon cost $1.25, and reservations were required.[24]

Once a woman had educated herself about current fashions, how did she go about clothing herself in them? Just as today, the options then available were made-to-order, ready-to-wear, or home-sewn clothing. Within this framework, however, women had a much broader range of choices than would be expected nowadays. In addition to purchasing French models or authorized copies of French designs, custom-made clothes could also be had from the better known dressmakers and fashion creators who worked in New York or other large cities. Women could also purchase, according to their means, fabrics and trims from retail shops and department stores and take them home or to their local dressmaker to make up. By the mid-1910s, acceptable ready-to-wear women's garments were no longer confined to pieces such as blouses, skirts, cloaks, and undergarments, which were either loose-fitting or easily altered. By the late 1920s, ready-to-wear clothing purchases, through mail order or from retail shops, far outnumbered those from other sources. Then, as now, second-hand clothing could also be purchased. It is likely that the wardrobes of all but the very wealthy and the very poor contained elements from at least a few of these categories.

Sewing presented women who had to work with a way to do so within the bounds of traditional feminine roles. Mary Brooks Picken, author of many books on sewing and dressmaking and director of the fashion and sewing program of the Woman's Institute of Domestic Arts & Sciences, advised women on how to earn a living with a needle. One could "conduct a dressmaking and tailoring establishment or simply a dressmaking shop…or specialize in sewing in some other way, as, for instance, sewing by the day…" She explained how to conduct a business of either plain sewing at home for others or going to clients' homes by the day or week. The importance of taste, cleanliness, and a good selection of current fashion magazines were all stressed.[25]

Evidence suggests that in many middle- and upper-class households it was common to have a local dressmaker come to the house twice a year or so to make up on the premises things that were needed for the coming season. This practice, wide-

spread in the pre-World War I years, probably continued for much longer than has previously been understood. Carolyn B. Reed, chairman of the Arlington branch of the American Red Cross in 1946, wrote a memoir of a day's shopping in 1910 for the *Boston Herald.* She recalled that "nearly every home had its dress form…and its semi-annual family dressmaker, augmented by a bi-weekly seamstress. These faithful visitors moulded and worked on the necessary and serviceable blue serge dress, or the broadcloths and silks to wear to church, as well as the beautiful satin brocades and moirés for evening wear. Dress materials such as these were the object [of the shopping trip]."[26] *Ladies' Home Journal* carried an advice article in 1917 with the pointed title "Sewing in Other People's Homes."[27] One North Carolina woman, now in her eighties, recalled having had dance dresses made up by her mother's favorite local seamstress as late as the early 1930s. A New England woman recalled from her childhood in the early 1910s that only basics – school skirts and blouses, nightclothes, and flannel undergarments – issued from the needle of the woman who visited twice a year, while special clothes were commissioned from Boston or a local dressmaker who kept a shop.[28]

Women could also sew for themselves and their families. Mary Brooks Picken's Woman's Institute ran correspondence courses in sewing and provided paperbound booklets containing instruction on the principles of design, advice on choosing patterns or reproducing simple garments, and illustrations showing the proper methods of putting the garments together. In addition, the final page of the booklet contained a list of examination questions, which the correspondent answered on a special sheet of paper and sent in for grading [fig. 82]. How-to-sew books and wardrobe-planning books were commonplace commodities: for example, *Dress and Look Slender,* and *Designing Women: The Art, Technique and Cost of Being Beautiful.*[29] Home-economics textbooks for high-school and college students also focused on sewing, choosing, and caring for clothes. One such book, *Textiles and Clothing* by Ellen Beers McGowan and Charlotte A. Waite, was first

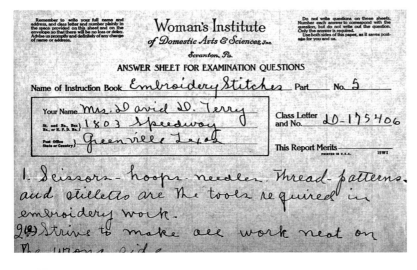

Fig. 82
Woman's Institute Correspondence Course Exam Paper (detail): many dressmaking schools and correspondence courses advertised in fashion and women's magazines. The *Providence City Directory* listed two such schools throughout the 1910s and 20s. Private collection.

published in 1919, but revised by the authors in 1931 to keep up to date with the increased use of synthetic fibers. Another textbook, *The Arts of Costume and Personal Appearance* by Grace Margaret Morton, was published in 1943. It should be remembered that home-economics classes were required for girls (and only for girls) in public junior and senior high schools until fairly recently and also that when higher education for women was still controversial, choosing home economics as a college major was one way to defuse the argument that attending college was unfeminine as well as unnecessary.

Many women's magazines carried patterns that home sewers could write in to request. *Vogue* maintained one of the largest services, by 1915 carrying patterns for suits, day dresses, coats, evening frocks, evening cloaks, blouses, lingerie, sleepwear, and collections of three to six different sleeve or collar styles combined in one set.[30] *Good Housekeeping* also had a pattern service, although on a smaller scale than *Vogue*, and it also had a shopping service for out-of-town readers [fig. 83]. The editors featured a selection of finished and "semi-made" dresses from New York shops, which readers could order through the magazine. Although no shop or manufacturer names were listed, the guarantee of New York's Fifth Avenue was perceived as an indicator of quality and style. The April 1929 issue shows fifteen dresses and ensembles over three pages, including sportswear and models for day and afternoon. A sleeveless, partially made, printed batiste dress was priced at $2.95, a polka-dot silk day dress at $15, and a two-piece checked silk dress with a suede belt at $35. The *Ladies' Home Journal* boasted in 1940 that "Journal readers want high fashion," offering as evidence that "226,706 readers ordered a pattern for a John-Frederics hat and handbag from a recent issue."[31]

Purchasing cut-out or partially made garments to sew at home was possible through other sources in addition to women's magazines. The Costume and Textile Department library at the Museum of Art, RISD, contains two catalogues from New York companies, Berth Roberts and Fifth Avenue Modes, who sold semi-made dresses by mail order.[32] The clothes were called "semi-finished" or

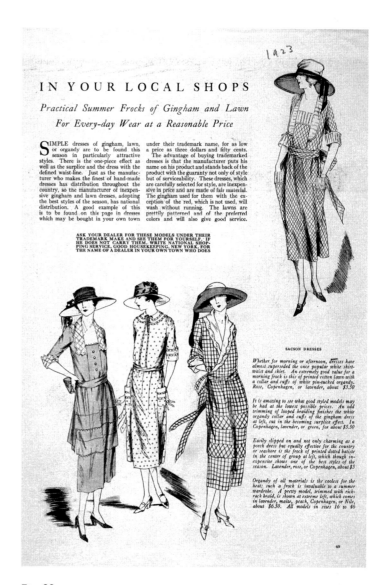

Fig. 83
"In Your Local Shops" page from *Good Housekeeping* magazine (1923): many magazines offered a variety of shopping services to readers (reproduced by permission). Advertisements for unaffiliated businesses were also published. Museum of Art, RISD, Department of Costume and Textiles, clipping file.

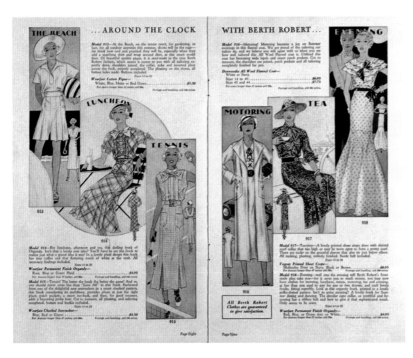

Fig. 84
Mail-order catalogue for *Berth Robert's Semi-Made Dresses* (April–June 1934): when time or skill was a factor for home sewers, they could turn to providers of partially made-up garments, a transitional step between the world of custom dressmaking and the triumph of ready-to-wear. Museum of Art, RISD, Department of Costume and Textiles, library.

"finish-at-home" fashions. The garments were said to be "cut-to-measure," meaning individually cut to the measurements sent in by the customer, as opposed to being cut to a standard size. All the detail sewing was done by the manufacturer, which generally meant that collars and cuffs, pleats, tucks, decorative stitching, multiple rows of gathering – almost anything other than straight seams – were already in place when the home sewer received the kit [fig. 84]. The purchaser was assured that "since all the difficult sewing is done in our Fifth Avenue shop, by the most skilled men-tailors, a 'Finish-at-Home' garment never looks 'home-made.'"[33] Depending on the model, prices averaged half that of a comparable "Budget" or "Moderate" ready-to-wear dress at the time. Both catalogues had back sections with a few pages of accessories, blouses, lingerie, and some dresses available as ready-to-wear. The Berth Robert publication included a finished maid's uniform and apron (along with a few sum-

mer menus), which raises some questions as to the social class of the market targeted by the firm.

In examining the dressmaking business of Anna and Laura Tirocchi, it is important to understand the context of both the Providence microcosm and the larger fashion world. The Tirocchi sisters were not the only dressmakers in Providence and may not have been either the most successful or the best. The evidence suggests that they were also not the only dressmakers to move from the made-to-order to the ready-made world. The *Providence City Directory* for 1911, the first year in which the sisters are listed under the heading "Dressmakers," filled eight and one half columns over five pages with the names of other dressmakers. This is in addition to listings for "Cloaks and Suits," "Clothing Dealers," "Clothing – Retail," "Department Stores," and "Dry Goods." As the nature of the clothing business in the United States changed, the number of dressmakers dropped, while listings for "Clothing Dealers – Retail" increased. By 1937, separate listings were required for "Men's and Boys" and "Women's and Misses" clothing.

It is worth noting that the names in the *Directory* listings changed from personal to corporate as the nature of the clothing industry evolved. Rose Carraer-Eastman, a Providence dressmaker active as early as 1896 (under her birth name of Carragher) and still listed under "Dressmakers" in 1918, had exchanged this heading for "Cloaks and Suits" by 1924. Given the names of the other listings under the "Cloaks and Suits" category, it seems that Eastman had shifted the focus of her business from custom dressmaking to ready-to-wear sales, although at least until 1930 she was still purchasing small quantities of specialty fabrics from the French manufacturer Soieries F. Ducharne. By 1937, the business was called Zarr Rose Eastman Inc. and was listed under "Clothing Dealers – Retail, Women's and Misses." It had also moved from the downtown district, formerly dense with dressmaking establishments, up the hill to Thayer Street on Providence's residential East Side, a shopping street with many other small retail establishments conveniently located to its clientele.

The large amount of material preserved in the Tirocchi Archive allows a glimpse into the business activities of the sisters. In most other instances, all that remains as evidence of a dressmaker's work are advertisements, or perhaps a single labeled garment in the collections of a museum or historical society. It is not always easy to ferret out additional information. For instance, a dress from about 1918 in the RISD Museum collection has a label reading "Dowling, Providence" [fig. 85]. A check of the *Providence City Directories* for 1917, 1918, and 1919 reveals three possibilities: Louise G. Dowling, Mary J. Dowling, and Nellie T. Dowling. The 1911 *Directory* lists the two latter, and two additional: M. A. and A. E. (together at one address), and Nellie L. The three listed in 1918 are also listed as late as 1932, but only Mary J. survives in the listings to 1937. It is possible that the Mamie J. Dowling listed in 1901 is the Mary J. Dowling of the later directories, just as the Helen T. Dowling at 24 Mansfield Street in 1924 may be presumed to have been the Nellie T. Dowling of 24 Mansfield Street in 1918. There has yet to be uncovered any trove of written documentation of any of the Dowling businesses that might allow attribution of the surviving dress to one or another of these women. The dress is a work of art, but in the absence of documentary evidence, the artist must yet be considered unknown. Several other dresses with labels from Providence dressmakers, including Rose Carraer-Eastman, may be found in the RISD collection. These examples testify to the existence of several producers of high quality work and, by extension, to the probable existence of no little competition among dressmakers to retain their clients. The diary of Harriet Sprague Watson Lewis (Mrs. Jack Lewis) in the Rhode Island Historical Society's collection provides evidence that at least one East Side society woman tried the Tirocchi shop for a season before returning to her previous dressmaker, Rose Carraer-Eastman.[34]

Custom-made clothes by dressmakers such as Carraer-Eastman, Dowling, and A. & L. Tirocchi were more common than either haute couture or ready-to-wear during the first two decades of the twentieth century. Custom dressmakers brought to their trade a wide range of both technical and artistic skills. To many, the word "dressmaker" connotes a technician. In fact, many custom dressmakers

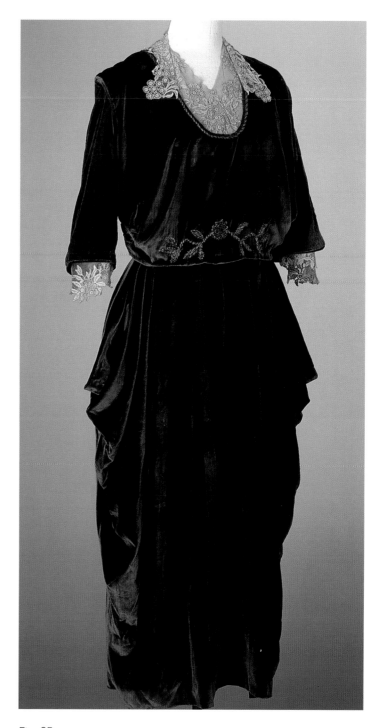

Fig. 85
A purple velvet dress, ca. 1918, with a square pink satin sachet label reading "Dowling, Providence" in silver printed letters. Museum of Art, RISD, gift of the estate of Elizabeth Claflin Rowe.

contented themselves with copying Paris models or interpreting styles from print sources in the client's choice of fabric and color. It takes something extra to turn a dressmaker into a designer. It is difficult now to gauge how original or creative individual dressmakers were. One is equally likely to undervalue as to overvalue their work. Even among the acknowledged designers, style leadership was not constant from year to year or season to season.

In that era when the names of French designers were elevated above all, who were the men and women who designed or styled for the American market? Were there, in either the custom or wholesale trades, those who had that extra something to deserve the appellation of designer? Was there a definable American aesthetic or style? Since the industry in this country was so large and reached across many price levels, the answers are difficult to find. Few American dressmakers have been studied by fashion scholars. Anonymity is a very real stumbling block, and issues of attribution arise in evaluating work. Many designers and stylists worked for specialty shops, department stores, or ready-to-wear manufacturers who preferred to cultivate client loyalty to a brand name or trademark rather than to a designer name. People who were well known for one type of garment sometimes moonlighted, anonymously, in other areas of the industry. Both custom and ready-to-wear houses are known to have purchased sketches of models designed by free-lance artists. Well known fashion personalities such as Hattie Carnegie and Maurice Rentner are often described as "editors" of ideas that emerged from an in-house stable of designers. In such cases, who gets the credit for the finished product?

Custom dressmakers may be assumed to have varied widely in skill, originality, and clientele. Certainly even a cursory examination of the classified listings in *Vogue* and *Harper's Bazar* from the 1910s, 20s, and 30s opens up avenues for further research. The issue of *Vogue* for October 15, 1915, lists twenty-six names in the classified ads for providers of "Gowns and Waists" made to order and six names for the same category of ready-to-wear. *Vogue's* "Address Book" in the January 15, 1935, issue still lists six names under "Dressmaking." Sample book no. 17 for Soieries F. Ducharne, probably from 1930 (in the Musée des Tissus de Lyon), lists among those who ordered yardage names from all over the United States, some well known, others unfamiliar. Representative names include Lucile Woods and Misses Perkins and Collins, Los Angeles; Mrs. E. H. Hills, Baltimore; Greer, Inc., Dot Gregson, Irene, Jean Schwartz, and RKO Studio, Hollywood; Stella L. Chapman, Minneapolis; Mrs. McFadden and Katir, Philadelphia; and Mme. Clara and O'Connor Moffat, San Francisco; not to mention the many purchasers from the sizable New York market. A detailed analysis of the names in the rest of the Ducharne records and order books from other companies might give quite an interesting picture of the purchase of French fabrics by American custom and wholesale dressmakers.[35]

Some dressmakers copied from legitimately imported and/or pirated Paris designs, and also, by the late 1920s, from American models of the top custom houses or high-end wholesalers. Many ads throughout these decades echo two from a 1936 issue of *Harper's Bazaar*: those of Mme. Lichtenstein at 286 Park Ave, who had "just returned from abroad,"[36] and Janet Rose, Importer, who was "just returned from the Paris openings." It seems to have been accepted in the early decades of the century that models illustrated in magazines were open to copying or interpreting in other fabrics and colors by individual clients of custom dressmakers,[37] although even in the early 1910s, many dressmakers also offered original designs. Madame Najla Mogabgab, with shops in New York, Palm Beach, Newport, and Hot Springs (Virginia) – the East Coast social centers – advertised herself as both importer and designer.[38] Other names offering both services, such as Joseph, Thurn, Stein and Blaine, L. P. Hollander, and Annette Mayer, may be found in advertisements, in the "Shoppers and Buyers Guide" pages of *Vogue*, and the "Where to Shop" listings in *Harper's Bazar*. A hierarchy existed within the high-end custom trade, based on whether the business was entirely custom, existed as part of a specialty shop or department store, or also produced ready-to-wear.[39]

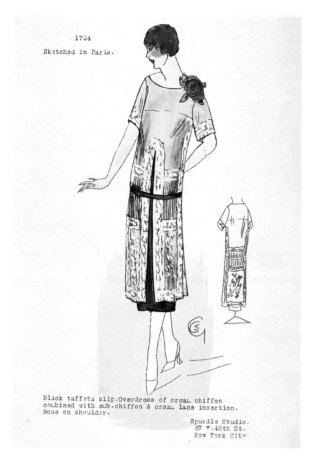

1724
Sketched in Paris.

Black taffeta slip. Overdress of cream chiffon combined with cmb·chiffon & cream lace insertion. Rose on shoulder.

Spurdle Studio.
67 W·46th St.
New York City

Fig. 86
Spurdle Studio, no. 1724, n.d.: sketches of garments from the Paris showings were often used by both custom and ready-made houses as "inspirations" for their own lines, which could translate as anything from line-for-line copying to using a detail of the original's cut, fabric, or trim. Tirocchi Archive.

Berley Studio and Spurdle Studio were two firms that produced books of "After designs," with sketches of Paris models annotated by indications of colors, fabrics, and trims [fig. 86]. Some designers (Elizabeth Hawes and Muriel King, for example) got their start in fashion as sketchers: those who would commit models from the Paris showings to memory and then draw them afterward on commission by wholesale houses in the U.S. or elsewhere in Europe. The sketches were used by many custom dressmakers and wholesale manufacturers to style their own lines of merchandise. These drawings were not always employed to create direct copies. They were also used to inform American manufacturers of the latest Paris trends. The final American products would feature original details or twists on the Paris silhouette.

High-end retailers with custom salons (Saks Fifth Avenue, Bergdorf Goodman, Bonwit Teller, Jay-Thorpe, Henri Bendel) would not only buy Paris models for reproduction, but also often had in-house designers to create originals for clients. Their work was sometimes seen in fashion magazines alongside that of the Paris couturiers. An early example of a shop that employed designers was Hickson's, Inc., a New York specialty house. In 1915, the store advertised not only Paris models," but "collaborateurs…who will meet patrons with the view of providing exclusive and unusual creations…" The advertisement went on to actually name the in-house design staff: Jean, Mr. Melville Ellis, and the Baron de Planta.[40] Other shops preferred to keep their in-house designers anonymous, conforming to an advertising style like that of Best & Company, which offered the "Newest modes…featuring the latest Parisian novelties…Including many original and distinctive effects, designed exclusively by us."[41] Bendel's also kept its custom design staff anonymous. As with much of American fashion before the mid-1930s, the individual remained submerged within the organization.

A few New York-based custom designers had important reputations during the 1920s and early 30s, such as Sophie Gimbel of Saks Fifth Avenue, Sally Milgrim, and Jessie Franklin Turner. By far the larger number, however, became known by name in the later 1930s and during the war years. People such as Fira Benenson of Bonwit Teller, Emmet Joyce of Saks, Wilson Folmar of Jay-Thorpe, Louise Barnes Gallagher, and Mabel McIlvain Downs enjoyed far more publicity after the fall of Paris in 1940 than they ever had before. Houses with large design staffs, such as Hattie Carnegie and Bergdorf Goodman, began to allow publicity to mention the names of the designers, not just of the house. Carnegie employed several designers at a time to come up with original models for her customers, both in the custom salon and in her ready-to-wear lines, which she began to produce in 1928. Many of Carnegie's house designers – Norman Norell, Pauline Trigère, Jean Louis, James Galanos, Gustave Tassell, Claire McCardell – would become well known in their own right. Bergdorf Goodman counted eight designers on its staff in the 1940s, each with a different specialty. Ethel Frankau and Leslie Morris were perhaps the best known: the rest of the staff included Peggy Morris, Mark Mooring, Mary Gleason, Philip Hulitor, Alice Gleason, and John Dean.

Jessie Franklin Turner, who worked for Bonwit Teller in the custom salon from 1916 to 1922, established her own couture business, which was successful for many years even though she did not advertise conspicuously. In her early career she also designed under the name "Winifred Warren, Inc."[42] Another important factor in American fashion during the 1910s and early 1920s was Lucile, an English import via Paris. When she opened her New York house in the early 1910s, she established her reputation by dressing young ballroom dancer Irene Castle,

an important style model for many young women at the time. During World War I, she was a leader in encouraging American silk manufacturers to produce better-designed goods and often used American-made silks in her work. In the Tirocchi Archive is an invitation from Lucile Ltd. to view a special "exhibition for dressmakers" from March 9 to 15, probably in 1916, although no year is mentioned. The invitation specified that this would be a "unique" event, "planned and carried out solely because of the present chaotic conditions in the world of fashion due to the war," and would show models "mostly of American-made goods" in aid of the "Made-in-America" movement.[43] She also hired American design talent and purchased sketches from free-lance designers. Howard Greer, later an important figure in Hollywood and Seventh Avenue fashion, spent a brief period as an employee of Lucile.[44]

Old newspapers and trade journals tantalize with names seemingly once well known, but no longer familiar. Ethel Traphagen won first prize for her entries in the 1912–13 *New York Times* competition to encourage American "style creators" and went on to run an important New York school for fashion design. Mollie O'Hara, another name from the 1910s and 20s, was influential enough in the custom field to have had a fabric named after her by H. R. Mallinson & Company: "Molly-O crepe." Another dressmaker, Marguerite (also called Madame Margé), who thrived between the wars in New York and Chicago, is documented in the Special Collections Library at the Fashion Institute of Technology, New York. There are scrapbooks of sketches from the 1920s embellished with trim samples [fig. 87] and newspaper clippings from 1937 discussing her success with a line using Indonesian batik fabrics. Her name appeared often in the *American Silk Journal* in the 1910s, when her work was featured for its use of American silks. Three times between 1915 and 1918 she won the Gossard Trophy for excellence in dress design from the Fashion Art League of America. H. R. Mallinson's *Blue Book of Silks* from 1921 displays photographs of Margé models made in Mallinson silks. She seems to have managed to run a successful business between the 1910s and late 1930s and was listed as a

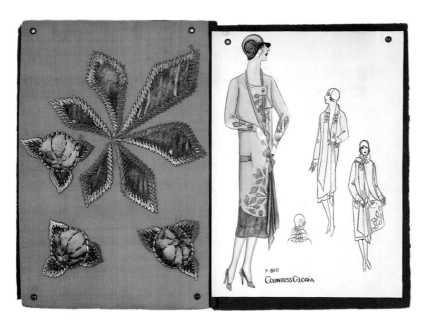

Fig. 87
Georgette and velvet afternoon ensemble, "Countess Gloria," by Madame Margé (from a model book, n.d.) available for $371, $395, $426, or $465, depending on the brand names of the fabrics used (label on the reverse of page): Madame Margé was a successful couturiere for more than twenty years in Chicago and New York. Courtesy Fashion Institute of Technology, Special Collections Library, New York.

customer in the records of Soieries F. Ducharne for the early 1930s, yet her name never appears in *Vogue* or *Harper's Bazaar*, nor has her story been published.[45] There were probably dozens of women like her, successful to varying degrees, who survived primarily through word of mouth, as the Tirocchi sisters did, and who in fact preferred to keep a low profile and an exclusive clientele.

The attribution of ready-to-wear designs is even more complicated. Some retailers sold under "house" brand names, with designs either by in-house stylists, free-lance designers, or perhaps by stylists employed by the wholesale firm that actually manufactured the product. The National Cloak and Suit Company, a mail-order manufacturer/retailer of women's and children's ready-to-wear, kept its stylists anonymous. In 1922, Franklin Simon trademarked its store-brand "Bramley" dresses, which were advertised not only in the store's catalogue, but also in the newspapers, with large ads introducing the styles for the new season or holiday wear. The Fall 1923 store catalogue describes these as "Originated by and exclusive with Franklin Simon & Co." and also warns, "Registered in the United States Patent Office – Our rights will be fully protected."[46] Best & Company had its in-house brands, including the 1926 "Shirtmaker" shirtwaist dress, as did Peck & Peck and other department and specialty stores. Best and Franklin Simon were among the first retailers to promote quality cotton dresses for activities other than keeping house. The originators of these styles are currently unknown and may be difficult to identify, given the scarcity of archival material related to defunct retail establishments. This type of everyday garment, adaptable to many of a woman's normal activities, remained popular, with variations, for decades. One wholesale manufacturer noted in the 1960s that "his firm turns out 150 to 200 styles in the course of a season, but works within two basic silhouettes, the sheath and the shirtwaist."[47]

In the 1930s, many previously anonymous ready-to-wear designers began to surface as important names in the fashion field. The occasional newspaper or trade-journal article mentions ready-to-wear designers by name [fig. 88]. "St. Louis'

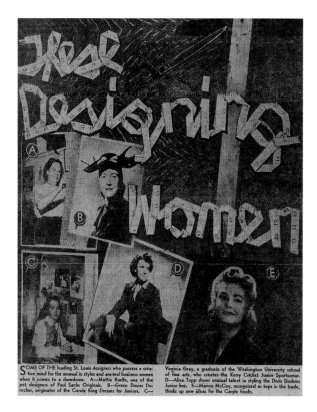

Fig. 88
Article in the *St. Louis Post Dispatch* (September 29 or 30, 1944) mentioning highly paid ready-to-wear designers: organizations such as The Fashion Group became possible when the number of women in positions of importance in the apparel industry reached critical mass (reproduced by permission of the *St. Louis Post-Dispatch*, ©1944). Museum of Art, RISD, Department of Costume and Textiles, clipping file.

Designing Women," an article from late 1939, is unusually interesting in that it gives the names and occasionally the salaries of some of the best designers in the St. Louis wholesale trade. Grace Ashley, Grace Durocher, Grace Davile, Bessie Recht (who also taught design at Washington University), Dorothy Garrison, and Marian McCoy are named as being among the best designers for the "Junior" market. Grace Davile is said to have earned $10,000 a year from her employer, the Doris Dodson Company. The Donnelly Garment Company in Kansas City (Missouri) started making their "Nelly Don" dresses in 1916. A twentieth-anniversary publicity booklet proudly stated that the company's "designers create Nelly Dons from…exclusive fabrics and original designs" and that they offer "important hidden values…lingerie strap[s], generous hems… and side seam allowance."[48] According to Elizabeth Hawes (admittedly not the most unbiased of observers), few ready-to-wear manufacturers concerned themselves with these types of quality dressmaker details.

Dorothy Shaver, an executive at Lord & Taylor, started in 1932 to campaign strongly for recognition for American designers. She began her promotion with three young women who were fairly new to designing, though not to the trade: Muriel King, Clare Potter, and Elizabeth Hawes. Many others followed, including Tina Leser, Bonnie Cashin, Tom Brigance, Vera Maxwell, and Helen Cookman. In response to a revived nationalist fervor for American design following the outbreak of World War II in Europe, Lord & Taylor opened The Designers' Shop in October 1940. The forerunner of many department-store designer boutiques, it was "a new American effort – featuring 10 of the most successful professional designers in the American fashion field – Frances Troy Stix, Charles Cooper, Bertha Altholz, Karen Stark, Vera Jacobs, Zelma Golden, Fritzie Hannah, Pat Warren, Vera Host and Will Saunders – who will create exclusive dresses for Lord & Taylor."[49]

Harper's Bazaar, Mademoiselle, Vogue, Fortune, Life; each of these magazines carried articles in the 1940s celebrating American fashion creators. *Harper's Bazaar* listed its top ten American wholesale designers in a feature entitled "They Have Designs on You," found in the issue of September 15, 1940. Vincent Monte-Sano of Monte-Sano and Pruzan, Nettie Rosenstein, Maurice Rentner, Jane Derby, Norman Norell and Jean-Louis Berthault of Hattie Carnegie, Anthony Blotta, Stella Brownie of Fox-Brownie, and Bruno of Spectator Sportswear made the cut. *Vogue* for February 1, 1940, listed not only wholesale but custom designers and came up with a different group of names. Obviously, there were many successful Americans from whom to choose.

Nettie Rosenstein was a ready-to-wear designer who had two careers in the industry. She retired in 1927 from the firm she had run for almost ten years, returned in 1930 to design for another company, and then re-established herself in 1931 under her own

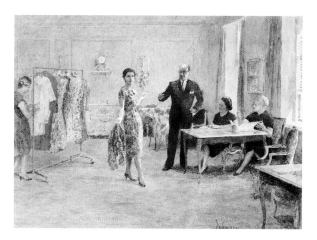

Fig. 89
Watercolor sketch, ca. 1958, of the Nettie Rosenstein showroom: the buyers' previews of the season's merchandise in ready-to-wear showrooms rarely had the theatrical quality of Parisian couture showings. Museum of Art, RISD, gift of Mr. and Mrs. Alfred T. Morris, Jr.

name [fig. 89]. In a *New York Times* interview for the "Women's Page" in March 1939, Rosenstein is said to have "bid for a restricted but sound patronage."[50] Her work was wholesaled to high-end retail shops, which, as late as 1934, still sold them under the label of the shop, not the name of the designer. As one article explained, retailers "usually endeavored to give their salons the Paris feeling…It would scarcely enhance that feeling if they were to announce that many of their most irresistible dresses were designed by Nettie Rosenstein in West Forty-seventh Street in New York…The name of Rosenstein, let alone being soft-pedalled, is not being pedalled at all."[51]

By the mid-1930s, Hollywood costume designers and the "sunshine culture" of California had proven to be a vital force in American fashion. Many designers either started out or ended up as couturiers in Los Angeles. The clothes that Adrian, Howard Greer, Irene, Travis Banton, and Edith Head put on the American movie screen were seen and absorbed by an enormous audience. Certain trends from film are well known: the Letty Lynton dress, versions of *Gone With the Wind* dresses [fig. 90], and the broad-shouldered Joan Crawford look created by Adrian. *Vogue* in 1932 acknowledged that

"The Hollywood influence – credit Marlene Dietrich in 'Shanghai Express' – has invaded Paris at last. The film was first shown at Mrs. Fellowes [sic] house in Paris, after which she appeared at almost every party in a different arrangement of coq...."[52] Several years later the *New York Times* observed that period dramas "had a particular impact on the mode" in a rotogravure feature illustrating actresses in costume for several upcoming films in 1938.[53] Articles from the *Times*, the *Christian Science Monitor, Fortune,* and *Nation's Business* attested to the growing importance of West Coast creators and markets in the overall American fashion scene.[54]

The casual outdoor California lifestyle and the clothes that actors and actresses wore in their personal lives also had an impact on American fashion. Not until Marlene Dietrich and Katharine Hepburn appeared in public in men's trousers did it begin to be possible for the average woman to appear in public in pants, although admittedly in restricted situations. Even women such as Amelia Earhart and her fellow female pilots of the late 1920s and 30s (Louise Thaden, Elinor Smith, and Bobbi Trout), who might have been expected to have a reason for appearing in trousers, rarely did so until late in the 1930s. A Hollywood men's tailor named Watson was apparently known for making trouser suits for "Garbo, Dietrich, Hepburn, Rosalind Russell, and all the knowing ones in the movie colony."[55] Bettina Ballard wrote of Marlene Dietrich, a fellow passenger on a transatlantic crossing in 1937, that "she wore slacks and a man's jacket and a fedora all day – the first woman I had ever seen wear pants in public."[56] In contrast, in Paris at the same time, according to Ballard, women went to Creed for the perfect ladylike (skirted) suit.

Stage celebrities appeared in ads for fashionable commodities in the 1910s. Hazel Dawn, star of *The Pink Lady* on Broadway, was used by H. R. Mallinson & Company in their silk ads of 1915. Many other stars of both stage and silent film followed for both Mallinson and other fabric and garment manufacturers. Irene Castle was an important promotional link for Corticelli Silks during the early 1920s [fig. 91]. "Irene Castle Corticelli Fashions," designed

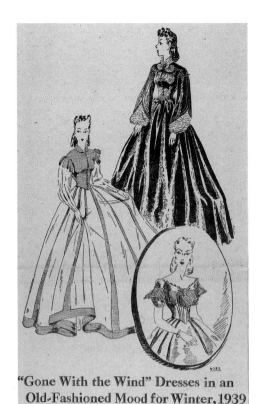

"Gone With the Wind" Dresses in an Old-Fashioned Mood for Winter, 1939

Fig. 90
Illustration from *Women's Wear Daily* (October 23, 1939), p.15: popular films and movie stars' wardrobes often provided fashion designers with inspiration and consumers with a desired look. Costumes from the film *Gone with the Wind* spawned a number of imitations, both licensed and unlicensed (reproduced by permission).

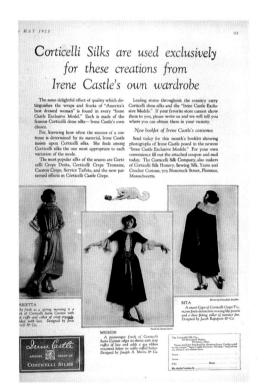

Fig. 91
Advertisement for Irene Castle Corticelli Silks in *Harper's Bazar,* vol. LVIII, no. 5 (May 1923), p. 111: celebrity connections and endorsements helped to sell products. Castle and Corticelli maintained a connection for at least three years in the early 1920s. Castle appeared in ads for Corticelli silk hosiery as well as dress goods (reproduced by permission).

by New York ready-to-wear firms Jesse Woolf & Company, Jacob Rappaport & Company, and Joseph A. Morris & Company, were available at "an exclusive dealer in each city."[57] The new attitude of the late 1930s toward original American design is shown in a newspaper ad for Best & Company from October 24, 1938. Day and evening dresses in "The Algerian Silhouette, sponsored by Gertrude Lawrence" featured a draped front and the proud claim, "Introduced by Best's."[58]

Clothes for actresses on the Broadway stage were often provided by well known dressmaking establishments in New York. Joseph, one of the more exclusive custom dressmakers in New York (producing both copies and/or adaptations of Paris models and original designs), made the costumes Louise Gunning wore in a play entitled *The Balkan Princess*.[59] Madame Margé received the Mallinson Cup for excellence in stage costume design for clothing Marilyn Miller of Ziegfeld Follies fame. Hattie Carnegie outfitted Gertrude Lawrence for her American stage appearances. Even Mainbocher, on his return to New York from Paris after the outbreak of war in 1939, made clothes for Broadway plays. This added a certain prestige all around: publicity for the designer, the actress, the play. It may have also been financially important, although it is unclear whether the designers provided the clothes for free, counting on the advertising value of the publicity, or were paid for their efforts. Hawes states in *Fashion is Spinach* that many producers expected to pay low prices for wardrobes for their stars and that most stars expected wardrobes that would strengthen their stardom, not their characterization.

Conversely, although some couturiers did create wardrobes for Hollywood films, it was more often the Hollywood costume designer who made a name in films and then established a business in custom or ready-to-wear design. Adrian is perhaps the best known of these, but there were many others. Omar Kiam actually started in New York's wholesale dress business, went into film work, and then returned to New York to design for Ben Reig. Howard Greer was courted by the Celanese Corporation in 1937 to create an "exclusive collection, in Celanese fabrics, designed by an American and specially conceived

for the great American sun season" [fig. 92].[60] Joset Walker, by 1940 the designer for wholesale dress manufacturer David Goodstein, had learned her craft ten years before, first in Saks Fifth Avenue's "Theatrical Department," then at RKO Studios in Hollywood. Norman Norell worked in film and stage costuming before joining Hattie Carnegie in 1928. It seems likely that the ease of movement between Hollywood or Broadway and Seventh Avenue fostered a kind of cross-pollination of ideas between the East and West Coasts. Perhaps this is one factor in the eventual recognition of an American style.

Much of the literature about fashion in the pre-World War II decades discusses the issue of exclusivity. Fault is found with expensive ready-to-wear clothing because, in order to be financially successful, a garment had to be sold in multiples, thereby increasing the probability that a woman

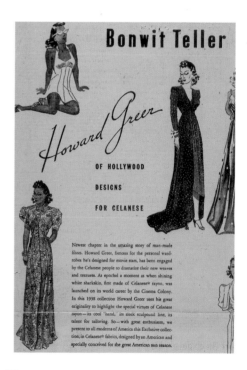

Fig. 92
Advertisement for Bonwit Teller in the *New York Times* (December 1937): Hollywood designer Howard Greer created a promotional line of clothing for the Celanese Company, manufacturers of rayon yarns and fabrics, evidence of the increased recognition of American designers in the late 1930s. Museum of Art, RISD, Department of Costume and Textiles, clipping file.

might see someone else wearing the dress she had purchased. Importers of model gowns from Paris also came in for criticism since their goal was to sell enough copies of a model gown to pay for the cost of importing it. Tied closely to exclusivity was originality. Original models designed in this country were common enough in advertisements. Most importers of Paris models also developed original designs in-house. Advertisements in fashion magazines indicate that even small dressmakers knew the value of the words "exclusive" and "original" in relation to their wares. In Providence, for example, Anna Tirocchi's stationery in the mid 1920s listed "line, color, detail, distinction, individuality" as attributes of her own business. The question in the fashion press seemed to be, however, whether American design was indeed original or followed Paris's lead so closely as to be indistinguishable, except for that extra degree of elegance and sophistication that was supposed to mark a Paris original.

For as long as there have been fashion creators, there have been fashion copiers. Fashion literature in the first half of the twentieth century is awash in denunciations of "design piracy," whether the pirating is the unauthorized copying of Paris styles by American manufacturers and custom dressmakers or of expensive American ready-to-wear by lower-price manufacturers. Organizations such as the French Chambre Syndicale and the American Fashion Originators Guild attempted to fight design piracy and extend copyright protection to apparel and textile designs.

The early 1910s saw the first concerted efforts on the part of the French couture to halt the copying of their designs. Agreements between London's Royal Worcester Corset Company and couturiers in Paris and Vienna kept the former from giving any advance information of the "new curve" in its Spring line of corsets and so made headlines in *Women's Wear* in early 1912.[61] In February and April 1912, leading Paris couturiers held their Spring models back from both the Auteuil and Longchamps races, traditionally events of great importance to both the designers and their customers. The mannequins attended the races, but wore furs from the winter collections. The reason given was specifically to keep the clothes from being "immediately copied by the smaller houses and wholesale dressmakers, who only vulgarize the models."[62]

Several months later, the *New York Times* also carried an article essentially denouncing the counterfeiting of Paris couture. In a practice that has parallels today, labels carrying the names of French couture and millinery houses were imported to the States and used in American-made products.[63] Jacques Worth and Paul Poiret headed attempts over the next four years to control how purchasers of models from the top couture houses were allowed to use them. In July 1914, the Couturier's Defense Syndicate was established with Worth, Poiret, Premet, Chéruit, Rodier, Paquin, Callot, Lucien Vogel et Compagnie, and Atuyer, Bianchini, Férier as the first subscribers. A tiered pricing system was suggested with the purpose of adding to the standard cost of a couture gown a copyright fee, payable by business customers who wished to reproduce the design for sale. Wholesalers and retailers were barred from the major couture openings unless specifically invited.[64] These moves were so controversial that the *Times* printed both the articles of the Syndicate and a speech by Poiret on the subject of design protection in January 1916, by which time it appeared that the Syndicate was near collapse.[65] The *Times* reported that many of the smaller houses had refused to abide by the Syndicate's rules with the result that the reputations of couturiers such as "Arnold, Germaine, Bulloz, Patou, Chanel, Royant, Bernard, and Mme Groult, Poiret's sister" grew rapidly.[66] The same article went on to state that

> these houses have already begun to show collections privately to the American buyers, so anticipating the 'openings' of the syndicate houses, which are mostly set for the first week of February. Realizing that no monopoly of styles was possible, these early birds boldly struck out on new lines, with the certainty of getting such a start on the former headliners that the latter would be compelled to follow where they used to lead.

It is a measure of how important the couture industry was to France that this debate could be sustained during some of the worst months of the Great War.

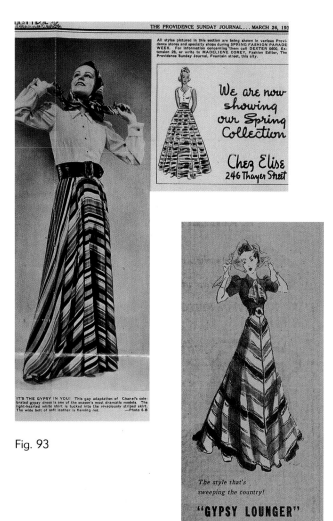

All styles pictured in this section are being shown in various Providence stores and specialty shops during SPRING FASHION PARADE WEEK. For information concerning them call DEXTER 0600, Extension 28, or write to MADELEINE COREY, Fashion Editor, The Providence Sunday Journal, Fountain street, this city.

We are now showing our Spring Collection

Chez Elise
246 Thayer Street

IT'S THE GYPSY IN YOU! This gay adaptation of Chanel's celebrated gypsy dress is one of the season's most dramatic models. The light-hearted white shirt is tucked into the vivaciously striped skirt. The wide belt of soft leather is flaming red. —Photo 6-B

Fig. 93

The style that's sweeping the country!

"GYPSY LOUNGER"

3.98 Special Anniversary Price!

Fig. 94

Fig. 93
From couture to bargain counter in a matter of weeks: the "Spring Fashion Parade" photogravure section of the *Providence Sunday Journal* (March 26, 1939) illustrated two knock-off versions of the many spawned by a Chanel "Gypsy" evening-dress design of spring 1939. One is a photo of an "adaptation," another is shown in an ad without acknowledgement by a small Providence shop called Chez Elise (reproduced by permission of the *Providence Journal*).

Fig. 94
Another version, the "Gypsy Lounger," a $3.98 special in the housecoat department at Bloomingdale's, New York, advertised in the *New York Times* (March 12, 1939), section L, p. 10 (reproduced by permission). It is no wonder that copyright protection and design exclusivity were of such concern to both designers and consumers.

In spite of the failure of the couture establishment to maintain a united front at this time, it seems that some of the rules were generally implemented. Another spate of press coverage in the early 1920s suggests that efforts were made to prohibit photographing or sketching a Paris model even at public social events or private showings for fear that the circulation or publication of the illustration would enable copying. In addition, admittance to the couture openings was limited to those who "are well known and have been honest in former transactions."[67]

In 1921, for the first time, American garment manufacturers began to discuss seriously the need for adopting Paris-style regulations to protect their own products. A member of the Cloak, Suit and Skirt Manufacturers Protective Association stated that "the garment in a new style is merely an idea, and its value depends upon how good that idea is… Therefore, the garment possesses something besides its intrinsic value, and it would be entirely proper for the manufacturers to get together and agree to protect their designs and to bar out those who rob them of what is probably the most valuable part of their product."[68] From this time on, a variety of trade organizations appear, lobbying for tighter or looser controls on copying, depending upon which side they represented: the copied or the copiers.

It is sometimes thought that the crusade against style piracy was fought by the Paris couture solely against the American ready-to-wear industry; however, it appears that the first court case to offer "protection to a sartorial idea or conception as such" was contested by Madeleine Vionnet in Paris, December 1921, against two smaller Parisian houses. Miler Soeurs and Henriette Bondreaux were accused of copying Vionnet originals and selling them to Franklin Simon, Bergdorf Goodman, and Saks Fifth Avenue.[69] December 1922 saw additional claims by Vionnet and others "of the most famous Paris couturiers" that piracy was rampant within the French industry.[70] Two years later, the couturiers were joined by other luxury-goods manufacturers in forming the Association for the Defense of Plastic and Applied Arts.[71] Elizabeth Hawes recounts her own activities as a clandestine sketcher of Paris models in the 1920s in *Fashion is Spinach*, implicating not only French copyists, but also American and European wholesalers and retailers. Copying was so lucrative for everyone – except the originator of the dress – that in spite of repeated efforts by the couture and other luxury industries to curb it, it remained a serious plague throughout the 1930s [figs. 93–94].[72]

Despite the apparent interest in the topic in the early 1920s, it took some time for the French complaint – that copyists hurt business by making new ideas commonplace – to take hold in the American industry. Maurice Rentner, an important New York manufacturer of high-end ready-to-wear from the 1910s, spearheaded the establishment of the Fashion Originators Guild in 1933. From twelve original members, it had grown by the end of its first year to sixty members, all high-price manufacturers. The Guild established a Design Registration Bureau following the French lead and asked retailers for "Declarations of Cooperation" in which they "agreed not to buy or sell copies of styles originated by Guild members" [fig. 95].[73] By late 1935, the Guild was being sued by the Federal Trade Commission for restraint of trade and warring in the press with retailers, particularly department stores, and with the Popular Price Dress Manufacturers Group Inc., the trade organization of moderate and budget dress wholesalers.[74] Ultimately, the Guild was forced to back down.

This was not, however, the end of efforts to protect original designs. Magazine and newspaper ads in the late 1930s, both those of manufacturers and of department or specialty stores, often added a copyright line at the bottom of the page, hoping in this way to at least provide legal recourse if garments were copied. A *New York Times* Bonwit Teller ad from 1938 with a copyright statement at the bottom also had captions for two of the dresses that read, "Like Molyneux" and "Suggesting Mainbocher."[75] One author suggested as the reason for the rise of wholesale dress manufacturers in St. Louis that "nowhere else…are style piracy regulations being as effectively enforced as here…The Style Piracy Bureau of the Associated Garment Industries of St. Louis has the co-operation of the Ladies Garment

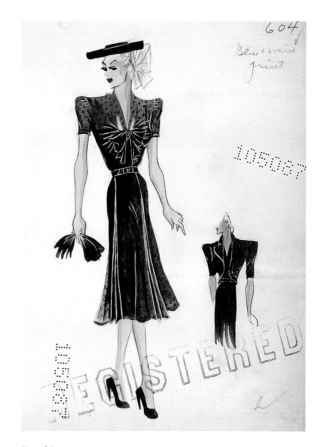

Fig. 95
Registered dress design, ca.1939, by an unidentified American manufacturer: the Design Registration Bureau marked submitted designs with a number and a stamp. This drawing is from one of a number of notebooks of registered designs left out on the street for trash collection in Manhattan in 1980, but no clues to the designers or manufacturers have been found. Private collection.

Workers Union. Members…refuse to work on a design that has been adjudged by a constantly sitting trial board to be a copy of another maker's design."[76] A 1930s study of the dress industry by Helen Everett Meiklejohn, quoted by Bernard Roshco in his 1963 book *The Rag Race*, summed up the issue. "It is this close relationship between copying and adaptation which suggests that the property right inherent in a dress design is difficult to establish and to protect…Dress designers conform to fashion trends and the most brilliant designers are 'adapters'."[77] Roshco wrote of his own time: "A manufacturer of low-priced dresses offers his idea of ethical copying: It's fair to exercise one's judgement of style by copying from higher-priced firms, but another matter to copy from direct competitors."[78]

It is difficult to evaluate and compare prices between custom and ready-to-wear, since ads and features for made-to-order imported or even American-designed models in *Vogue* and *Harper's Bazar* rarely included prices. Store and manufacturer ads for ready-to-wear usually listed prices, however, and the range for ready-to-wear is considerable, even as it is today.

A *Vogue* article from 1915, "Frocks and Gowns Made To Order," gave estimates from dressmakers on producing day, sports, and evening wear. *Vogue* cautioned that "the out-of-town reader should perhaps be warned, however, that these are New York prices and that really good work of this kind is very highly paid. The well-known dressmakers of today seldom make even a simple costume for less than $150, and the prices rise from that to $500." The article went on to suggest that careful attention to ready-made clothing could provide the basis for a "smart" wardrobe, but that "when distinction and individuality are required in a dress, however, it is better to have it made to order." Prices quoted from smaller dressmakers for a silk day dress (still New York prices) averaged $50 to $60.[79]

Elizabeth Hawes explained the pricing of a custom-made dress as of 1938 in *Fashion is Spinach*. The labor of the workers who made an average garment requiring fifty-five hours of work came to $44. Cutting the fabric and fitting the dress added $16.45. A moderately priced fabric might cost $5 a yard, and an average dress might take seven and a half yards for a total cost of $37.50. In addition, a charge of $16.71 for direct "production overhead, workroom manager's salary, stockroom costs, muslin, pins, sewing machines…" and $15 for the design had to be added. Hawes estimated that indirect overhead costs such as rent and utilities, sales staff, clerical help, etc., added about a third again to the price of the dress, or $59.61 on her example. This gave a total of $189.27, which Hawes stated would be rounded up to a selling price of $195. A dress or suit requiring more labor or material might easily cost $400.[80] By the late 1930s, when Hawes was writ-ing, it was not only the custom-made dress that might cost upwards of $200, but expensive ready-to-wear as well.

Ready-to-wear pricing must, of course, have followed the same basic structure of computing direct and indirect costs to come up with the price for a dress. In addition, however, ready-to-wear manufacturers had to figure in the hefty markup by the retailer. As Hawes pointed out, "the cheap wholesaler gets his profits by selling a very large volume, multiplying his 50-cent profit over and over again."[81]

A random sampling of prices in *Vogue* and *Harper's Bazar* over three decades indicates that moderate-priced, ready-to-wear silk day dresses could be had for around $29 in the 1910s and 1920s, while the price drops somewhat in the early and mid-1930s before rising again by 1939. During the 1930s, however, the dress was more likely to be made of rayon or acetate than silk. Cottons and linens were less expensive than silk; woolens about the same. Suits and ensembles, coats, and evening dresses were all higher priced. Sportswear was the least expensive category of clothing. In 1915, Spalding sportswear outfits were sold for $75 made-to-order and $35 plus for ready-to-wear. *Vogue*'s "Seen in the Shops" feature quoted prices of $29.50, $35, and $49.50 for ready-to-wear dresses, while Mazon's, a company established in 1899 that purchased Paris models to sell "after they have been shown to illustrate the Parisienne modes," offered model sizes only within the range of $20 to $75. Franklin Simon & Company, New York, offered ready-to-wear suits in 1916 at $29.50 or $39.50. In 1924, Best & Company offered ready-made copies of French dresses for $38 and $55. Other retailers in that year advertised ready-to-wear dresses at a wide range of prices: "Queen Make" washable linens, voiles, and ginghams ranged between $7.95 and $13.50, Stewart & Company's linen dresses could be had at $19.50 or $24.50, and R. H. Macy's linen frocks at $11.74, $13.74, $14.74 or $16.74. Barbara Lee silk day dresses cost $39.50 with the added attraction that they were "shown exclusively" at one department store only in each city. In 1935, ads for ready-to-wear in *Harper's Bazaar* included a Bergdorf Goodman original evening gown for $160, silk sports dresses for tennis and golf from Lord & Taylor for $16.95, and day dresses from Bonwit Teller for $49.75. In addition, Bullock's Wilshire (Los Angeles) touted authorized copies of an Irene original day dress. Bullock's copies sold for $35 for linen, $45 for solid-color crepe (whether silk or rayon is not clear), and $55 for printed crepe. The original Irene cost $145. In 1938, Russeks (a New York specialty store) offered a topcoat and suit ensemble for $50, or $25 each for the suit or coat. The following year, "scrupulous copies of our own Paris imports" of six coat styles by Mainbocher, Molyneux, Schiaparelli, Paquin, and two by Alix sold at $135 each. It is unusual to find mentions of copies of an American designer: the Irene day dress is the exception to the rule.[82]

How did pricing in the Tirocchi shop match up with prices for comparable garments elsewhere? A black dress by Premet, purchased in 1924 for $89 from Maginnis & Thomas, importers of French gowns, was sold to a client for $145. The same client purchased a Drécoll gown from the Tirocchis for $125 a few months prior. That gown, too, came from Maginnis & Thomas for a price of $89. A three-piece day ensemble from Callot Soeurs sold in 1925 for $175, a modest markup from its purchase price to the Tirocchis of $140.[83]

As many fashion writers and designers have pointed out, custom dressmakers made their money on clients who ordered several garments at a time and also looked to the same shop for accessories; buying hats, gloves, and handbags to complete their outfits. The woman who came in and ordered a single dress was almost more trouble than her order was worth. The client ledger in the Tirocchi Archive bears this out. Many of the most faithful clients would order several new garments and remodeling of one or two older dresses at the same time.

When the Tirocchi sisters first set up their custom dressmaking business, women of a certain social and economic class expected to spend both time and money on being well dressed. The concern with exclusivity that echoes through magazine and newspaper articles of the 1910s could only work to

the benefit of the Tirocchi shop and its Providence competitors. Drawing from the same illustrations of new modes as New York shops, the Tirocchis and their clients could interpret these modes in different color combinations or graft a detail from one design onto the silhouette of another. With her knowledge of the lifestyles and needs of her clients, Anna Tirocchi may also have truly designed garments for them: garments original both in conception and execution and, therefore, truly exclusive.

As the pace of life quickened in the 1920s and ready-to-wear clothing began to be better made and better fitting, many women who formerly had submitted to and even enjoyed the rituals of ordering a custom-made wardrobe began to incorporate ready-to-wear into their lives. As Bergdorf Goodman and Hattie Carnegie did in the 1920s, the Tirocchis began to carry ready-made garments in the shop to augment the custom trade and to encourage clients to spend more of their clothing allowance within the walls of a single shop. Perfumes, hats, handbags, and jewelry were made available. The Tirocchis even stocked imported table linens, catering to yet another need of the social class they served. Still, models from the Paris couturiers were also purchased by Anna Tirocchi to copy and sell.

On a much larger scale than the Tirocchis, most custom dressmakers and department or specialty stores who maintained custom salons depended on the ready-to-wear departments to actually pay the bills. Volume of merchandise sold and the markup on that merchandise were extremely important to the bottom line. Apparently, Bergdorf's custom salon lost money for the store almost every year after 1929. It was "maintained for prestige," not income.[84] Given the apparent vagaries of Anna Tirocchi's many business interests, her dressmaking shop perhaps provided her with an elevated social status that she was loath to discard in favor of more profitable, but less grand, ventures.[85]

The Tirocchi dressmaking shop was not unique in its inception or in its demise. All of the tricks and schemes that larger dressmaking concerns and retail shops used to stay abreast of the times and maintain some profitability were used by the Tirocchis. At this time, however, the volume and variety of documentary evidence surviving the closure of the shop remain unique. In total it indicates the need for a reevaluation of American dressmakers and the American dress industry in the first half of the twentieth century.

1. "Who's Who in the Mode: A Tale of Two Cities," *Vogue*, vol. 61, no. 1 (January 1, 1923), pp. 70–71 ff. This article in the thirtieth anniversary issue of *Vogue* gives an overview of both New York and Paris fashion between 1892 and 1923. It is a useful starting point for understanding the fashion hierarchy of the early part of this century.

2. Bettina Ballard, *In My Fashion*. New York: 1960, pp. 72, 259.

3. Bernard Roshco, *The Rag Race: How New York and Paris Run the Breakneck Business of Dressing American Women*. New York: 1963, p. 57.

4. Leslie Woodcock Tentler, *Wage-Earning Women: Industrial Work and Family Life in the United States, 1900–1930*. New York: 1979, p. 109. For a fuller discussion of the changes in American women's activities, see Dorothy and Carl J. Schneider, *American Women in the Progressive Era, 1900–1920*. New York: 1993.

5. Elizabeth Hawes, *Fashion is Spinach*. New York: 1938, p. 233.

6. The Fashion Group, Inc., *New York's Fashion Futures*. New York: 1940, p. 10.

7. Edna Woolman Chase, *Always in Vogue*. New York: 1954, p. 289.

8. *Ibid.*, p. 32.

9. Royal Pattern Company (285 Fifth Avenue, New York), *Le Costume Royal*, vol. 16, no. 10 (July 1912), copy in the Museum of Art, RISD Department of Costume and Textiles [hereafter, RISD Museum, Dept. Costume/Textiles] library (see "Note on the A. & L. Tirocchi Archive, Collection, and Catalogue," p. 23).

10. Betty Kirke, *Madeleine Vionnet*. San Francisco: 1998, p. 224.

11. I am deeply grateful to Joy Emery and Whitney Blausen for sharing their research on dress patterns with the author for the purposes of this essay. The information on McCall's Couture, Vogue Couture, and Butterick's Starred patterns was conveyed to the author by personal communication with Joy Emery, November 18, 1999.

12. The library of the RISD Museum, Dept. Costume/Textiles, contains several copies of these three magazines, mostly from the 1910s. *Le Bon Ton* was established in 1851, *Le Costume Royal* and *Elite Styles* in the 1890s. Single pages from *Elite Styles* from the late 1920s also exist in the department files.

13. Thanks to Diane Hamblin for drawing the author's attention to *Inspiration* and its companion magazine for men, *Ambition*.

14. This practice is noted in various *Providence Sunday Journal* articles from the 1930s in the clipping files of the RISD Museum, Dept. Costume/Textiles. Corey's first name is spelled "Madeliene," not the conventional "Madeleine." She was a graduate of RISD (1933) and a fashion writer for almost fifty years.

15. Chase, *op. cit.*, p. 295. Many fashion writers have used the term "fashion Ford" to indicate a highly popular, best-selling style that crosses the boundaries of social class and income level.

16. *Ibid.*, p. 108. Bettina Ballard describes the erosion of this policy in the post-World War II era, *op. cit.*, pp. 303–05. Elizabeth Hawes gives her opinion on the intertwining of advertising dollars and editorial space in *Fashion is Spinach* (previously cited), pp. 177–88.

17. RISD Museum, Dept. Costume/Textiles files contain vol. VII, no.3 of Filene's *Clothes* (September 1929). The publication span of the quarterly is currently unknown.

18. The Bergner name is also listed on the title page and at the bottom of a corset advertisement in the complete issue. This issue contains as well an article on new Paris designers called "The Rise of the Smaller Dressmaker," illustrated with sketches by Muriel King, who became an important New York couturier in the 1930s. King was also the cover artist for the 1926 issue.

19. "Dress War," *Time* (March 1936), pp. 70–76.

20. Both booklets exist in the files of the Department of Textiles, National Museum of American History, Smithsonian Institution, Washington, D.C.

21. *Vogue*, vol. 61, no. 1 (January 1, 1923), p. 136. Milgrim is also listed as fashion editor of the *New York Tribune* Syndicate Service.

22. *New York Times* (January 8, 1924), n.p.; clipping in the RISD Museum, Dept. Costume/Textiles files.

23. *Women's Wear* (January 30, 1915), sect. 1, p. 12; and *Women's Wear Daily* (July 8, 1937), sect. 1, p. 3.

24. *Providence Sunday Journal* (September 24, 1939), photogravure section, n.p.; clipping in the RISD Museum, Dept. Costume/Textiles files.

25. Mary Brooks Picken, "The Dressmaker and Tailor Shop," *Harmony in Dress: Woman's Institute Library of Dressmaking*. Scranton: 1924, chap. IX, p. 121.

26. Carolyn B. Reed, "A Day of Shopping in 1910," *Boston Herald* (undated clipping with 8/46 written across the face), p. 12; clipping in the RISD Museum, Dept. Costume/Textiles files.

27. M. Tuttle, "Sewing In Other People's Homes," *Ladies' Home Journal*, vol. 34 (January 1917), p. 20.

28. Eleanor Rogers, Columbus, North Carolina, in a personal communication with Julia Turner of Providence, Rhode Island, October 1999. Mary Campbell, Cohasset, Massachusetts, in a

personal communication with the author of July 1988. Mrs. Campbell also recalled having disliked her new, itchy wool-flannel petticoat enough to discard it in the bushes outside her home on her way to school, resuming it before she re-entered the house in the afternoon.

29. Jane Warren Wells (probably a pseudonym for Mary Brooks Picken, judging from inscription in the book's flyleaf), *Dress and Look Slender.* Scranton: 1924; and Margaretta Byers with Consuelo Kamholy, *Designing Women: The Art, Technique and Cost of Being Beautiful.* New York: 1938.

30. See, for example, *Vogue*, vol. 46, no. 8 (October 15, 1915), pp. 77–90.

31. The Fashion Group, Inc., *op. cit.*, p. 17.

32. *Berth Robert's*, 1239 Broadway, New York (April, May, June 1934); *Fifth Avenue Modes – The Magazine of Fashion*, 74 Fifth Ave, New York (Fall 1933).

33. *Fifth Avenue Modes, op. cit.*, p. 4.

34. The author is grateful to Susan Hay, RISD's Curator of Costume and Textiles, for sharing her research on Mrs. Lewis's diary.

35. The author is grateful to Jean Lewis Keith of Providence for sharing her research of the Soieries F. Ducharne records for the purposes of this essay. Susan Hay pointed out the location of this information in the Musée des Tissus de Lyon.

36. *Harper's Bazaar*, vol. LXX, no. 9 (September 1936), pp. 46, 48.

37. See, for example, *Vogue*, vol. 45, no. 8 (April 15, 1915), pp. 60–61, "Frocks And Gowns Made To Order." Caption to far right illustration on p. 61: "Chéruit also originated this model which makes striking use of gold embroidered black net over Nattier blue net, with Nattier blue ribbon and pink roses. Many other combinations are possible and the resulting gown may be simple or very elaborate."

38. Advertisement in *Vogue*, vol. 38, no. 9 (May 1, 1911), p. 107.

39. For an explanation of these distinctions at that time, see "Who's Who in the Mode," *Vogue*, vol. 61, no. 1 (January 1, 1923), p. 196.

40. *Vogue*, vol. 46, no. 7 (October 1, 1915), p. 4.

41. Advertisement for Best & Company in *Vogue*, vol. 37, no. 7 (April 1, 1911), p. 9.

42. See Patricia Mears, "Jessie Franklin Turner: American Fashion and 'Exotic' Textile Inspiration," in *Creating Textiles: Makers, Methods, Markets. Proceedings of the 1998 Symposium of the Textile Society of America.* Earleville (Maryland): 1999, pp. 431–40.

43. The invitation was extended to a "limited number of the first class dressmakers of America." The admission fee was $10, and no sketching was allowed. Attendees could order models for copying in their own shops, but no model would be sold to more than one dressmaker in the same city. Exclusivity was still uppermost in the minds of fashion consumers at this level.

44. "The Thrilling Romance of Smart Clothes," *Boston Herald* (November 6, 1934), n.p.; clipping in the RISD Museum, Dept. Costume/Textiles files.

45. Much of the information on Marguerite comes from an unpublished paper by Filomena D'Elia of Washington, D.C. The author is grateful to her for sharing her research for the purposes of this essay.

46. *Franklin Simon Fashion Catalog* (Fall 1923). New York: 1993 (reprinted), p. 2 (inside front cover of original edition).

47. Roshco, *op. cit.*, p. 48.

48. Donnelly Garment Company, *Fashions To Live In From The House That Nelly Don Built.* Kansas City: 1936, pp. 4, 11; in the RISD Museum, Dept. Costume/Textiles files.

49. Advertisement for Lord & Taylor in *Harper's Bazaar* (October 1940); clipping in the RISD Museum, Dept. Costume/Textiles files.

50. Kathleen McLaughlin, "A Brilliant Business Career Found its Birth in Boredom," *New York Times* (n.d., but from other bylines, probably March 18, 1939), n.p.; clipping in the RISD Museum, Dept. Costume/Textiles files.

51. "The Dressmakers of the U.S.," *Fortune* (1934), p. 40; clipping in the RISD Museum, Dept. Costume/Textiles files.

52. "Parisian Cocktail," *Vogue*, vol. 80, no. 5 (September 1, 1932), p. 92. The quote refers to Mrs. Reginald (Daisy) Fellowes and a black dress trimmed with *coq* feathers worn by Dietrich in the film.

53. *New York Sunday Times* (January 29, 1939), rotogravure picture section, n.p.; clipping in the RISD Museum, Dept. Costume/Textiles files.

54. See, for example: "K. Howard and G. Walters Stress Growing Importance of Hollywood as a Source of Inspiration," *New York Times* (September 15, 1936); "Hollywood's Fashion Parade," *Christian Science Monitor* (January 22, 1936); "Cinema Fashions," *Fortune* (January 1937); E. L. Hampton, "1200 Mile Style Parade: World's Style Capital Moved to Hollywood," *Nation's Business* (April 1937).

55. *Harper's Bazaar* (January 1939), n.p.; clipping in the RISD Museum, Dept. Costume/Textiles files.

56. Ballard, *op. cit.*, p. 91.

57. Advertisement in *Harper's Bazar*, vol. LVIV, no. 3 (March 1924), p. 125. Ads exist in *Harper's* at least back to 1921. Corticelli also offered several free fashion booklets to readers by mail. The March 1924 ad listed "Irene Castle Corticelli Fashions," "The Correct Color Hosiery For Every Shoe and Occasion," and "Spring Secrets in Corticelli Silks."

58. Advertisement copyrighted 1938 by Best & Company, probably from the *New York Times* (clipping dated in pencil, October 24, 1938); clipping in the RISD Museum, Dept. Costume/Textiles files.

59. "Gowns of a stage princess," *Vogue*, vol. 37, no. 7 (April 1, 1911), pp. 40–41.

60. *New York Times* (n.d., probably December 12 or 13, 1937), n.p.; clipping in the RISD Museum, Dept. Costume/Textiles files. Celanese manufactured rayon fabrics.

61. "Corsets," *Women's Wear*, vol. 4, no.22 (January 26, 1912), p. 12.

62. "Hold Back the New Styles," *New York Times* (February 25, 1912), sect. III, p. 1. The author is grateful to Pamela A. Parmal for sharing her research on copying and the Paris couture for the purposes of this essay.

63. *New York Times* (October 27, 1912).

64. "Paris Dressmakers in Protective Union," *New York Times* (October 24, 1915), sect. III, p. 9.

65. *New York Times* (January 23, 1916), sec. VI, p. 2.

66. "Predict Failure of Poiret's Plan," *New York Times* (January 15, 1916), p. 5.

67. "Against Style Piracy," *New York Times* (August 28, 1921), sec. II, p. 6.

68. *Ibid.*

69. *New York Times* (January 1, 1922), p. 3; and Betty Kirke, *op. cit.*, p. 221.

70. "Mode Designers War Against Paris Pirates," *New York Times* (December 2, 1922), p. 17.

71. "War on 'Fashion Pirates'," *New York Times* (December 24, 1924), p. 24.

72. See Kirke, *op. cit.*, pp. 221–25, for a fuller discussion of copyright disputes in France.

73. "Dress War," *Time* (March 23, 1936), pp. 70–76.

74. For articles related to this suit, see the *New York Times* throughout February 1936; *Business Week* (December 28, 1935; February 29, 1936; March 14, 1936; March 28, 1936; April 25, 1936); and *Newsweek* (April 4, 1936).

75. *New York Times* (n.d., probably late February 1938), n.p.; clipping in RISD Museum, Dept. Costume/Textiles files.

76. Marguerite Martyn, "St. Louis' Designing Women," *St. Louis Post-Dispatch* (December 4, 1939), n.p.; clipping in the RISD Museum, Dept. Costume/Textiles files.

77. Roshco, *op. cit.*, p. 57.

78. *Ibid.*, p. 51.

79. *Vogue*, vol. 45, no. 8 (April 15, 1915), pp. 60–61.

80. Hawes, *op. cit.*, p. 235.

81. *Ibid.*, p. 240. The quote continues: "The specialty shop profits by its large markup. …The couturiere profits chiefly in the satisfaction of being able to eat while she has the pleasure of dressing stylish ladies in beautiful clothes."

82. Prices have been taken from the following sources: *New York Herald Fashion Magazine* (April 2, 1916), p. 5; Bonwit Teller advertisement copyrighted 1938, *New York Times* (possibly February 26 or 27, 1938), n.p.; *New York Times* (September 17, 1939), sec. L, p. 6; the above all clippings in the RISD Museum, Dept. Costume/Textiles files. See also *Vogue*, vol. 46, no. 7 (October 1, 1915), p. 125; *Vogue*, vol. 63, no. 11 (May 1, 1924), p. 8; *Harper's Bazaar*, vol. LXIX, no. 5 (May 1935), p. 13.

83. See Pamela A. Parmal's essay in this volume (pp. 25–49) for an in-depth look at the Tirocchis' pricing.

84. Roshco, *op. cit.*, p. 138.

85. See John W. Briggs's essay in this volume (pp. 79–102) for discussion of Anna Tirocchi's other business interests.

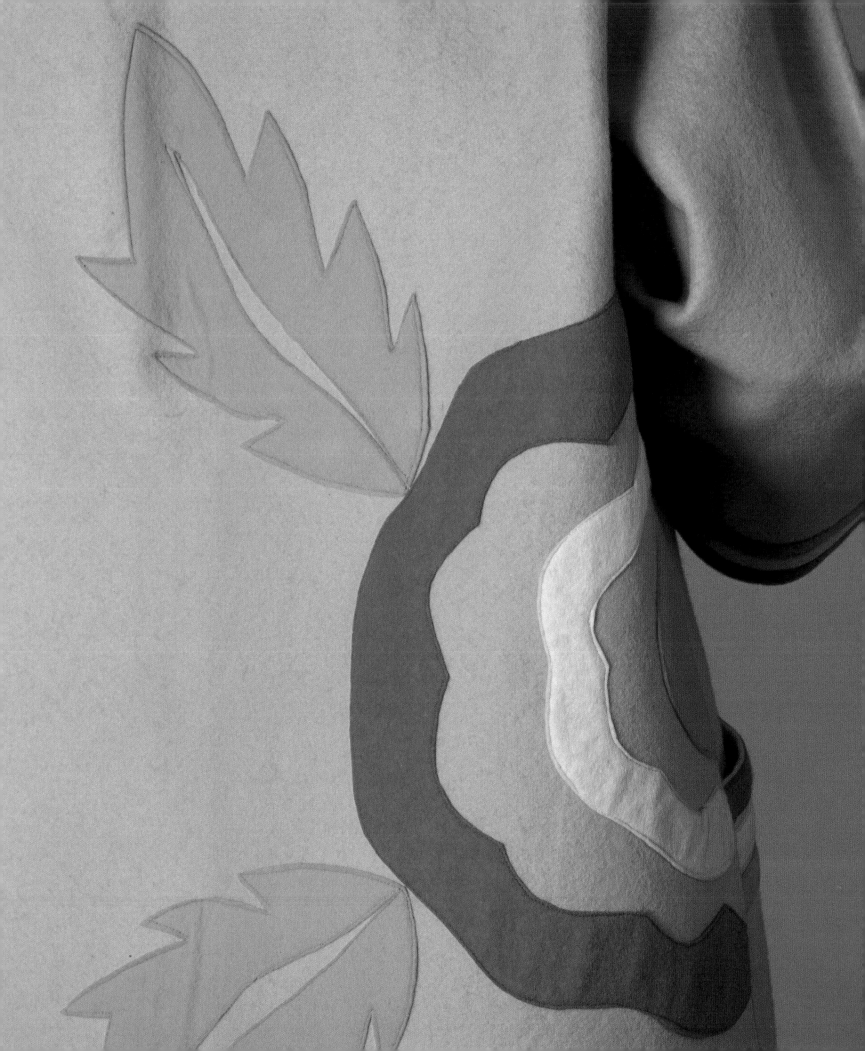

SUSAN HAY
Curator of Costume and Textiles
Museum of Art, Rhode Island School of Design

Paris to Providence:

French Couture and the Tirocchi Shop

The period between the turn of the twentieth century, when Anna and Laura Tirocchi were being trained as dressmakers in Italy, and the Second World War, which marked the end of their business in Providence, was a time of tremendous artistic ferment. In Paris, the origin of fashion for the Tirocchi sisters and their clientele, modernism was bringing a fresh breath of air to all the arts, including the couture. It seemed that everyone looked to Paris for fashion, for art, for contemporary life. Now, artists in all media were flocking to Paris from around the world, forever changing art, as well as fashion, which converged as never before during these years.

"Paris was where the twentieth century was," wrote American Gertrude Stein about the excitement generated by early modernism in the world of art and ideas. A perspicacious observer and participant in the Paris art scene, Stein came to Paris in 1903. She soon became friendly with Picasso, who arrived from Spain the next year and met Stein in 1905. Other young modernist painters, such as Georges Braque, Fernand Léger, Sonia and Robert Delaunay, Francis Picabia, and Marie Laurençin, as well as poet and critic Guillaume Apollinaire, frequented the salon that Stein hosted at her house in the rue de Fleurus on the Seine's left bank. Pablo Picasso and Henri Matisse met one another for the first time there.[1] American photographer and gallery owner Alfred Stieglitz, Spanish cubist painter Juan Gris, and American writer Carl Van Vechten were frequent visitors in the 1910s, testifying to the inclusiveness and international character of the art world. After the demise of the salon in 1913, Stein befriended the Americans novelist Hemingway and modernist composer Virgil Thomson, and the Frenchmen sculptor Jacques Lipschitz and poet

Fig. 96
Wool felt beach coat with *"moderne"* flower (detail of fig. 140, p. 167), a prominent motif decorating fashions sold by A. & L. Tirocchi: here, the flower components have been cut out and applied to the coat like a cubist collage. Museum of Art, RISD, gift of L. J. Cella III.

and designer Jean Cocteau. In the 1940s, she counted among her friends couturier Pierre Balmain.

Gertrude Stein immediately recognized that fashion was an integral part of art and literature and a major factor in the electrifying ambience of Paris. "There is no pulse so sure of the state of a nation as its characteristic art product which has nothing to do with its material life," she wrote. "Fashion is the real thing in abstraction."[2] To her, fashion reflected the revolutionary ideas and excitement of the modernist movement without theorizing or fussing: it just *was*.

In Gertrude Stein's Paris, early modernism in the art world revolved about the concept of abstraction [fig. 96]. In 1905, Matisse and his fellow artists had shocked critics with their paintings. For their use of bold color in ways unrelated to realism, an unsympathetic critic dubbed them "*fauves*" ("wild beasts"). By 1911, Braque and Picasso were painting realistic forms abstracted by converting them to geometric components, by using nonlinear perspective, and by portraying them from several viewpoints at once. Cubism's iconoclastic vision and revolt against tradition gave impetus to many other artists, including the Russian Vasili Kandinsky, who, in an analogy to music, painted purely abstract geometric forms with no relation to actual objects. Futurists Filippo Tommaso Marinetti and Gino Severini in Italy, Piet Mondrian and other artists of the De Stijl movement in Holland, and the Russian constructivists employed abstraction in many media, including architecture, painting, and printmaking.

Artists in other forms also embraced abstraction in the early years of the twentieth century. Composers such as Frenchman Erik Satie, who wrote music without bar lines or key signatures, and German Arnold Schoenberg, who replaced the traditional octave by a twelve-tone scale, were in open revolt against nineteenth-century romanticism. Guillaume Apollinaire was composing poetry with nontraditional capitalization and punctuation as early as 1910. At the same time, Marcel Proust was writing his great novel cycle *À la Recherche du temps perdu* (*Remembrance of Things Past*, published between 1913 and 1927), embracing the revelations

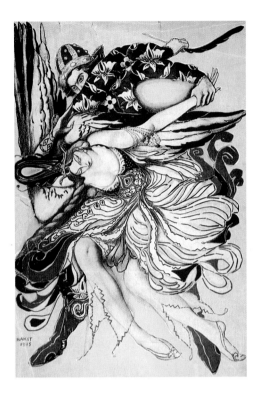

Fig. 97
Design by Léon Bakst illustrating Stravinsky's *Firebird* ballet, produced by the Ballets Russes in 1915; published in *Harper's Bazar* (February 1916; reproduced by permission). Tirocchi Archive.

of Freudian theory by calling forth his subconscious memories – the only way, he believed – to achieve a true representation of the past. James Joyce, who came to Paris from Ireland in 1920, presented the innermost thoughts of his protagonist through an original stream-of-consciousness style in his novel *Ulysses*. For Ezra Pound, the American poet, or British poet T. S. Eliot, also living in Paris, modernism was free verse and verse as collage. Painters were poets, poets painters: Francis Picabia, Max Jacob, and Jean Cocteau were among them. Literary magazines encompassing contemporary poetry and illustration arose and disappeared in the years between 1910 and 1930.

Modernist artists in France were collaborating on works in all media, ranging from theatrical and related arts to illustration and textile and fashion design. The Ballets Russes arrived in Paris in 1909, creating a sensation with the choreography of Michel Fokine and brightly colored sets and costumes by

Léon Bakst [fig. 97]. The group's founder and impresario, Serge Diaghilev, began to employ modern artists in musical and design collaborations, an idea that would influence dance and theater across the entire twentieth century. Claude Debussy, Paul Dukas, Sergei Prokofiev, Maurice Ravel, Erik Satie, Richard Strauss, and Igor Stravinsky all wrote music for him. Jean Cocteau and Hugo von Hoffmansthal wrote librettos, while Natalia Gontcharova, Mikhail Larionov, André Derain, and Pablo Picasso formed an international group of set and costume designers. In 1917, Picasso provided sketches for the costumes and décor to be used in the celebrated Ballet Russes work *Parade* with music by Erik Satie and concept by Jean Cocteau. These were realized in the ateliers of couturiere Jeanne Paquin. In the 1920s, the Ballet Suédois, resident in Paris, would commission modernist artists to compose music and design sets and costumes for such modern ballets as *Skating Rink*, 1922, with "cubist" costumes by Léger, and *Relâche*, designed by Francis Picabia in 1924. The Ballets Suédois also employed modern poets, including Paul Claudel, Blaise Cendrars, and the ubiquitous Cocteau. In the new medium of moving pictures, Léger's *Ballet méchanique* of 1924 had no scenario and consisted of only rhythmic images taken with a prismatic camera (recommended by Ezra Pound) and music by composer Georges Antheil.[3]

The presence of other modernist artistic centers in Berlin, Vienna, Glasgow, and elsewhere guaranteed the movement an international outlook. Anything and everything was possible. French couture benefitted from this explosion of creativity and collaboration, joining the worlds of art and fashion in a way that had never been seen before and would scarcely be seen thereafter. Couturiers Paul Poiret, at the beginning of the period spanned by the Tirocchi shop, and Elsa Schiaparelli, at the end of it, were particular foils for and participants in the artistic community. Jeanne Lanvin, Madeleine Vionnet, Jean Patou, Gabrielle Chanel, and others also undertook collaborations with modern artists at some time in their careers. In France these connections with the art world were taken as a matter of course, and because of them, the forms that

French couture took in the early years of the century must be seen against the philosophical and aesthetic background of art in French culture generally.

When the first couturier, Charles Frederick Worth, arrived in Paris from London in 1846, he found that the couture was already recognized as one of the decorative arts and was represented in the frequently held government-sponsored exhibitions. Worth himself took first place for his white silk court train at the Exposition Universelle of 1855. By 1860, he had become a supplier to the Empress Eugénie, and his fame was growing. In 1867, Bostonian Isabella Stewart Gardner became a Worth client. In her wake came New Yorkers Mrs. J. Pierpont Morgan, Mrs. William Astor, Jr., and novelist Edith Wharton. When Worth retired, his sons took over the business, in their turn contributing to the Exposition Universelle of 1900. The French government, which had been protecting and promoting France's luxury industries since the time of Louis XIV, awarded Gaston Worth membership in the Légion d'honneur and recognized the House of Worth as an "*ancien notable commerçant*" ("historic notable business").[4] By the turn of the century, French couture was known worldwide, and American women who came to Paris were flocking to the ateliers of Worth, Doucet, and Paquin [fig. 98]. In the 1890s, John Wanamaker of Philadelphia and later New York was the first businessman to import French fashions to sell in his store, then fitting them to the

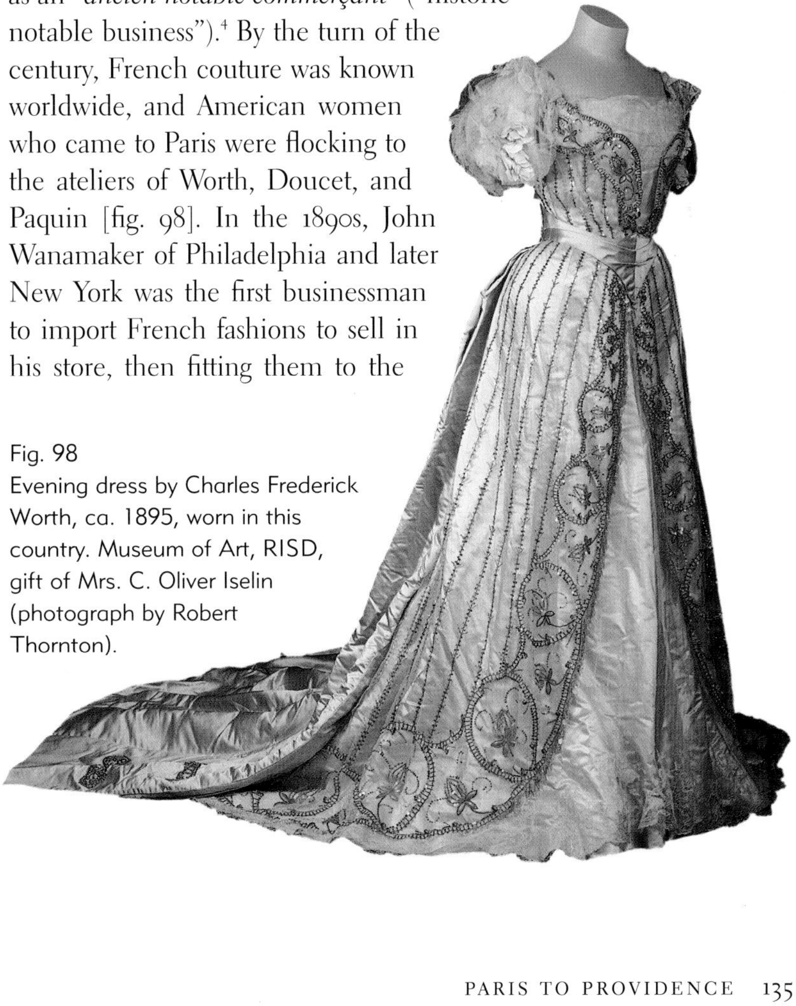

Fig. 98
Evening dress by Charles Frederick Worth, ca. 1895, worn in this country. Museum of Art, RISD, gift of Mrs. C. Oliver Iselin (photograph by Robert Thornton).

measure of his clients. Marshall Field & Company in Chicago followed suit. Poiret, Schiaparelli, and many other couturiers soon came to be well known to fashionable women everywhere.

Paul Poiret, born in 1879, began his career with a brief stint at the House of Worth. Poiret was a quintessential Parisian who saw himself as a modernist, moved in artistic circles, patronized artists and collected their work, and thought about the issues and controversies of the contemporary art world. Through the publicity apparatus he developed by his employment of artists, his encouragement of the fashion press, and his highly visible and flamboyant lifestyle, he greatly influenced the development of modern dress.

To understand how natural was the connection of the world of fashion to the world of the arts, it is instructive to look at Paul Poiret's upbringing. The household of his father, a textile merchant, was situated in Les Halles, the great market district through which pulsed the lifeblood of Paris. Poiret discussed his childhood in perhaps the most charming section of his autobiography, *En Habillant l'époque*.[5] As a boy he enjoyed that most Parisian pastime of people-watching in the streets and at cultural events. Paris, with its wide spaces and elegant gardens, the Palais Royale and the Tuileries, seemed like a stage setting for fashionable women, whose elegant toilettes he admired. As an adolescent he haunted the amphitheater of the Comédie Française, where students paid one franc to see the classics, played by the celebrated actresses Réjane and Sarah Bernhardt (both dressed on and off the stage by couturier Jacques Doucet, for whom Poiret would work after his two years with Worth). Poiret attended the Théâtre Gymnase and the Vaudeville, where he was struck by the beauty of the women and their giant leg-of-mutton sleeves. He went to art galleries, attended openings, and showed his incipient avant-garde sensibilities by preferring Impressionist paintings at a time when they were still new and unappreciated by his family, at least.

As a young couturier, he became fascinated by modern art, befriending students of the École des Beaux-Arts and cultivating the company of painters, with whom he had an excellent rapport. "I have always liked painters," he said. "It seems to me that we are in the same trade, and that they are my colleagues."[6] Before his marriage in 1906, he was already friendly with fauvist painters Francis Picabia, Maurice Vlaminck, and André Derain, who shared his love of bright color. In 1910, he met illustrator Jean-Louis Boussingault and painter André Dunoyer de Segonzac, who became his friends and collaborators. After 1910, Poiret began to purchase modern paintings. He was Dunoyer de Segonzac's first patron, and the artist remembered seeing "a Picasso still-life [hanging] next to van Dongen nudes, Matisse paintings [along] with mine," placed on the walls according to Poiret's personal style. His collection, sold in 1925, also included works by Derain, Dufy, Rouault, Utrillo, and Vlaminck. Poiret had a marked effect on the artists whose pieces he collected and with whom he was close. Dunoyer de Segonzac wrote, "As important as his collecting was the active support he lent to artists throughout his lifetime. He related to them at a profound level and he delighted in their company."[7] Ironically, Poiret also patronized Charles-Édouard Jeanneret, who designed a seaside villa – never built – for the couturier during or immediately following the First World War. In later years, as the architect called Le Corbusier, Jeanneret was the foremost exponent in France of an anti-ornamental purist philosophy, which stood in opposition to Poiret's brilliant achievements in the decorative arts.[8]

Poiret's youthful addiction to the theater served as a springboard for his use of dramatic presentation in the promotion of his fashions. From his earliest days as a couturier, he recognized the publicity to be gained by costuming famous actresses in stage productions, as did many other couturiers. Between 1898 and 1900, while still serving his apprenticeship with Doucet, Poiret designed costumes for Réjane in the melodrama *Zaza* and for Sarah Bernhardt in *L'Aiglon*, in which she played a young son of Napoleon I. Poiret's costume made the aging diva look like an adolescent, emphasizing her still-slim figure, and was a forerunner of his future embrace of the Empire silhouette. Throughout his career, he used the theater to promote his designs, even during the long decline of his couture house's later years.

A larger-than-life figure with a larger-than-life ego, Poiret's flamboyant lifestyle also attracted publicity and added to his renown. In a city and an era famed for its banquets and parties, his stood out: each "*fête*" was an elaborate costume drama with decorations by modern artists and an historical theme. He assigned roles to his friends. They were required to play characters of all periods from ancient times to the seventeenth century and to dress the part. "Sets" were provided by his artist friends. His most famous party, in 1911, was entitled "The Thousand and Second Night" and was based upon the classic tales told by Scheherazade in *A Thousand and One Nights*. Three hundred guests were invited to attend in "ancient Persian" costume. Dufy and Dunoyer de Segonzac painted a huge vellum awning to hang over the buffet table, and Oriental rugs covered the floor. Dufy designed the program. Guests included photographer Edward Steichen, whom Poiret employed to take photographs of his collections; painters Kees Van Dongen and Guy-Pierre Fauconnet; the actor Édouard de Max; and Lucien Vogel, founder of the avant-garde fashion magazine *Gazette du Bon Ton*, which he was to establish in 1912 and which employed the illustrators Poiret also patronized.[9] Poiret also gave lavish dinner parties that were likely to be attended by Picasso, Apollinaire, and Dufy, as recorded by fellow guest Marie Laurençin.[10]

Other artists had similar backgrounds and took part in similar activities. Isadora Duncan, as a young woman in Paris, provided herself with an education in the cultural world of the capital. Together with her brother, she attended the Louvre, the theater, the Exposition Universelle of 1900 with its Oriental temples and exotic music. Nearly penniless at first, they got to know the city by walking its streets and elegant public spaces. Her career began in earnest when she was asked by Parisian intellectuals to dance at their salons, which she did barefoot wearing only a Greek tunic. Some years later, when she was famous and the mistress of the wealthy Paris Singer, heir to the Singer Sewing Machine fortune, she held her own lavish parties, one of which took place at Versailles. There in the park were marquees with every sort of refreshment from caviar and champagne to tea and cakes. After this prelude, in

an open space on which tents had been erected, "the Colonne orchestra…gave us a programme of the works of Richard Wagner…After the concert, a magnificent banquet…lasted until midnight, when the grounds were illuminated, and, to the strains of a Vienna orchestra, every one danced until the small hours."[11] Duncan became one of Poiret's better clients, putting aside her Greek tunics in favor of his high-waisted, slender gowns, which she wore, like her tunics, without a corset. She also employed him to design the interior of her studio in Neuilly in 1908.

Poiret's theatrical background also helps to explain his great interest in the Ballets Russes, whose first appearance in Paris in 1909 impressed him so much. The boldly designed costumes by Bakst, their bright colors echoing Russian peasant art, expressed for him not only the exoticism celebrated by painters such as Picasso, but the appeal of spontaneity, a concept at the heart of much modern art. Immediately Poiret began including Oriental motifs in his dresses, and the turban he created for his wife, Denise, became a classic. For "The Thousand and Second Night" event he created an "Oriental" costume for his wife that included harem trousers topped by his famous "lampshade tunic." Oriental motifs continued to be part of his designs until the end of his career [fig. 99].

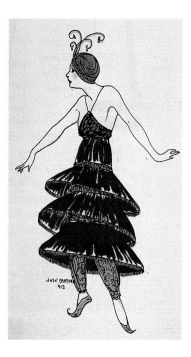

Fig. 99
Illustration by José Lamora of Paul Poiret's costume for the stage play *Le Minaret* of 1913, typical of his gift for designing in an "Oriental" mode; published in the *Gazette du Bon Ton*, no. 6 (April 1913), p. 185.

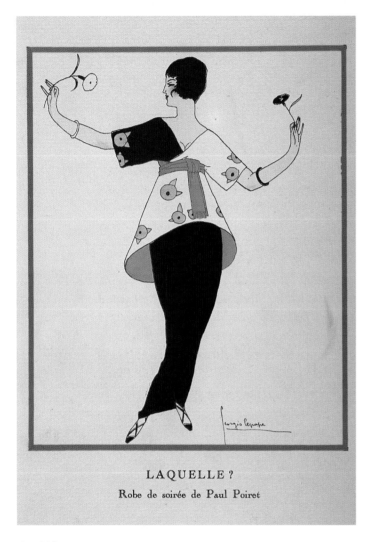

LAQUELLE?
Robe de soirée de Paul Poiret

Fig. 100
Illustration by Georges Lepape of an evening dress by
Paul Poiret with "lampshade" tunic; published in
Gazette du Bon Ton, no. 11 (September 1913), pl. 5.

Poiret's innate sympathy with artists, his employment of them, and his support of the artistic and fashion press gave couture, and his own designs, a new exposure. The perfecting by illustrators of the *pochoir* printing technique – in which colors were brushed onto the paper through thin zinc or copper cut-out stencils – was an important boost for the art of fashion illustration, and Poiret was one of the first to realize its possibilities. In 1908, he hired the young printmaker Paul Iribe, whose works in the *pochoir* technique appealed to the couturier because their simple line and broad, flat, abstract expanses of bright color perfectly captured the Empire dresses he was then making [see fig. 156, p. 181]. Iribe executed ten images of Poiret gowns, which were reproduced by *pochoir* in an edition of 250 copies, called *Les Robes de Paul Poiret, racontées par Paul Iribe* (Paris: 1908). It was the first time a couturier had looked to modern art to represent his creations, and it sounded the call for a redefinition of fashion illustration, while making a name for Iribe, who went on to a career in the graphic and decorative arts. In 1911, Poiret again published a brochure of his designs, this time created by another young artist, Georges Lepape, who had been trained in the atelier run by Fernand Cormon, where Toulouse-Lautrec, Van Gogh, Sérusier, Matisse, and Picabia had all studied.[12] *Les Choses de Paul Poiret, vues par Georges Lepape* appeared in a larger edition: one thousand copies were printed (Paris: 1911). Lepape, too, had absorbed the lessons of bright color taught by the Ballet Russes, and his *pochoir* prints of Poiret's still high-waisted fashions in this brochure and later in the *Gazette du Bon Ton* used line drawings with large areas of blues, greens, reds, pinks, and yellows [fig. 100]. Photography was only just becoming a tool of the fashion press. The technology of reproducing a photograph on the same page as text had been perfected in the 1890s, but Poiret exploited it innovatively by hiring Edward Steichen to record his collections.

Poiret was also close to the fashion press as it developed in the early twentieth century. Lucien Vogel, a publisher of art books and a friend of Poiret who had been one of the guests at the "The Thousand and Second Night," was inspired by

Poiret's brochures and by other works of young artists to begin a new kind of fashion magazine illustrated by modern artists. As an art publication, it would be totally different from other contemporary fashion publications, such as *Vogue*, which included literature and articles of interest to women on other subjects such as architecture, society goings-on, and travel. Vogel's *Gazette du Bon Ton* emphasized fashion and art with fine *pochoir* illustrations by Jacques and Pierre Brissaud, as well as Lepape and others.

Vogel, like Poiret with his Empire-waisted dresses, was looking back to the end of the eighteenth century and the beginning of the nineteenth, when such fashion magazines as *Galerie des Modes* and *Journal des Dames* were charmingly illustrated. In the first issue of the *Gazette du Bon Ton*, Henri Bidou summarized the atmosphere in which it appeared: "Today, as at the end of the 18th century, the entire public pays attention to Fashion…Painters collaborate with couturiers. The dressing of women is a pleasure to the eye that is not judged inferior to the other arts."[13] Each number was to have fashion designs by modern artists, in addition to drawings by these artists of fashions designed by couturiers like Poiret, Paquin, Lanvin, and others who agreed to collaborate with the magazine. The *Gazette du Bon Ton* became a magnet for young illustrators, including Georges Barbier, André Marty, Charles Martin, Lepape, and in later years the Russian Erté. All of these artists produced fashion illustrations, but were variously talented as painters, commercial artists, and stage, furniture, or textile designers: yet another example of the close connections of art and design in the first decades of the century.

Other magazines in the same vein as the *Gazette du Bon Ton* appeared in 1912. *Le Journal des Dames et des Modes*, published between 1912 and 1914, used many of the same illustrators – as did the journal *Modes et Manières d'Aujourd'hui* (1912–22) – and published short articles on fashion by many modern writers, including Claude Roger Marx, Jean-Louis Vaudoyer, and Jean Giraudoux, among others. Although many of these journals lasted for only a short period of years (the *Gazette du Bon Ton* merged with *Vogue* in 1925), they utterly shifted the direction of fashion illustration. Mainstream journals like *Vogue*, *Harper's Bazar* (which ultimately hired Erté), *Vanity Fair*, *Les Feuillets d'Art*, and *L'Illustration* continued to publish fashion images by modern artists after the demise of the smaller journals. As Elsa Schiaparelli has pointed out, until the Second World War such magazines encouraged the connections of fashion designers and artists in a way that has not been seen since, and she felt that their editors were among her main supporters. "It was not a matter of pure advertising interests: of who bought and how widely a model could be reproduced," she said, "but how creative the presentation of fashion could be."[14]

In 1911, Poiret established Barbazange, a gallery for the fine arts in the ground floor of his showrooms in the rue d'Antin, where he intended to display avant-garde artworks. A story recounted by Roger Shattuck about this gallery in his wonderful book on early modernism in France, *The Banquet Years*, illustrates perfectly the interpenetration of the arts at this period and the degree of involvement of Poiret himself. In March 1920, an event took place in Poiret's gallery that expressed all the creativity, all the experimentation, all the excitement, and all of the good humor of the days of early modernism. Actor Pierre Bertin sponsored a concert with music by Russian composer Igor Stravinsky and by Les Six, the group of French composers surrounding Erik Satie. Also on the program was a play by Max Jacob with "furniture music" by Satie and Darius Milhaud to be played during the first intermission. The program directed the audience to treat the music "as if it did not exist, as if it were a chair on which one is or is not seated." When the musicians began to play, however, the audience sat down and began to listen. At this, Satie "rushed around the gallery exhorting them to appropriate behavior. 'Talk, keep on talking. And move around. Whatever you do, don't listen!'"[15]

Although Poiret is the best known and most documented of the couturiers with strong connections to the art world, there were many others who were not only collectors, but also friends of artists and collaborators with them in the design of couture or in other artistic projects, especially for the ballet and the stage. Before Poiret, and no doubt an inspiration to him in his own collecting, was Jacques Doucet, Poiret's mentor, whose family fortune, supplemented with the profits from his hugely successful couture house, had enabled him to become a major art collector. Doucet had begun collecting eighteenth-century art in the late nineteenth century and by 1910 had amassed a large group of furnishings and textiles, as well as painting and sculpture. Concurrently, Doucet put together a library of books, reproductions, photographs, engravings, drawings, sale catalogues, and other documents for the study of art history.

In 1912, he sold his art collection and gave his library, which he had opened to scholars, to the University of Paris. Soon thereafter, he began commissioning decorative arts by such young modern artists as Paul Iribe, Eileen Gray, Marcel Coard, and Pierre Legrain for his apartment in Paris, and, later, his studio in Neuilly, while purchasing paintings by Manet, Cézanne, Van Gogh, Derain, Braque, and Picasso. Interested in literature since 1896, when he had become involved briefly with the group of symbolist poets surrounding Paul Valéry, Doucet now had the idea of forming a library for the study of the origins of modern literature. He began collecting manuscripts and issues of small, short lived, but important modernist literary reviews and commissioning regular reports from poets such as Max Jacob, Pierre Reverdy, and others then in cubist circles. Jacob's letters to Doucet, kept intact in this second important library, which was also eventually given to the University of Paris, are now of great importance for the study of literature at the beginning of the twentieth century.

Doucet hired essayist André Suarès as his library's curator. Suarès was succeeded in 1920 by the surrealist poet André Breton. Breton, in the modernist spirit, believed that literature and art were intimately connected, so closely connected that they could not be separated. He advised Doucet to add to his collection of paintings what Breton considered to be the great landmarks of modern art: Seurat's *Le Cirque*; Picabia's *La Musique est comme la peinture*; *La Charmeuse de serpents* by Douanier Rousseau; Marcel Duchamp's *Deux Nus*; and

paintings by Matisse, Max Ernst, and Giorgio DiChirico, among others. Breton also guided him to the purchase of African art. Perhaps the most famous acquisition Breton counseled Doucet to make was Picasso's controversial *Les Demoiselles d'Avignon* with its images derived from African art (now in the collection of the Museum of Modern Art, New York).[16] Following Breton's departure as curator, Doucet continued to add to the collection until his death in 1929. Much of it was sold in the 1930s. Exceptions were made for Rousseau's *La Charmeuse de serpents*, promised to the Louvre in accordance with the wish of Robert Delaunay, from whom Doucet had purchased it, and a substantial legacy to his nephew, which now forms the collection of the Fondation Angladon-Dubrujeaud in Avignon. Doucet's library of modern literature, however, went to join the Library of Art and Archaeology at the University of Paris.

Doucet's contemporary, Jeanne Paquin, while never a patron of modern painting, collected old master artworks, which she left to the Louvre after her death. She did, however, acquire contemporary jewelry, mostly by Cartier and Lalique, and employed Louis Süe to design her villa at St. Cloud, called Les Treillages. Robert Mallet-Stevens built her villa at Deauville, and Lalique did the interior decoration of her dining room in Paris as late as 1931.[17] Paquin in turn designed and executed costumes for the theater and the ballet. Very prolific before World War I, she produced costumes for more than thirteen works in 1913, including *Jeux*, choreographed for the Ballets Russes by Vaslav Nijinsky to Debussy's music with costumes designed by Léon Bakst.[18]

Paul Poiret's sisters Nicole Groult and Germaine Bongard also designed clothing and possessed the Poiret family's interest in the art world. Nicole, the wife of André Groult, a designer of modern furniture and a member of the Artistes Décorateurs, had a couture salon in the rue d'Anjou, where she created "artistic" fashions. Her brother accused her of "borrowing" his designs. An article in American *Vogue* in April 1912 made her famous in the United States. Through her husband, she knew the *coloriste* artists: cubist painters, architects, and designers including Van Dongen, Laurençin, and Picabia. Dufy, Martin, and Süe also belonged to the circle around André Groult. Van Dongen, Laurençin, and Süe each painted Nicole Groult's portrait.[19] After World War I, Groult reopened her salon in 1919, commissioning her friend Gabrielle Picabia, estranged wife of the painter, to introduce her creations in the United States. By coincidence, the future couturiere Elsa Schiaparelli, then a struggling young mother who had just been abandoned by her husband, met Mme Picabia in New York and assisted her in selling Groult's designs. Like her brother, Nicole Groult also designed theater costumes. Groult's couture business continued throughout the Depression years, while her brother's was in desperate straits. Her clients were an international "who's who," including Dorothy Parker; Virginia Woolf; the Comtesse Marie Laure de Noailles, perennial best-dressed of Frenchwomen; and the actress Madge Garland.[20]

Despite the war, Germaine Bongard set up a couture salon for children in 1916. At this time, cubist painter Juan Gris commissioned an outfit from her for his wife, offering a painting of Bongard's choice in exchange. With her connections to the avant-garde and the assistance of purist painter Amédée Ozenfant, she opened her salon to exhibitions of paintings for the benefit of "the painters at the Front," like Léger, whom she counted among her friends, along with Derain and Ozenfant. After the war, she established an avant-garde art gallery, which she managed in addition to her couture house. In 1921, she constructed the costumes Picasso had designed for the ballet *Cuadro Flamenco*. She herself composed a ballet that was to have music by Francis Poulenc and costumes by Marie Laurençin. The project did not come to fruition, but it demonstrates once more the degree of openness to collaboration that was one of the most novel and exciting characteristics of early modernism.[21]

Another couturiere who collected modern art was Jeanne Lanvin. One of the favorite designers of the Tirocchi clientele in the 1920s, she collected impressionist and fauvist paintings. The portrait she commissioned from Édouard Vuillard shows her at her worktable and is now in the collection of the Centre Georges Pompidou, Paris. In the 1920s, Lanvin employed architect Paul Plumet to design her town house, for which she purchased furniture by Armand Rateau and Jean Dunand, now in the Musée des Arts Décoratifs, Paris.[22]

Madeleine Vionnet, endowed with a great sensitivity to geometry, in 1921 hired Italian futurist artist Ernesto Michelle, called Thayaht, to illustrate her designs in the *Gazette du Bon Ton*. In these works, he employed an American system called "dynamic symmetry," which used geometrical formulas based on the golden mean of the ancient Greeks to produce pleasing proportions for depictions of the natural world and the human figure. Vionnet also employed him to design surface ornament for her simple chemise gowns in the 1920s.[23] Like Lanvin, she patronized modern artists for furniture for her salon, purchasing items from Dunand, Lalique, and Boris Lacroix.[24]

In this period of experimentation, artists in various media and from many European countries designed items of dress. In 1913, the same year that his costumes for *Jeux* were made in Paquin's workshops, Bakst also collaborated with her to produce dresses for the couture [fig. 101]. Russian émigré

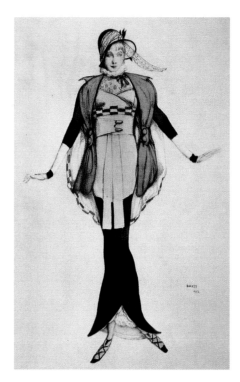

Fig. 101
Illustration by Léon Bakst of his dress realized by Paquin; published in *Gazette du Bon Ton*, no. 6 (April 1913), pl. 1.

painters Sonia and Robert Delaunay were designing "reform" costumes as early as 1914, using the abstract theories of color placement they called "simultaneous Orphism" [figs. 102–103]. In an article in *Mercure de France*, Apollinaire described Robert Delaunay's "red coat with blue collar, green vest, sky blue shirt and red tie," next to Sonia Delaunay's violet suit with bright "color zones" on the jacket ranging from rose to blue to scarlet.[25] Sonia Delaunay's "simultaneous fashions" in abstract prints and embroideries to her design were displayed at the famous decorative arts exhibition of 1925.

Elsewhere in Europe, Russian constructivists and Italian futurists both tackled apparel from the point of view of ideological reform, seeking "sanity in dress" and designing many variations for both men and women. Madeleine Vionnet produced Thayaht's invention, the *tuta*, a futurist "overall" for men. The artists of the Wiener Werkstätte also designed clothing, and the fashion department was the most commercially successful of all their varied enterprises. At the same time, all were participating in many other aspects of art and design, including painting, sculpture, book and magazine illustration, theater design, decorative arts, textile design, and even advertising art.

Couturiers traditionally participated in events that showcased the decorative arts. Doucet, Paquin, Poiret, and Delaunay all showed their work at the exhibitions of the Société des Artistes Décorateurs, founded in 1901 for the promotion and display of French decorative art. It was this body that originated the idea for an international exposition to showcase modern French design in all areas of the decorative arts. The eventual result was the Exposition Internationale des Arts Décoratifs et Industriels Modernes of 1925.

French design and the superior craftsmanship employed in its realization had always guaranteed access to the world's luxury markets for all of the decorative arts, including the couture. At the beginning of the twentieth century, however, revival styles were common in France, and even art nouveau, created in the 1880s in an attempt to develop a French style competitive with the English arts and crafts aesthetic, was suffering from the omnipres-

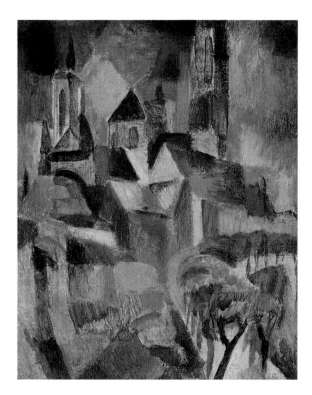

Fig. 102
Robert Delaunay's oil painting on canvas of the *Tours de Laon*, ca. 1914. Museum of Art, RISD, Jesse H. Metcalf Fund and Chace and Levinger Foundations (photograph by Cathy Carver).

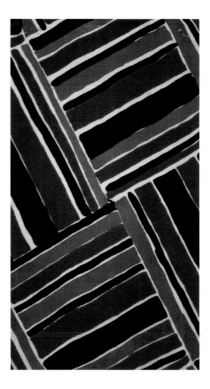

Fig. 103
Silk textile designed by Sonia Terk Delaunay. Courtesy Musée des Tissus de Lyon.

ence of cheap machine-made copies. Moreover, French artists feared that French design was beginning to be overshadowed by decorative arts from Germany, particularly those produced by the Vereinigten Werkstätten für Kunst im Handwerk (United Workshops for Art in Handwork) of Munich and the Austrian artists of the Wiener Werkstätte (Vienna Workshops). Founded in 1897, the Munich Workshops aimed to bring designers and manufacturers together to develop decorative arts of a truly modern German style for industry. Products created by the workshops in what came to be known as Jugendstil were modeled on English arts and crafts principles of simplicity and appropriateness, but their output was based on machine manufacture. Their ensembles of practical, inexpensive furniture showed how interiors could look when all elements were designed with a single aesthetic in mind, even when made industrially.

The artists of the Vienna Workshops, of like mind with the founders of the Munich Workshops, wanted to develop a national style particularly expressive of Austria. They looked back to the Biedermeier period of the early nineteenth century as the last period of genuine Viennese design accomplishment. Unlike the Munich Workshops, however, the Vienna Workshops' concept was basically that of hand craftsmanship, in which the artist maintained complete control over what was produced, even though machines were used in its manufacture. The Wiener Werkstätte established textile and fashion departments in 1910, which would both borrow from and exert an immediate influence upon French design. These workshops were visited by Paul Poiret soon after their founding, and he brought back examples of their work for resale in his salon.[26]

It was in response to the challenges of Germans and Austrians that French designers banded together to form the Société des Artistes Décorateurs in 1901. Like the German and Viennese workshops, its members numbered artists in many media, including the couture. This gave the designers more visibility through annual exhibitions and provided a forum where they could meet to discuss their interests vis-à-vis Germanic theorists and practitioners. After 1910, when the Munich Workshops exhibited at the Paris Salon d'Automne, showing decorative arts with brilliant color schemes accompanied by contemporary German paintings, pressure on French designers increased. By this time, both the annual exhibitions of the Société des Artistes Décorateurs and the Salons d'Automne had assimilated the German practice of showing ensembles designed according to a single aesthetic, but French designers and critics continued to argue over the matter of style. One camp, which included mostly older artists and craftsmen, developed an approach based on the sinuous curves and muted colors of art nouveau and looked to the late eighteenth century prior to the Revolution as the last genuine French period of style. Their ensembles were luxurious and formal, appealing to aristocratic taste.

A second group included younger artists such as Süe, André Mare, and André Groult, all of whom knew Paul Poiret and his sisters and were patronized and encouraged by them. This group favored bright colors to create the ambience for their rooms: many designers of furniture, textiles, and architecture participated in making eclectic ensembles. They placed themselves within the French artistic tradition by looking to the Directoire, Empire, and Louis-Philippe periods as the last "true styles," to which they were the successors. Their sources ranged from French peasant and provincial art to cubist painting, and by 1912 they were collaborating outright with painters to produce an atmosphere conducive to the appreciation of cubist paintings, such as those which hung in Mare's Maison Cubiste at the Salon d'Automne of 1912. Collaborating on the projects of these so-called "*coloristes*" was a circle of young artists that included Laurençin, Raymond Duchamp-Villon (designer of the façade of the Maison Cubiste), Léger, Dunoyer de Segonzac, Albert Gleizes, Jean Metzinger, and others with impeccable cubist credentials.[27]

Paul Poiret was well aware of these issues when in 1907 he designed his first loose, elegant dresses with high waistlines and no corsets beneath, which looked back to the Empire period for inspiration. He claimed to have instigated the demise of the corset in these dresses, but the antecedents for this were many. Dress reformers had been urging the abolition of the corset since the mid-nineteenth century, but the movement did not penetrate high fashion, and the failure of the reviled bloomer is well known. "Reform dress," as it was called, did make headway among the pre-Raphaelites in England, and the loose gowns depicted in their paintings came to be known as "aesthetic dress." By the turn of the century, women were wearing at-home gowns, or tea gowns, with minimal corseting and a long, slim shape. Fashion designers took up this new, classicizing simplicity. In 1900, Paquin designed a ball gown in the Empire style and exhibited it at the Exposition Universelle, for which she was chairman of the couture pavilion. Variants of the Empire line were seen in 1905 in New York as well as Paris. By 1907, when Poiret released his versions, the Venetian painter Mariano Fortuny had already developed the pleated "Delphos" tea gown that clung to a woman's uncorseted body like the tunic of the famed Attic sculpture, the (male) *Charioteer of Delphi.* Fortuny pioneered the use of sheer silk-velvet coats that fell straight from the shoulder [fig. 104]. Isadora Duncan's corsetless tunics were also forerunners of the trend, as couturiere Madeleine Vionnet acknowledged in explaining her own uncorseted designs, which she launched in 1906 just before Poiret's designs appeared.[28]

Between 1908 and the end of the 1930s, the tubular silhouette, with its emphasis on slimness and the natural motion of the body, remained fashionable and, indeed, with the exception of some silhouettes of the 1940s and 1950s, has remained in fashion throughout the twentieth century, reflecting the persistence of modernism in the arts and its expansion into the general culture, as well as the changing role and status of women. The best end-of-the-twentieth century example of this style is perhaps the work of American couturier Geoffrey Beene, which is based on the same themes that inspired couturiers at the beginning of the century: the liberation of the body, the simplification of its contours to their constituent geometries, and the importance of motion. All these themes emerged in the early years of the century, promoted by Callot Soeurs, Doucet, and especially Poiret, then taken up by younger couturiers like Patou, Chanel, and Vionnet.

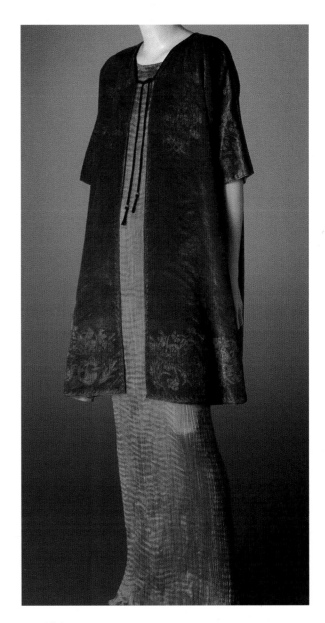

Fig. 104
Mariano Fortuny's pleated silk "Delphos" gown and printed velvet tunic, early twentieth century: Fortuny's slim gowns were a return to the "classical" silhouette, first appearing in 1906. Museum of Art, RISD, gift of Warren E. Teixeira (dress) and gift of Mrs. Robert Fairbanks and Mrs. Donald Crafts (jacket).

Poiret dominated the world of couture between 1907 and the First World War as no personality had done since Worth, but by 1914 there were ominous signs that his work was not universally appreciated in France. In a controversy that revealed the extent to which the couture could be viewed as a serious and influential art, critics on the extreme right used criticism of Poiret's work to attack the whole panoply of early modernism as it had been developing in Paris.[29] In a climate rife with war-driven anti-German feeling, newspapers published diatribes against cubism, the Ballets Russes, contemporary music, and other manifestations of the avant-garde, which were called "Germanic" and "barbarian," a repudiation of all that was "French." Cartoons appeared in the press ridiculing Poiret's fashions for precisely the Orientalist details that had made them so popular. The "lampshade tunic" that Madame Poiret had worn at the "Thousand and Second Night" fête in 1911 was particularly recognizable and thus a symbol of all Poiret's work [see fig. 100, p. 138]. His well publicized sorties into Austria, Germany, and Eastern Europe to show his collections also made him an easy target. Beginning in 1915, the journal *La Renaissance* attacked Poiret for "boche taste." The fact that his creations were favorites in Germany was used to "prove" his sympathy for the enemy, the same argument used to place cubist art in the realm of "foreign snobs and indigenous neurotics," i.e., the avant-garde.[30] After several reiterations of this calumny, Poiret sued, which only served to perpetuate the scandal and remind people further of his connections with Germany. In the end, *La Renaissance* apologized publicly to Poiret, whose "subversive" work merely reflected the internationalist, cosmopolitan character of all modern art before World War I. Artists banded together to defend Poiret, but the damage was done.

After the War, Poiret fought to reestablish his reputation in France, aided by letters from the artists who knew and supported him. Dunoyer de Segonzac wrote an especially telling missive in which he praised Poiret as "a child of Paris," possessing "all the independence of spirit, fantasy, and candor" that implied. "In many ways, 'Revolutionary' France has become more conservative than

'Medieval' Germany," he concluded, recognizing that the slander of Poiret was not only an attack on fashion, but an offensive against all the arts.[31] In his perceptive book *Esprit de Corps*, Kenneth E. Silver has shown how these threats eventually intimidated French artists with their calls for a "return to order" and chilled the character of artworks produced after the War. Poiret approached the struggle to restore his name with his usual élan. Returning from the Front, he continued to produce his Orientalist fashions, and, during the Exposition of 1925, rented huge barges to show his works on the banks of the Seine, a grandiose gesture funded entirely by himself. Its outrageous cost, combined with the negative publicity generated by his critics, doomed his efforts to continue business in his pre-War style. Although some of his most beautiful creations date from this period and his popularity was at its height in the United States, he was forced to close his couture house entirely in 1929 [figs. 105–106].

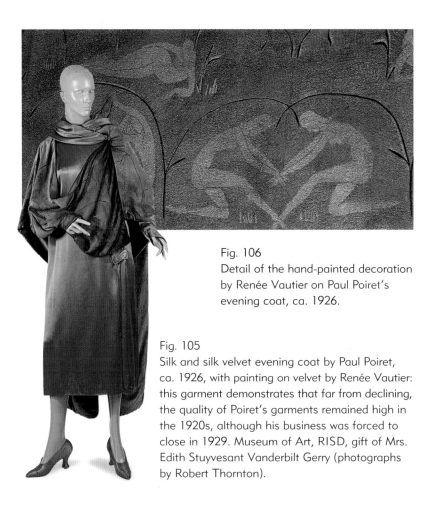

Fig. 106
Detail of the hand-painted decoration by Renée Vautier on Paul Poiret's evening coat, ca. 1926.

Fig. 105
Silk and silk velvet evening coat by Paul Poiret, ca. 1926, with painting on velvet by Renée Vautier: this garment demonstrates that far from declining, the quality of Poiret's garments remained high in the 1920s, although his business was forced to close in 1929. Museum of Art, RISD, gift of Mrs. Edith Stuyvesant Vanderbilt Gerry (photographs by Robert Thornton).

The First World War brought many changes to the couture. Men like Paul Poiret and the young Jean Patou were drafted into the military, and their houses closed. Commerce was curtailed between France and the United States, and, although the Lyon silk industry remained in operation, many of its weavers, as well as its clients, were called into the army. Meanwhile, new personalities appeared, including the young Gabrielle Chanel. In 1915, Chanel was in Deauville producing hats and making her first essay into the couture with loose-fitting chemise dresses belted at the hip. By 1916, she was making casual pleated skirts from the practical Rodier wool jersey that had been used primarily for men's underwear before the war. She topped the skirts with Breton sailors' sweaters in the "sportswear" mode that had begun to appear in *Vogue* and the *Gazette du Bon Ton* several years earlier and that was to become so important in the 1920s. Chanel was still little known in the United States.

The French government regarded support of the couture industry to be essential during the War. It sent to the Panama Pacific International Exposition of 1915 in San Francisco a selection of apparel by the "old masters": Paquin, Doucet, Lanvin, Chéruit, Callot Soeurs, Doeuillet, de Beer, Premet, and Martial et Armand. Most had long full skirts with tucked-in waists, while tailored suits had long jackets with loose belts [fig. 107]. One or two designs even returned to corseting. All of these houses dated from early in the century. A mere handful of references to them appear in the Tirocchi record books of the 1920s. Only Lanvin, well represented by several models in the San Francisco exposition, was still a force among the Tirocchi clientele by the mid-1920s.

During the War, fashion began to simplify, as Poiret's Ballets Russes dresses disappeared with his induction into the army and as their extravagant decorations began to seem inappropriate. A sober, even retrograde, mood prevailed. In the face of wartime shortages, Chanel's practical, albeit expensive, jerseys seemed an instant modern classic, appealing to wealthy clients because, in the words of historian Valerie Steele, "they made the rich look young and casual."[32] Couturiers like Paul Poiret

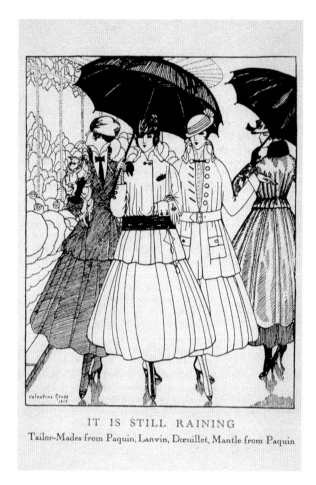

IT IS STILL RAINING
Tailor-Mades from Paquin, Lanvin, Doeuillet, Mantle from Paquin

Fig. 107
Illustration by Valentine Gross; published in *The 1915 Mode: as Shown by Paris. Panama Pacific Exposition of 1915*. New York: 1915, p. 21.

returned from the War to find that the aristocratic society lauded by the promoters of the San Francisco exposition as "that aristocracy of diplomates [*sic*]" no longer existed. Russian nobles who had fled to Paris after the Revolution of 1917 were living in penury, having been deprived of their incomes. Once well-to-do Russian women were earning their livelihoods by decorating dresses by Patou and Chanel with the traditional embroidery that they had learned as a female accomplishment in their former lives. Balkan and Eastern European monarchies had disappeared altogether. Many French and English aristocrats had been killed in the great battles of World War I, and the postwar cycles of depression and inflation created instability and financial uncertainty.

When Paris did revive, it awoke to a younger society with a different style and an American tinge. The spacious stage setting that had been Paul Poiret's Paris in the Belle Epoque once again served fashion, as the newly wealthy installed themselves in the Hotel Ritz and patronized cafés like the avant-garde Le Boeuf sur le Toit or Le Jardin de Ma Soeur, the nightclub that Elsa Maxwell created for couturier Edward Molyneux. Artists and designers, resuming their quest for an overarching French style, found it in the coalescing of what was then referred to as the *"moderne"* (renamed "Art Deco" long after the Exposition des Arts Décoratifs et Industriels Modernes of 1925, which was the source of the name). Technological innovations had changed life physically as well: the electric light, the radio, the motion picture, the automobile all came into common use. Life accelerated. Everything was in motion. Women drove cars, went out to work, played tennis and golf, and learned ballroom dancing. Some agitated for the vote and for complete equality with men. In Providence after 1920, when women were granted the franchise, Tirocchi client Harriet Sprague Watson Lewis found it important to record in her "Line A Day" diary each time that she went out to vote.

Clothing changed with women's evolving roles in modern society, particularly with the idea of increased freedom for women. Although society matrons of a certain age continued to wear conservative garments, forward-looking and younger women now made sportswear their dress of choice. The formal mood of the pre-War world was giving way to a more casual approach. The tubular dress of Paul Poiret had metamorphosed into a similar but shorter silhouette with pleated, gathered, or slit skirts, making ease of motion the rule in women's fashion for the first time in its history.

If Anne Hollander is correct, however, there is much more to be said about the emergence of the 1920s chemise, which, topped with the cloche hat, became the uniform of the early to middle years of the decade. Hollander maintains in *Seeing Through Clothes* that "developments in fashion are like changes in pictorial art; in clothes, as in pictures, technical inventions and social change are secondary to visual style." According to Hollander, garments on the body please not so much because they serve specific uses or circumstances (although they do), but rather because they resemble "a current pictorial ideal of shape, line, trim, texture, and motion."[33] Developments in art and fashion during the years from 1906 onward had accustomed the modern eye to the abstract by the early 1920s. The challenges that cubism presented in the Armory Show of 1913 in New York had now been assimilated. The tubular, slim silhouette proposed by Poiret, Fortuny, and Vionnet had now become the norm. The cylindrical silhouette of the body and the ovoid of the head accented by close-cropped hair and cloche hat are the geometries of Picasso, Léger, Duchamp-Villon, and others throughout the first two decades of the twentieth century [figs. 108–109; compare fig. 104, p. 144, and fig. 128, p. 161].

When the long-awaited Exposition des Arts Décoratifs et Industriels Modernes finally did occur in 1925, instead of introducing *"moderne"* fashion, it simply confirmed what Tirocchi clients had already accepted. The Exposition had been conceived some years before World War I as a way to renew French domination of the decorative-arts industries. It was postponed because of the War; and had to be put off further due to the straitened circumstances of the French government and postwar scarcity and economic depression. Finally, the exhibition opened in the various national and international pavilions that occupied the area from the Grand Palais to the Invalides, including the banks of the Seine. After the War, the economic need was even greater than in 1913 to reestablish the French luxury industries, and the Exposition emphasized opulence at the expense of modest but well designed decorative arts that could be produced industrially.

Fashion – perhaps the quintessential luxury industry – took a prominent place in the displays. The Exposition, extensively reported in America, threw the spotlight on the chemise and cloche, presented by designers ranging from the unknown Genevieve O'Rossen to the well-known Jean-Charles Worth, Callot Soeurs, Sonia Delaunay, and Paul Poiret, all of whom exhibited clothing in the tubular silhouette. In the end, the Exposition of 1925, instead of celebrating the advent of the overarching

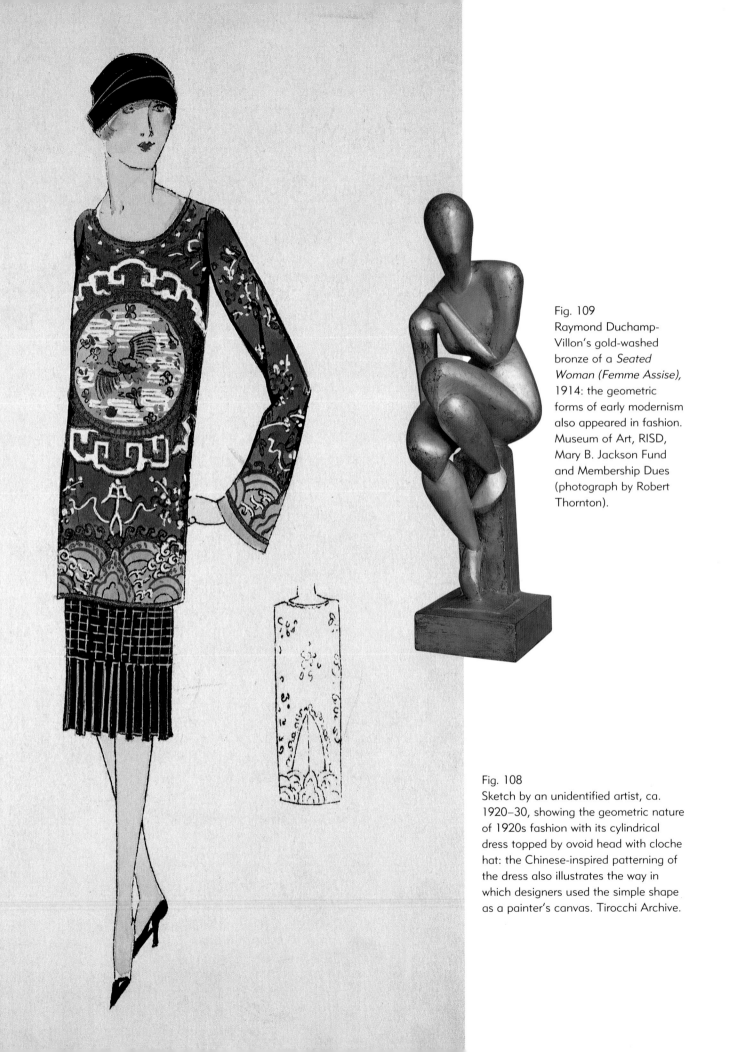

Fig. 109
Raymond Duchamp-Villon's gold-washed bronze of a *Seated Woman (Femme Assise),* 1914: the geometric forms of early modernism also appeared in fashion. Museum of Art, RISD, Mary B. Jackson Fund and Membership Dues (photograph by Robert Thornton).

Fig. 108
Sketch by an unidentified artist, ca. 1920–30, showing the geometric nature of 1920s fashion with its cylindrical dress topped by ovoid head with cloche hat: the Chinese-inspired patterning of the dress also illustrates the way in which designers used the simple shape as a painter's canvas. Tirocchi Archive.

French style sought by artists, marked the beginning of the decline of the *"moderne"* or Art Deco style. The presence among the ensembles of such designers as Ruhlmann, Süe, and Mare, and Poiret's boutique Martine of several "streamlined" creations, appropriately enough, for railway cars and steamships, and of a "purist" pavilion by Le Corbusier that rejected both styles, showed the direction in which art was moving – from *"moderne"* ornamentation to "machine-age" simplicity to the emerging "international style" advocated by the Bauhaus and promoted in France by Le Corbusier.

During and after the Exposition of 1925, decorative artists such as Ruhlmann, Dunand, and Paul Folliot were still producing luxury *"moderne"* interiors and individually handcrafted objects that only the wealthy could afford; and Le Corbusier continued to criticize them for their refusal to make beautiful, functional objects that could be mass-produced by machine for the benefit of ordinary people. In 1929, this purist, anti-ornament faction withdrew from the Société des Artistes Décorateurs to form the Union des Artistes Modernes, appropriating for themselves the adjective "modern." The two distinct factions would remain in contention until the Second World War. Perhaps put off by these controversies, and having been shown the folly of political engagement in the art world by the tribulations of Paul Poiret, couturiers had less and less to do with decorative arts organizations during the 1920s, although they still responded to the same artistic trends. By 1925, with the *"moderne"* style reflected so beautifully in the clothing shown by couturiers at the Exposition, a simplifying, classicizing trend also became visible, together with another trend welcomed by American clients: an explosion of sportswear.

By 1921, Madeleine Vionnet's unstructured styles were making a quiet revolution with their attention to cut and simple elegance, rather than ornament. Working between 1921 and 1925 with Thayaht (the son of an Italian friend of Vionnet), who had studied under Jay Hambidge at Harvard in 1920, Vionnet collaborated on an effort to design modern clothing according to Hambidge's princi-

ples of "dynamic symmetry," a system derived from classical proportions and based on a geometrical analysis of the Parthenon. Hambidge believed that the system could be applied in any field of art to objects of any style to assure the most beautiful results [fig. 110]. The Main Gallery of the RISD Museum, designed by American architect William Aldrich, is an example of "dynamic symmetry" applied to a classical-style building [fig. 111].[34] Thayaht used the theory of "dynamic symmetry" in creating some surface designs for Vionnet, and in one dress, Vionnet experimented with actually cutting the silk according to Thayaht's ideas.

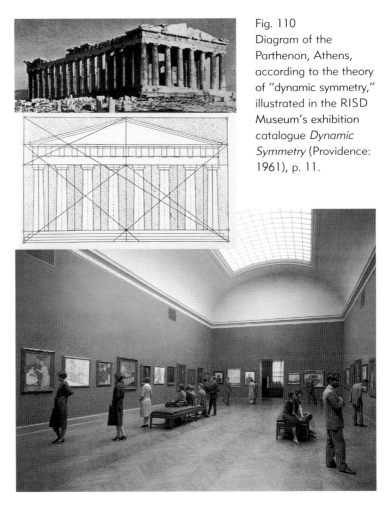

Fig. 110
Diagram of the Parthenon, Athens, according to the theory of "dynamic symmetry," illustrated in the RISD Museum's exhibition catalogue *Dynamic Symmetry* (Providence: 1961), p. 11.

Fig. 111
The RISD Museum's Main Gallery, designed by architect William Aldrich (brother-in-law of Tirocchi client Mrs. Stuart Aldrich) according to the principles of "dynamic symmetry"; ca. 1926. Museum of Art, RISD, photograph archive.

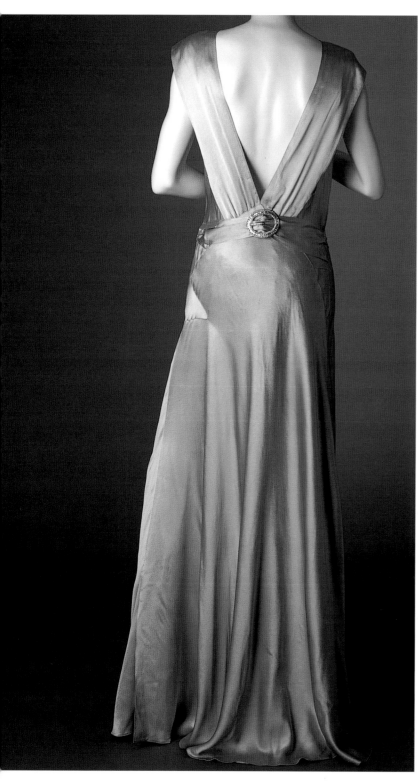

Fig. 112
Dramatic silk evening dress with intricate cut [see fig. 144, p. 169] and bias draping after Madeleine Vionnet, ca. 1931, imported by the Misses Briganti, New York. Museum of Art, RISD, gift of Dr. Louis J. Cella, Jr.

Betty Kirke believes that from that time forward, Vionnet, having assimilated the ideas of "dynamic symmetry," used them in her innovative cuts, which combined straight grain with bias to create elegantly draped clothing of superb fit that clung to the body beneath it.[35] "The couturier should be a geometrician, for the human body makes geometric figures to which the materials should correspond," Vionnet told Jacques Griffe, revealing her instinctive understanding of the importance of geometry in the design of clothing in the 1920s.[36] *Vogue* christened these dresses "anatomical cuts" in an article of 1925, and they were very successful in America. Vionnet's clothing based on the principles of geometry harmonized with the aesthetic of the machine, which was developing in America for everything from locomotives to decorative arts. This was also in line with what French purist artists Ozenfant and Le Corbusier were advocating, in that her dresses were classically simple, unornamented, and possessed of the shiny surface and perfect curves of the newest machines [fig. 112; compare fig. 144, p. 169]. It took an especially fine figure to wear one of these creations, and only six of Anna Tirocchi's clients tried. As usual, the chic Mrs. Byron S. (Isabel) Watson led the way by purchasing a blue velvet afternoon dress by Vionnet in 1926.

Even more important to the Tirocchi clientele was Jean Patou, who had worked as a tailor before World War I and had established his own fashion house on being demobilized in 1919. At first he produced loose dresses with sheer panels, as did many other couturiers, for a clientele that included both French and English aristocrats. In 1920, however, Patou's sister married French tennis champion Raymond Barbas, who introduced Patou to tennis star Suzanne Lenglen. In 1921, Lenglen appeared at Wimbledon in Patou's knee-length pleated skirt and sleeveless cardigan sweater, setting a fashion copied by many other women on and off court. The similarity of Patou's concept to that of Chanel's skirts and sweaters is unmistakable, but this is less a case of Patou copying Chanel than of the arrival in force of sportswear on the fashion scene. At first, Patou was aiming at a different clientele from that of Chanel: sports clothing for players of sports, wherever they found themselves [fig. 113]. For these women, simplicity was not only a design virtue, but a necessity, as Patou learned from Suzanne Lenglen.

A friend of Dunoyer de Segonzac and patron of André Mare and Louis Süe (who designed his salons in the rue St. Florentin), Patou was well aware of artistic trends. After 1921, he adapted the two-piece sweater-and-skirt format in luxurious wool jersey for morning dresses or sports suits, employing cubist ornament and collage principles to decorate them. For all the renown of Chanel (Valerie Steele calls her " the acknowledged dominatrix of fashion during the period between the wars"),[37] the Tirocchi clientele preferred Patou to Chanel by an overwhelming margin. In the 1920s and 30s, purchases of fashions and accessories by Patou outnumbered those by Chanel sixty-four to thirty-four, a definitive vote of confidence in the debonair young couturier who would die so prematurely in 1936. No labeled Patou was found among the dresses remaining in the Tirocchi shop, but several refer directly to his design principles [see fig. 34, p. 46].

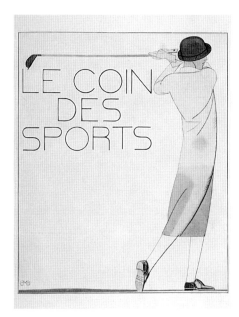

Fig. 113
"Le Coin des Sports" ("The Sports Corner"), an illustration of Jean Patou's solution for active sports clothing: simplicity and ease of movement, the essence of sportswear. Anna Tirocchi picked up this brochure from Patou's couture showing on her trip to Paris of either 1924 or 1926–27. Tirocchi Archive.

In step with the "return to order" that infused a post-war classicism into all the arts, the clothing of Patou, Chanel, and others represented a new idea, one that suited the range of possibilities now opening before the modern woman: "classic" clothing that was never out of style, easily cared for, and constructed for ease of movement. Clothing based on "classical" models was a theme visited off and on throughout the modern period, beginning with Fortuny's Delphos dresses of 1906–07, which continued to be made all throughout the period and are still obtainable today. The Empire silhouettes of the 1910s also relate to this theme, and a draped satin opera coat of 1931 from the Tirocchi shop [fig. 114] marks the continuation of the trend. "Classic" clothing, however, had nothing to do with antiquity; rather, "classic" clothing meant clothing that could be worn over and over again, clothing without copious ornament or complicated silhouette to date it [fig. 115]. The "classic" was epitomized in a simple sports dress by Patou, a black lace dinner dress by Chanel, or an exquisitely fitted black dress by Molyneux or Mainbocher.

Both Molyneux and Mainbocher specialized in a kind of slim, fitted apparel that perhaps seemed simple when compared to the extravagances of the 1920s, but was wholly satisfying in its beautiful tailoring and quiet elegance. Richard Martin, in his book *Contemporary Fashion*, declared that Molyneux, a friend of author Noel Coward (who himself embodied classic, elegant style of the most refined manner), produced "spartan clothing" in an "early and intended version of the International Style,"[38] and this is surely what "classic" clothing is meant to be. With the coming of age of the anti-ornamental purist element in art after Le Corbusier's breakthroughs in the late 1920s and the growth in philosophical importance of Germany's Bauhaus school, fashion's own "return to order" was the "classic" clothing of the 1930s.

Mainbocher, an American from St. Louis who combined his first and last names once in Paris, was beloved for his pure, uncomplicated, simply cut designs – what *Harper's Bazaar* called his "deceptive plainness" – that clients viewed as investments for the long haul.[39] Made famous by his selection as

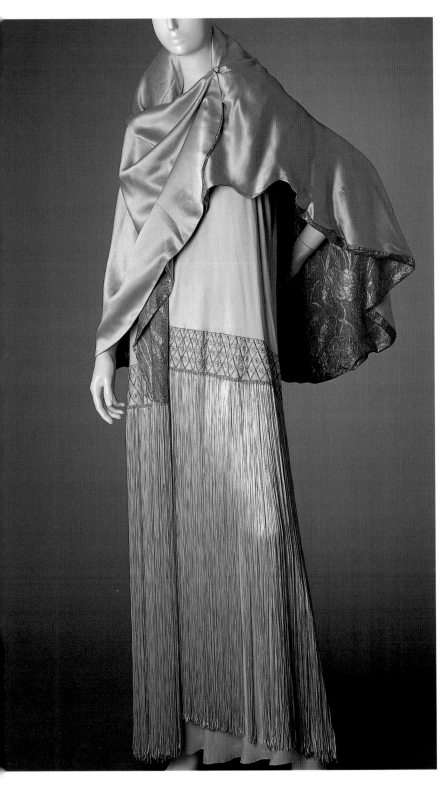

Fig. 114
Elaborate silk opera coat expressing "classical"
principles of line and draping. Museum of Art,
RISD, gift of L. J. Cella III.

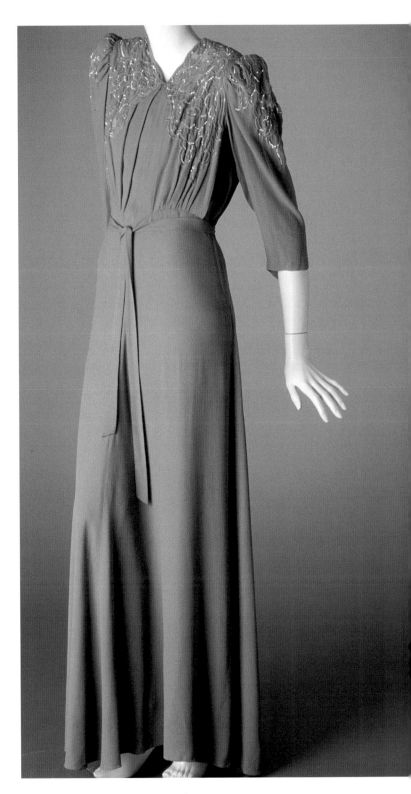

Fig. 115
"Classic" rayon evening dress with simple silhouette,
ca. 1930, in crepe and sequins. Museum of Art, RISD,
gift of Edward Cella.

designer of the Duchess of Windsor's wedding gown in 1939, Mainbocher came to the attention of the Tirocchi clientele too late to have much impact on the shop. A search of Tirocchi records turned up thirteen references to garments by Molyneux, the first purchased as early as 1924, while only one outfit by Mainbocher was supplied to a client – the always fashionable Mrs. Byron S. Watson – in 1939.

Sportswear also qualifies as "classic," and its simple utility further identifies it with the International Style. For American women, sportswear took off immediately and became the style of the century. Nothing shows this more clearly than the Tirocchi records. In no record does the word "sport" appear before 1918, and only seven mentions were found in 1918 and 1919. Between 1920 and 1930, more than one hundred and sixty-six entries record sport suits, sport dresses, sport skirts, sport sweaters, sport coats, etc. From 1930 onwards, sports dressing remained popular among clients of all ages; peaking in 1931; remaining steady between 1932 and 1936; then falling off only in proportion to the decline in client numbers in the late 1930s.

In 1927, a new designer of a younger generation took the stage with an intuitive knowledge of the place of fashion late in the decade. Elsa Schiaparelli understood instinctively the relationship between the "classic" and the modern. For her, modernity was rooted in classicism and in respect for the human body. More than any couturier since Paul Poiret, Schiaparelli was involved in and inspired by the world of art. In her 1954 autobiography, written partly in the third person, she credits her appreciation of the "surroundings of beauty" that inspired her clothing designs to her upbringing in a well-to-do and intellectual family in Rome. "She felt that clothes had to be architectural; that the body must never be forgotten and it must be used as a frame is used in a building," Schiaparelli wrote. "The Greeks, more than anybody else except the Chinese, understood this rule, and gave to their goddesses…the serenity of perfection and the fabulous appearance of freedom."[40] Her first evening gown was "a plain black sheath of crepe de Chine down to the ground, with a white crepe de Chine jacket with long sash that crossed in the back but tied in front. Stark

simplicity; That was what was needed."[41] She also understood the fact that fashion, as well as art, was moving toward the "classic" and the purist. Even her very first success, a sweater with knitted-in *trompe-l'oeil* bow at the neckline and a simple black pleated skirt, fit the definition, since it followed the lines of the body, while the knitted-in neckline trimming remained flat. It was the sweater of the future. Schiaparelli made many of them, and they were widely copied, to her great satisfaction [fig. 116].

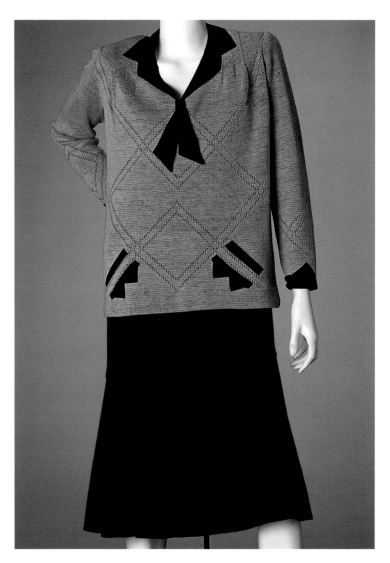

Fig. 116
Wool-jersey two-piece sport dress with *trompe-l'oeil* bow, pocket flaps, and cuffs, ca. 1928, after Elsa Schiaparelli. Museum of Art, RISD, gift of L. J. Cella III.

In the early 1930s, Schiaparelli's bread and butter was these sweaters, for which she used cubist, geometric, and *trompe-l'oeil* patterning, and her simple, slim-silhouette black dresses, suits, and coats. Because the effects of the Depression were quickly felt in France, Schiaparelli knew that she needed to mobilize the worldwide markets that had opened to French couture in the 1920s. Her cause had already been taken up by *Harper's Bazaar* and the New York press, and in 1928 she was selling her sweaters and jersey shorts through Saks Fifth Avenue. Although the simple classic blacks and tailored wools seem plain when compared to her later work, Schiaparelli was slowly letting her surrealist wit begin to show. In the early 1930s, she designed long black evening gowns with black cock's feathers protruding at the shoulders and black suits with buttons shaped like cicadas. In the early 1930s, her styles appeared frequently in *Harper's Bazaar* and *Vogue*, and by 1934, these designs were being illustrated by Jean Cocteau and Christian Bérard and photographed by Man Ray. Two years later, she was collaborating outright with surrealist artists, designing the "Desk Suit," a fitted, tailored suit of perfectly "classic" outlines, with drawer pulls on its many pockets, from a sketch provided by Salvador Dali. In 1937, a collaboration with Dali resulted in her "Tear Dress," again a perfectly classic shape with unexpected *trompe-l'oeil* decoration [fig. 118]. A linen jacket of around the same time (now in the Philadelphia Museum of Art) is but one of Schiaparelli's collaborations with Jean Cocteau [fig. 117].

Schiaparelli's surrealist ideas paralleled the increasing popularity of surrealist art and the use of surrealist imagery in the decorative arts, particularly in photography and magazine illustration. Surrealism continued to grow in popularity throughout the 1930s. The Paris Exposition Internationale des Arts et Techniques dans la Vie Moderne of 1937 was a case in point: the couture industry's Pavillon d'Élégance was surrealist in decor. Schiaparelli herself took part in the Exposition with an installation provoked by the ridiculous mannequin she was assigned (or so she claimed in her autobiography). In surrealist fashion she transmogrified the inappropriate mannequin into sculpture by placing it on the ground

and hanging the creations it was meant to display on a line nearby, as if on washing day.[42]

The Exposition Internationale of 1937 anticipated the Société des Artistes Décorateurs salon of 1939, the last salon before World War II, which was presented in the guise of a surrealist street at night. Sponsored by the Parisian electric power company, the exhibition had lighting designed by Man Ray and was meant to be a fantastic contrast to the evil events in the real world, where Hitler was on the march. Surrealism flourished in the late 1930s as the Second World War loomed over the horizon. In 1938, the largest surrealist exposition to date took place in Paris, and Americans saw Dali's water ballet at the 1939 World's Fair in New York.

Throughout the existence of the Tirocchi shop, its clients adopted stylish French silhouettes. The records, photographs, design books, and extant garments give an excellent overall view of fashion's changing lines and surface designs over the thirty-plus years up to 1941, when the customer base

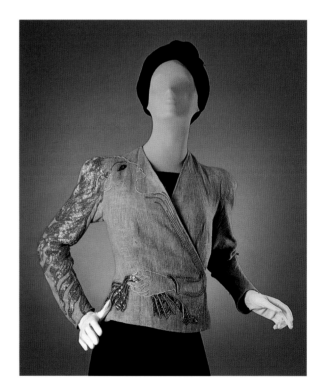

Fig. 117
Evening jacket by Elsa Schiaparelli, ca. 1937, in collaboration with Jean Cocteau. Courtesy Philadelphia Museum of Art, gift of Mme Elsa Schiaparelli.

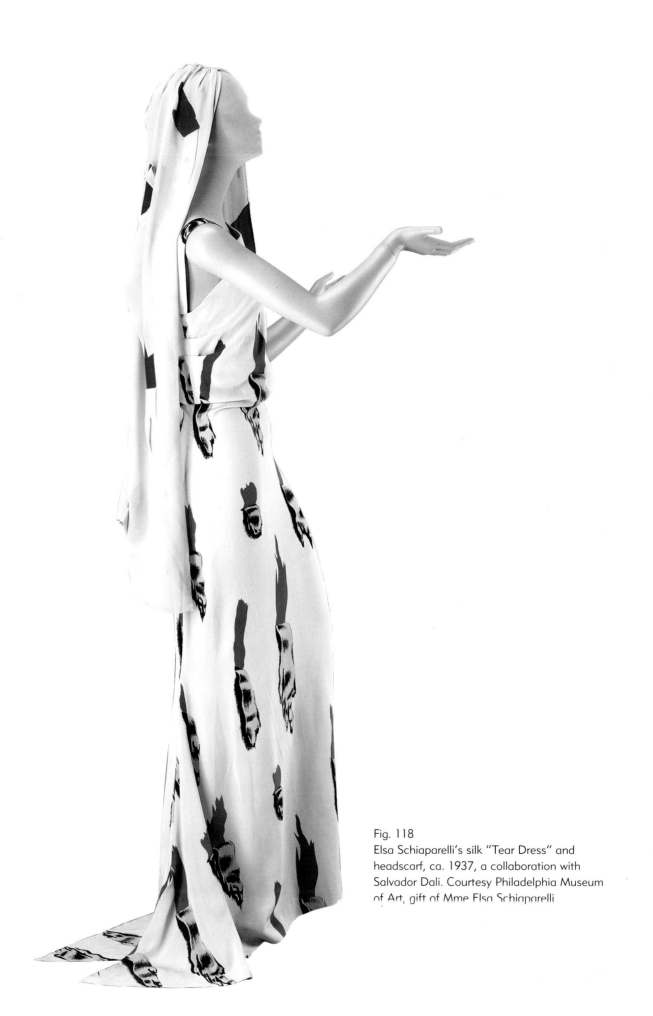

Fig. 118
Elsa Schiaparelli's silk "Tear Dress" and
headscarf, ca. 1937, a collaboration with
Salvador Dali. Courtesy Philadelphia Museum
of Art, gift of Mme Elsa Schiaparelli

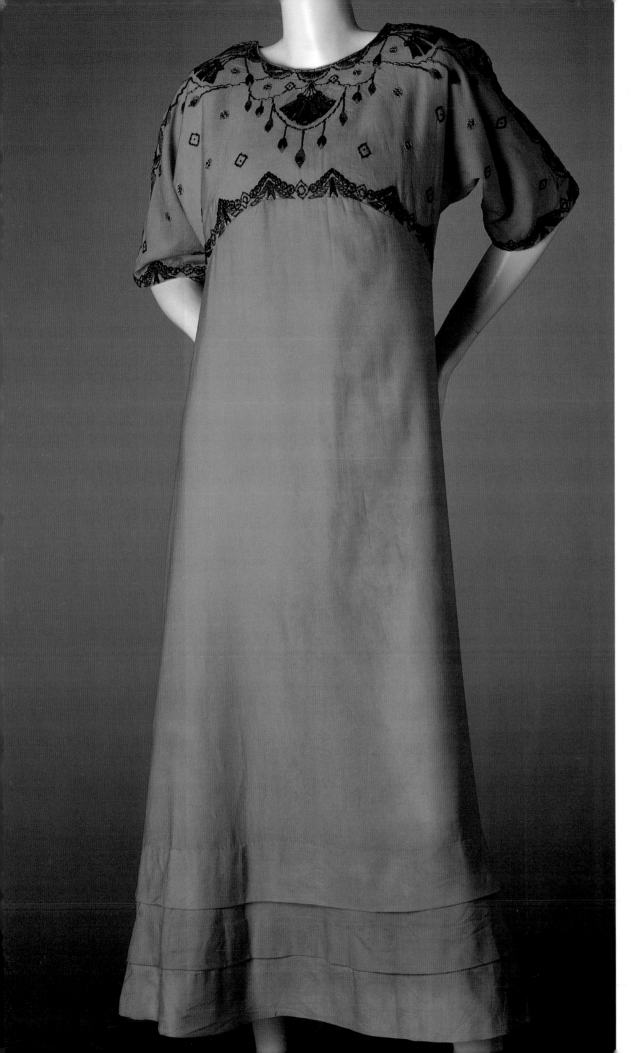

Fig. 119
Wool-and-cotton dress,
probably ca. 1910–20, with
silk embroidery displaying the
"Oriental" peasant-inspired
decoration espoused by
modern artists and adopted
by couturier Paul Poiret after
1907. Museum of Art, RISD,
gift of L. J. Cella III.

declined sharply. Little clothing remained from the 1910s in the shop itself in 1990, but the paper records and the design books referred to by Anna Tirocchi and her customers illustrate the advance of modernism. From about 1912 onwards, the records show a progression from the loose, liberating Empire styles of the 1910s through the chemise dresses of the 1920s to the restrained elegance of the streamlined, "classic" apparel of the 1930s and early 40s.

Among the earliest of the Tirocchi garments is a dress with high waistline, free-falling form, and gaily colored peasant embroidery strongly reminiscent of those Paul Poiret was designing in the 1910s. Found in the family quarters at 514 Broadway, this much worn dress [fig. 119] tempts the speculation that it belonged to Laura Tirocchi Cella herself – who then would have been just the type of slim young girl that Poiret used as his models – and was lovingly preserved first by her and later by her daughter Beatrice.

Dating from about 1918, an exquisite evening dress of pink gauze with silver paillettes appliquéd to the net bears the pin tag used by the Tirocchi sisters to indicate a dress included in the inventory they took of stock around 1920. The inventory itself reveals that no. 434 was "Flesh & Spang. robe 30.00," probably indicating that the sisters made the dress from a ready-to-cut, pre-embroidered dress-length called a "robe" in the trade. These pieces were a French tradition dating back at least to the eighteenth century for mens' waistcoats and ladies slippers, and at least to the nineteenth century for women's garments. The dress remained unpurchased, but was never disposed of by the sisters. In later years some of this early clothing was sold to clients for fancy dress; they were referred to by the Tirocchi bookkeeper as "ancient dresses" and were often altered to suit new occasions. Several garments from this period show the popularity of folk motifs such as those employed by Poiret in the early teens. Peasant embroidery, smocking, and the use of brightly colored fabrics are trends of the time represented in clothing in the Tirocchi collection [figs. 120–121].

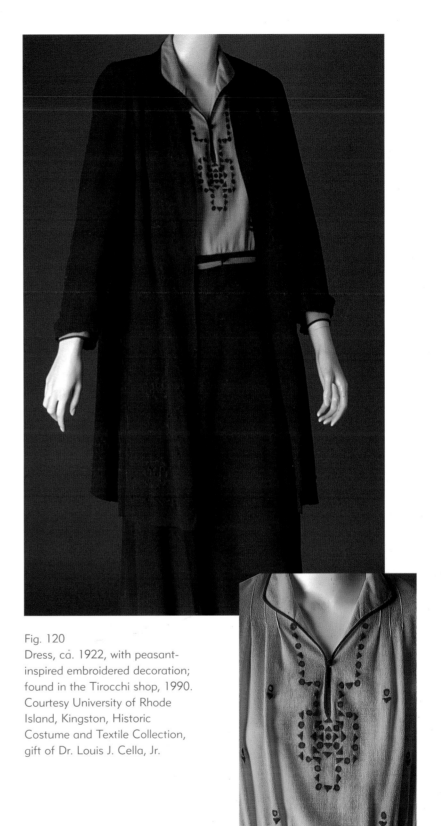

Fig. 120
Dress, cá. 1922, with peasant-inspired embroidered decoration; found in the Tirocchi shop, 1990. Courtesy University of Rhode Island, Kingston, Historic Costume and Textile Collection, gift of Dr. Louis J. Cella, Jr.

Fig. 121

Few couturiers' names can be associated with client purchases of this period, but several design books from various suppliers are preserved from this date. One, from B. Altman & Company, shows dresses for which materials and a photograph could be purchased from the New York department store. In 1919, three Tirocchi clients ordered dresses from B. Altman sketches: Mrs. William F. Chapin, Jr., purchased a serge dress, Altman's no. 2379, while Miss Helen Harris bought a blue embroidered serge, and Mrs. Barnes Newberry ordered a dress to be made based on B. Altman's sketch entitled "Tosca" in henna chiffon [see fig. 17, p. 34]. Tirocchi clients also made use of such fashion magazines as the widely available *Harper's Bazar*, to which the sisters subscribed, or *Vogue*, and could order a dress made after one of their sketches. *Vogue* illustrated as many as thirty-three models from Paris in each issue and about twice as many American dresses in the "Seen in the Shops" section. In addition, each issue contained pages of line drawings of its patterns, a service the highly skilled Tirocchi dressmakers did not use. Advertisements provided many more images.

In America, *Vogue* not only provided sketches and patterns of fashions derived from Paris models, but also actively promoted the French couture. In 1909, the magazine published a ground-breaking article about Paul Poiret with plates from the 1908 booklet *Les Robes de Paul Poiret, racontées par Paul Iribe* and in 1913 closely followed his trip to America. In April 1910, following another article on Poiret, it presented a piece on Lucile, Lady Duff-Gordon, who, although a British-born designer, worked in Paris. The issue of January 1923, the magazine's thirtieth anniversary year, was full of Paris. With a cover designed by French artists Pierre Brissaud and Georges Lepape, it contained articles entitled "So this was Paris, 1904–1911"; "Thirty Years of the Mode" (meaning "the mode that originates in Paris"); and a page of photographs and illustrations by "Our French Artists in Paris," including Lepape, Brissaud, Martin, Marty, Édouard-Garcia Benito, and others who were illustrators for the *Gazette du Bon Ton* and various magazines that began to appear in 1912.

Typical of the imagination that went into *Vogue's* promotion of French couture was a special feature, "The Six Characters in a Delightful New French Comedy, entitled A Prize Contest Staged by Vogue and gowned by ???? [*sic*]": seven pages of illustrations by *Vogue's* French artists of unidentified gowns by couturiers Worth, Lanvin, Chéruit, Poiret, Jenny, Doucet, Premet, Beer, Doeuillet, Patou, and Martial et Armand and the question "…for you to decide, Madame, is which couturier has dressed each lady?" A correct answer with a statement of the contestant's reasons for matching the couturiers with their gowns brought a first prize of any one of the original models illustrated. Ironically, the second prize was an evening gown from Henri Bendel in New York, and the third an afternoon gown from Thurn dressmakers, the most famous New York shop of the time (perhaps *Vogue* assumed that the second and third prizes would be copies of Paris fashions).

In the same issue, *Vogue* printed many of the accolades it had received from French designers. Doeuillet wrote: "Everywhere the name of *Vogue* is synonymous with chic, and…I think of the way in which your organization has always upheld the interests of the *haute couture française* and enhanced its prestige throughout the whole world."[43] Paul Poiret was more direct: "[*Vogue*] is today one of our best methods of communication with a distinguished clientele." His remark revealed how essential it was for him to reach American customers at this stage of his career. Thanks to these fashion magazines and an enthusiastic response from the United States, French couture itself was changing. By the 1920s, the industry was well on its way to world-wide distribution.

Because of the onslaught of publicity about Paris designers and the availability in local department stores of good ready-to-wear models that were advertised in *Vogue* and *Harper's Bazar*, Tirocchi clients changed their ways. More and more they asked for clothing by couturiers, rather than designs sewn and trimmed by the Tirocchi dressmakers themselves. By 1920, the Providence elite were placing their confidence in Paris. Anna Tirocchi turned this development to her own advantage by making a conscious decision to offer her customers copies of Paris couture from supply houses in New York. The

New York companies purchased models in Paris; paid for the right to copy them in the same materials as the original (although illegal copying was rife and bitterly resisted by the couturiers); and stitched up copies to order for retailers like Anna.

Several of the design books for ordering purposes sent to the Tirocchis by New York importer Maginnis & Thomas have survived, and these may be compared with Anna's customer ledgers to suggest something of the Tirocchi clients' tastes. In spring 1925, Mrs. A. T. Wall purchased a black satin chemise designed by Chéruit with elaborate ruching and a shoulder boa [fig. 122]. Tirocchi clients also liked the new designers who appeared after the First World War. Their all-time favorite was Jean

Patou. One example of a design by Patou sold in the shop is a sophisticated brown crepe satin chemise with uneven hem and cubist-influenced contrasting shiny and dull satins [fig. 123], ordered by Mrs. Charles (Ruth Trowbridge) Smith in in 1924, shortly after her marriage. Its tight band around the hipline could only have been worn by a young woman with a perfect figure.

Chanel was the second most favored designer of the Tirocchi clientele in the 1920s. Maginnis & Thomas's interpretation of Chanel is to be seen in a series of designs ordered by Mrs. Charles D. Owen in April 1925, which shows her taste for tailored day wear over frilly evening gowns and provides a glance at what Maginnis & Thomas considered the

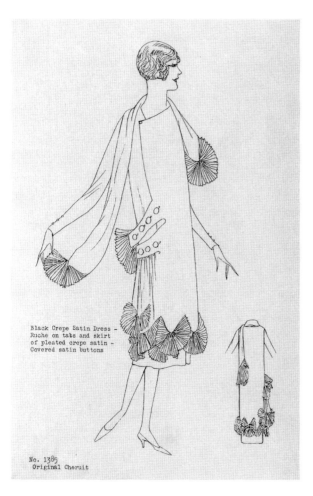

Fig. 122
Maginnis & Thomas sketch, no. 1385, after a Chéruit original of Spring 1925. Tirocchi Archive.

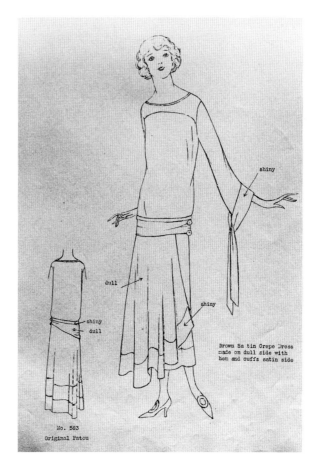

Fig. 123
Maginnis & Thomas sketch, no. 583, after a Jean Patou original of Fall 1924. Tirocchi Archive.

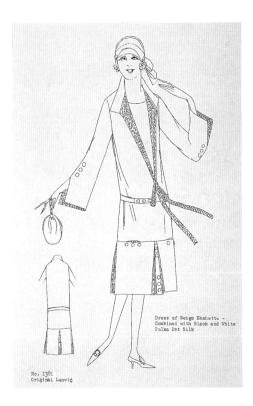

Dress of Beige Kashette –
Combined with Black and White
Polka Dot Silk

No. 1381
Original Lanvin

Fig. 124
Maginnis & Thomas
sketch, no. 1381,
after a Jeanne Lanvin
original of Spring 1925.
Tirocchi Archive.

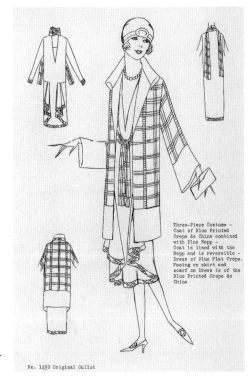

Three-Piece Costume –
Coat of Blue Printed
Crepe de Chine combined
with Blue Repp –
Coat is lined with the
Repp and is reversible –
Dress of Blue Flat Crepe.
Facing on skirt and
scarf on Dress is of the
Blue Printed Crepe de
Chine

No. 1430 Original Callot

Fig. 125
Maginnis & Thomas
sketch, no. 1430,
after a Callot Soeurs
original of Spring 1925.
Tirocchi Archive.

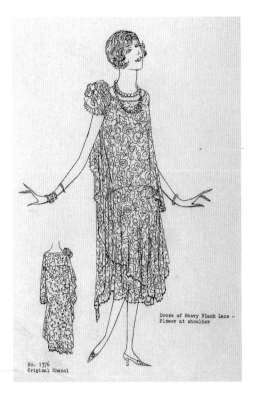

Dress of Heavy Black Lace –
Flower at shoulder

No. 1376
Original Chanel

Fig. 126
Maginnis & Thomas
sketch, no. 1376,
after a Gabrielle Chanel
original of Spring 1925.
Tirocchi Archive.

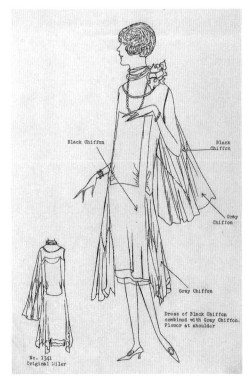

Black Chiffon

Black
Chiffon

Gray
Chiffon

Gray Chiffon

Dress of Black Chiffon
combined with Gray Chiffon.
Flower at shoulder

No. 1341
Original Miler

Fig. 127
Maginnis & Thomas
sketch, no. 1341,
after a Miler Soeurs
original of Spring 1925.
Tirocchi Archive.

Figs. 124–128
Apparel ordered by Tirocchi client Mrs. Charles D. (Alice) Owen for her spring wardrobe, April 1925.

best from several French couturiers. A Lanvin suit of beige "Kashette," probably a knock-off of Rodier's famed "Kasha" cashmere fabric, was combined with a black and white polka-dot silk lining that showed on the garment front, sleeves, and skirt pleats [fig. 124]. The three-quarter line of the middy-style chemise is emphasized by a seam just above the knee, to which a box-pleated skirt is attached. In the drawing the suit is worn with a turban, still popular after its arrival on the scene in the early 1910s with the Orientalist styles of Paul Poiret. An original by Callot Soeurs, a three-piece outfit of blue crepe and blue printed crepe de chine, has a plain blue dress with a skirt facing and a plaid scarf [fig. 125]. The coat is the three-quarter length that Mrs. Owen clearly found becoming and that allows the facing on the skirt to show. It combines plaid with plain and, a couture touch, is reversible. For evening, Mrs. Owen chose a heavy black lace dress with floating panels, typical of the "little black dresses" produced by its designer, Chanel [fig. 126], and a chemise with many draped panels of sophisticated black and gray chiffon by the now-forgotten designers Miler Soeurs that must have looked wonderful on the dance floor [fig. 127]. Last, and perhaps most interesting, is a three-piece costume with a green dress and a three-quarter coat of embroidered chintz [fig. 128]. In this case, the coat was sold to Mrs. Owen after the dress had been purchased by Mrs. Watson. This transaction was a coup for the Tirocchis, who ordered the dress and coat at wholesale for $65, and shows how dressmakers did not hesitate to charge whatever the market would bear. Mrs. Watson paid $88 for the dress, and the coat brought $79 from Mrs. Owen.

Surviving dresses from the 1920s discovered in the shop continue the theme of chemise and variations. The many beaded dresses purchased by the Tirocchis, perhaps more than any other form found in the shop, express the many facets of the art world that concerned artists and designers in the 1920s. This is because the chemise was a perfect foil for surface design. Taking advantage of the plain tubular shape by using it as a painter's canvas, each garment could be highly decorated in any of the numerous ways available to the "moderne" style. The Tirocchis' choices reflect their appreciation of

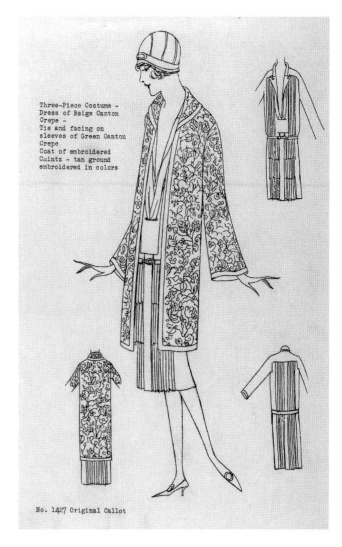

Fig. 128
Maginnis & Thomas sketch, no. 1427, after a Callot Soeurs original of Spring 1925. Tirocchi Archive.

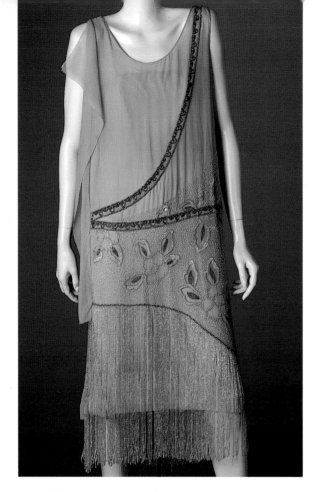

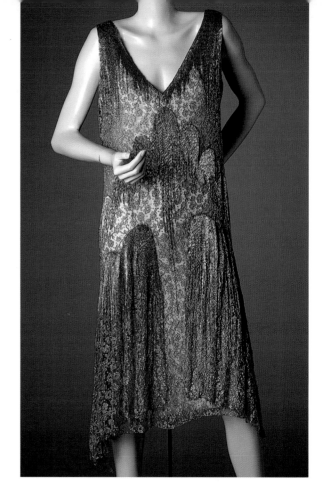

Fig. 129
Beaded silk chemise, ca. 1926, with decoration based on the "*moderne*" flower, by John Poynter for the House of Redfern. Museum of Art, RISD, gift of L. J. Cella III.

Fig. 130
Beaded silk dress, ca. 1926, with decoration in the Japanese taste. Museum of Art, RISD, gift of L. J. Cella III.

such garments. Quintessentially "*moderne*" floral ornament appears often on these dresses [fig. 129]. Oriental and exotic sources remained popular: one exquisite pink-and-white beaded dress has a flower pattern in the Japanese taste [fig. 130]. Others have Persian or Egyptian imagery or motifs derived from textiles made at the Wiener Werkstätte [figs. 131–132]. French designers were still looking in large part to international sources for early modern ornamentation, despite the upheavals of World War I.

The Tirocchis also sold opera coats, of which Anna apparently was especially fond, since several survived in the shop. Dating to about 1926 is a coat attributed to Paul Poiret with Persian patterning [figs. 133–134]. Anna marked several creations on the program of Poiret's salon, which she visited when she went to Paris in 1926–27, but she apparently did not purchase this coat at the time. It was probably

sewn in Providence from a "robe" made in New York from a Poiret design, judging from the fact that the back panel of the coat has been incorrectly placed. It is upside-down, a rare example of an outright mistake on the part of the Tirocchi sewing staff [fig. 133]. A glamorous coat by Lucien Lelong from about 1926 has a fur collar and is made from an exquisite silk velvet printed with futurist swirls [fig. 135], while an elaborately sequined coat in pinkish beige dating to about 1926 has the shiny, metallic "machine-age" look [fig. 136].

Daywear from the 1920s is particularly interesting, since so little of it survives from this period in museum collections. A staple of Tirocchi sales was the lace or voile afternoon dress. These were actually imported from France, rather than copied in New York, where the hand-finishing required for transparent fabrics could not be done in a cost-effective

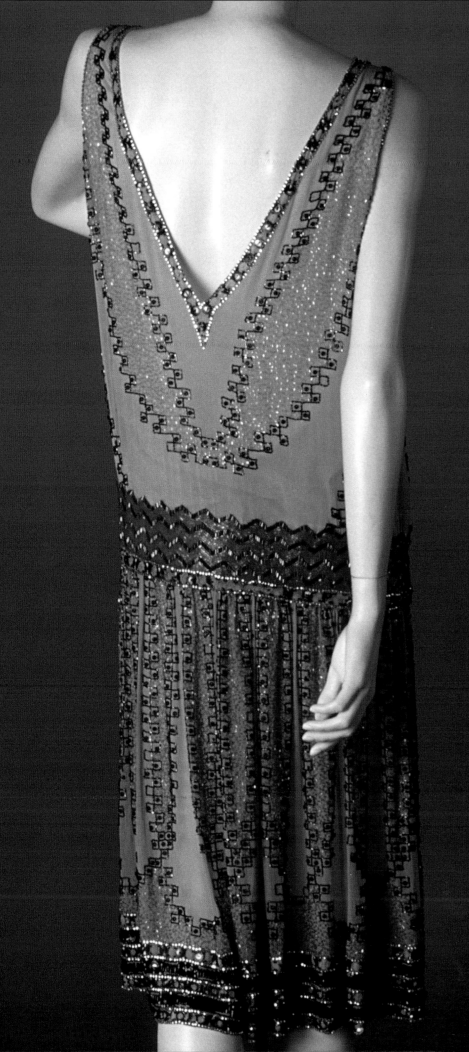

Fig. 131
Sequined and beaded silk dress with decoration inspired by textiles of the Wiener Werkstätte; found in the Tirocchi shop, 1990. Courtesy University of Rhode Island, Kingston, Historic Costume and Textile Collection, gift of Dr. Louis J. Cella, Jr.

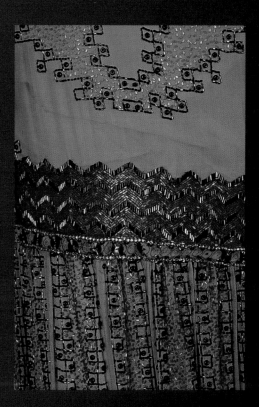

Fig. 132

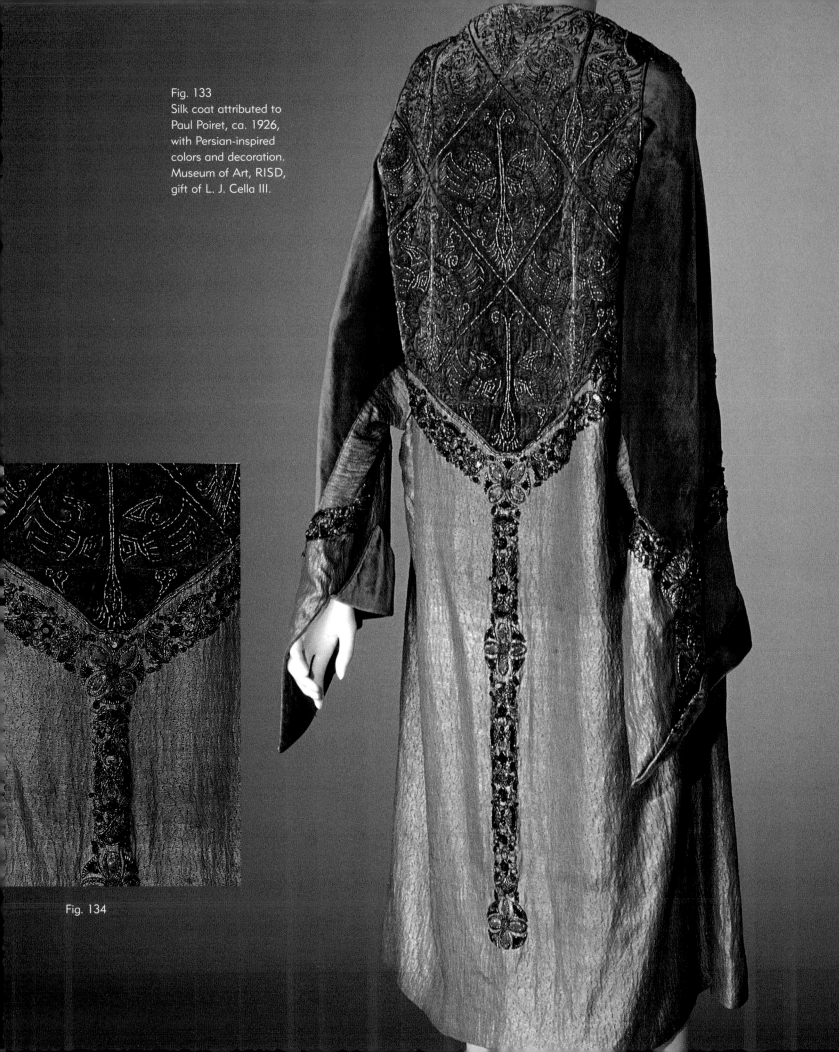

Fig. 133
Silk coat attributed to
Paul Poiret, ca. 1926,
with Persian-inspired
colors and decoration.
Museum of Art, RISD,
gift of L. J. Cella III.

Fig. 134

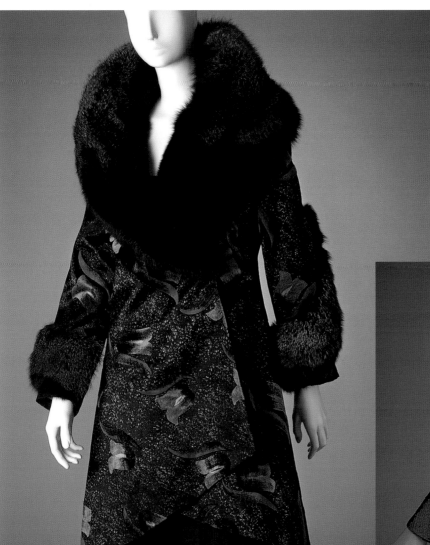

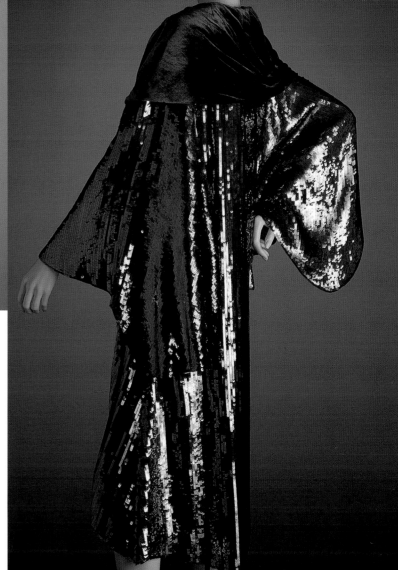

Fig. 135
Silk-velvet evening coat with futurist swirls and fur collar by Lucien Lelong. Museum of Art, RISD, gift of L. J. Cella III.

Fig. 136
Opera coat, ca. 1926, entirely covered with machine-applied pink sequins, giving it a hard-edged look typical of "machine-age" design. Museum of Art, RISD, gift of Dr. Louis J. Cella, Jr.

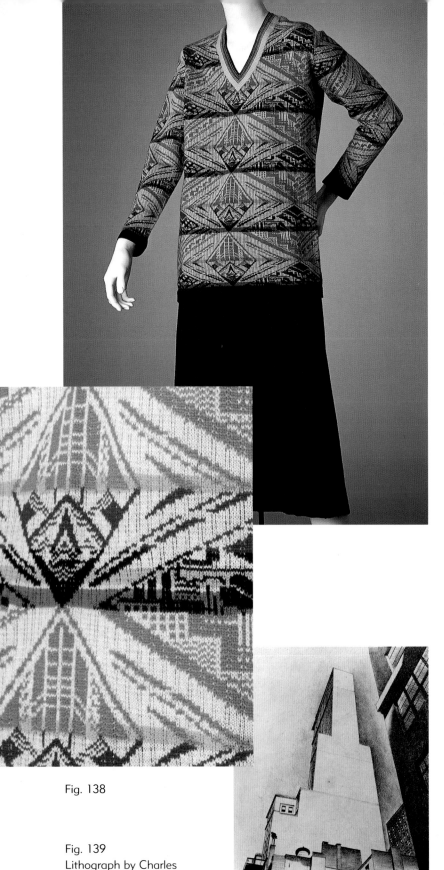

Fig. 137
"Machine-age" imagery reflected in a two-piece wool dress with jersey skirt and knitted overblouse in an intricate pattern of skyscrapers, factories, and smokestacks, ca. 1926, with label "Vienna Knit Art." Museum of Art, RISD, gift of L. J. Cella III.

Fig. 138

Fig. 139
Lithograph by Charles Sheeler of the *Delmonico Building New York*, 1926. Museum of Art, RISD, Museum Works of Art Fund.

way. Knitwear was also a prime seller and appeared in large numbers in the 1920s. The two-piece jersey sport dress popularized by Chanel and, above all, Patou, could also employ motifs that reflected contemporary art, and geometric, cubist-inspired motifs appeared often in these knits. In 1928, just after Elsa Schiaparelli brought out her famous *trompe-l'oeil* sweater paired with black skirt, the young Kathleen Fielding-Jones rushed to A. & L. Tirocchi to buy just such an outfit, surely a knock-off made in New York [see fig. 116, p. 153]. For her sweater, Schiaparelli had developed a new technique, that of using a flat, Armenian stitch that did not stretch and would hold the shape of a knit-in pattern. A 1930s sweater-and-skirt outfit found in the shop is made with a similar technique. Although machine-knit, it too holds its shape without stretching. The wonderful pattern is typical of the "machine-age" images of skyscrapers and of factories belching smoke, composed in a stepped design that reflects artworks of the time and echoes the forms of skyscrapers themselves [figs. 137–139].

Sports dressing became more popular in the 1920s, and the 1930s saw a diversification of forms from the simple two-piece jerseys of Patou and Chanel to specific garments for specific activities such as dancing, tennis, golf, and swimming. A wonderful example of a wool-jersey bathing suit from 1930 survived in the Tirocchi shop. Patterned with contrasting yellow and green areas, the suit has a felt jacket and large straw hat to match, both trimmed with huge "*moderne*" flowers in felt [fig. 96, p. 132; figs. 140–141]. This contemporary motif in bright, sun-filled colors reflects the lifestyles of the Tirocchi clients, who went off to their beach houses in summer or to the Caribbean in winter. A group of

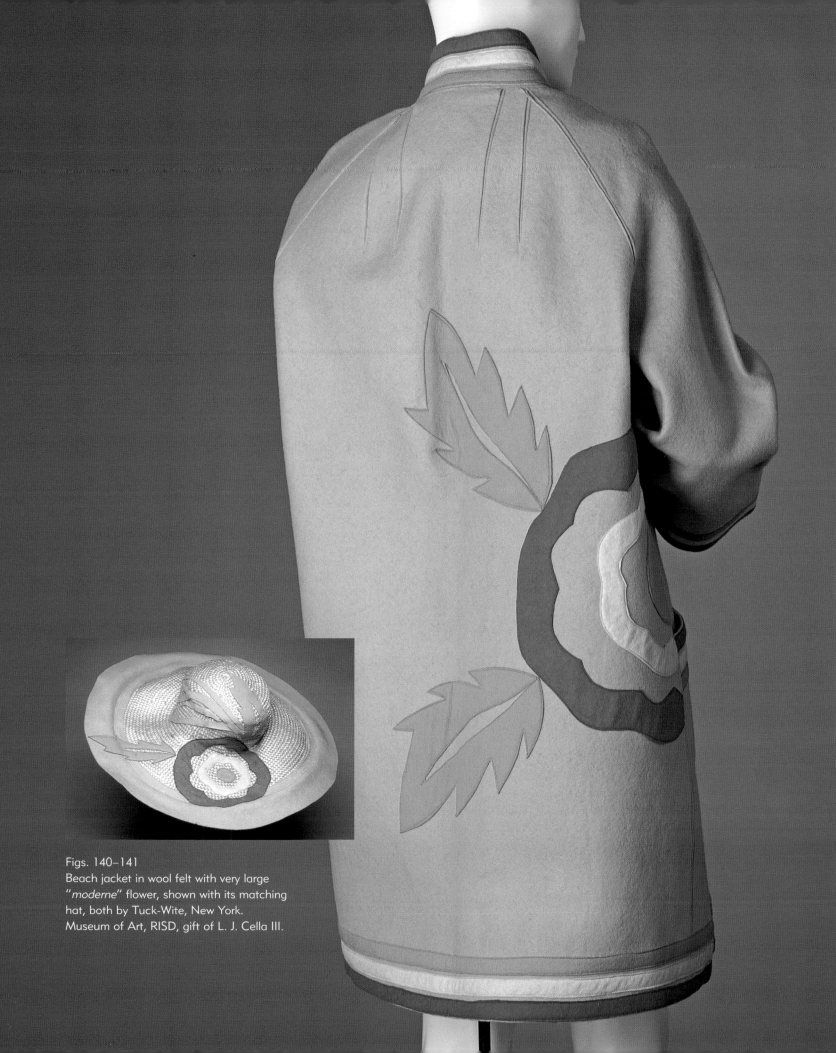

Figs. 140–141
Beach jacket in wool felt with very large
"*moderne*" flower, shown with its matching
hat, both by Tuck-Wite, New York.
Museum of Art, RISD, gift of L. J. Cella III.

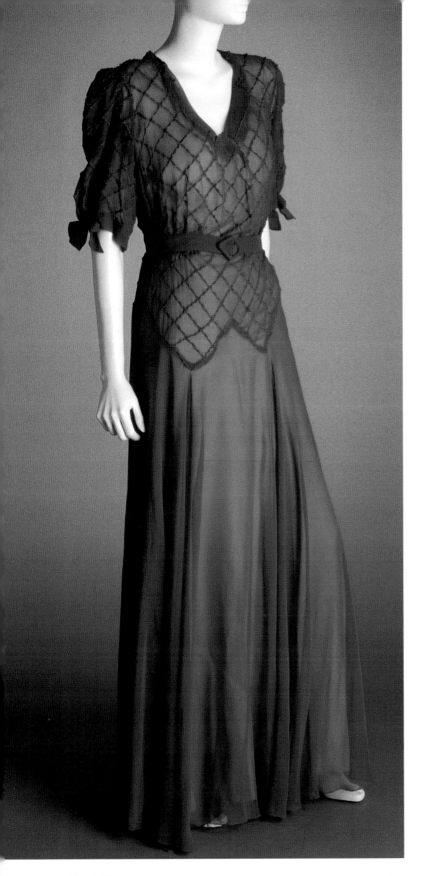

Fig. 142
Dancing dress in red silk chiffon, ca. 1930, influenced by the popularity of South American dances such as the tango. Museum of Art, RISD, gift of L. J. Cella III.

Fig. 143
Bell-bottom wool pants and wool top purchased by the Tirocchi sisters in 1933 from New York supplier Russell, copied from a design by Paris couturier Edward Molyneux. Museum of Art, RISD, gift of L. J. Cella III.

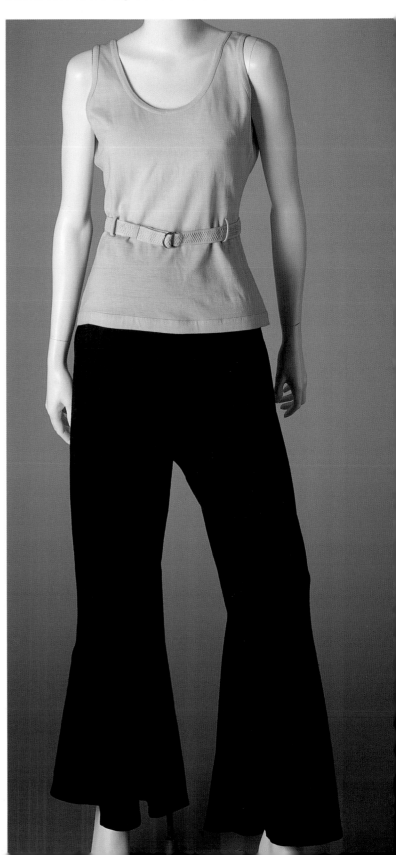

evening dresses found in the shop point to another side of the woman in motion. A handful of long, wide-skirted, narrow-waisted, colorful gowns of chiffon and other lightweight materials fairly scream "tango," bringing to mind the South American dances popular in the mid-1930s [fig. 142].

Reflecting streamlined 1930s design, as well as women's new social permission to wear trousers, is an outfit attributed to Molyneux, purchased with its own white sweater and jacket from the New York supplier Russell in 1933 [fig. 143]. The bell-bottomed pants and sweater were preserved in the shop, but the jacket was not to be found. Perhaps it was sold separately when the entire outfit failed to appeal to any client. Streamlined design is epitomized in the elaborately cut satin and velvet evening dresses of the 1930s. These pieced dresses are collages in themselves. Several examples of these cuts popularized by Madeleine Vionnet in the late 1920s and early 30s remained in the shop. All are stylishly svelte and gleamingly reflective, those two attributes of "machine-age" styling that applied to all the arts [figs. 144–145; see also fig. 112, p. 150, and fig. 123, p. 159].

The Tirocchi records become less and less informative about style during the mid-1930s. The bookkeeper stopped recording designers and couturiers, except on rare occasions, more often naming only the importer. Rodier wool dresses and suits increased in popularity throughout the late 1930s. Liberty "loan" (lawn, a light-weight cotton fabric) dresses become popular for summer wear. By 1933, the effects of the Depression began to be seen, as clients delayed payment and canceled orders. The client base shrank over these lean years from the heyday of the 1920s until finally, by 1941, only the faithful few were left. Mrs. Frederick Stanhope Peck, Mrs. Harold J. Gross, and Mrs. Byron S. Watson remained from the early days. One of the last entries in the customer ledger is Mrs. Watson's visit in May 1939, when the bookkeeper suddenly abandoned her policy of not recording designers' names. Chic as always, Mrs. Watson purchased a print dinner dress by Mainbocher, a Chanel suit, a fitted dinner dress in wine-colored silk by Molyneux, and a Jay-Thorpe hat. In 1944, only Mrs.

Fig. 144
Detail of the silk satin dress after Madeleine Vionnet in fig. 112 (p. 150), showing an intricate cut inspired by cubism. Museum of Art, RISD, gift of L. J. Cella, Jr.

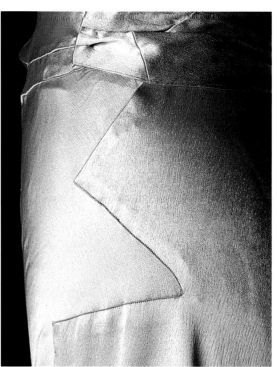

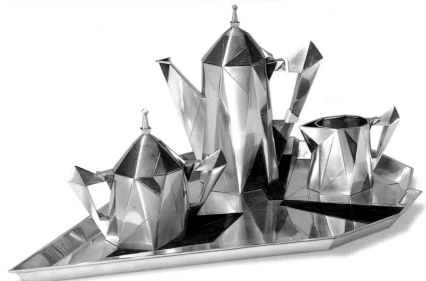

Fig. 145
"Cubic" Coffee Service, 1927, designed by Erik Magnussen for Gorham Manufacturing Company, Providence: the planes are accentuated by different finishes, highlighting the cubist geometry, much as the dress after Madeleine Vionnet with differing orientations of the satin fabric achieves similar effects [fig. 144]. Museum of Art, RISD, gift of Textron Inc. (photograph by Cathy Carver).

Peck was being dressed by Anna, who by then was ill and probably unable to handle a larger clientele.

Even if the records in the Tirocchi Archive do not reveal in visible detail every dress that passed through the shop or every sport suit purchased by its clients, they explicitly document the changing silhouettes and styles of decoration between 1915 and 1941. The dresses, coats, bathing suits, and evening wraps found in the shop, if arranged chronologically, chart for the observer not only the different silhouettes of fashion, but also the overall aesthetic of modernism as it developed through the years. From the chemise and cloche in a cubist mode of the 1920s to the evening dresses of the late 1930s with their body-skimming silhouettes and "machine-age" reflective surfaces, each garment has a particular relationship to the art of its time.

Raymond Loewy, the industrial designer of everything from the Pennsylvania Railroad's stream-lined Broadway Limited train to the Studebaker Champion Cruising Sedan, made this point unforgettably in his "Evolution Chart of Design."[44] He compares the changes in architecture, from the ornate houses of earlier centuries to streamlined modern architecture up to the 1930s, with developments in female dress, starting with the seventeenth century's long, full, enormous skirts, full sleeves, and high coiffures and ending in 1934 with the svelte, form-fitting evening gown, exactly reflecting the silhouette of gowns found in the Tirocchi shop [fig. 146]. In the same chart, using a woman clad in a bathing suit, he shows how the very ideal of a woman's figure changed from the plump form of the 1890s to the thin, long-legged creature of 1935.

Fashion designers conceived each of their garments in the context of the greater art world, and were themselves recognized as decorative artists familiar with the concerns of their time. The question they attempted to answer – what does it mean to be modern? – is as much in contention now as it was at the beginning of the twentieth century. The concepts of modernism are still present in the Western aesthetic at the beginning of the twenty-first century. The search for elegance in fashion at the start of the new millennium reflects the concerns and debates of the early modern period as they are revealed in fashions from the Tirocchi shop. Although their elaborate Art Deco fabrics and often exuberant ornamentation may have come to look less and less "modern" as the century progressed, among them are many garments that could be worn with great pride today.

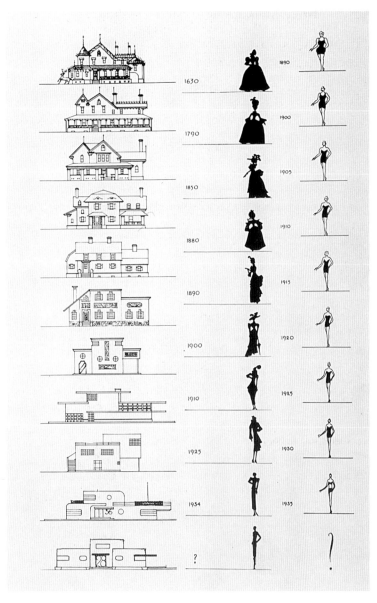

Fig. 146
Raymond Loewy's "Evolution Chart of Design"; published in his book *Industrial Design*. Woodstock (New York): 1988, pp. 74–76 (reproduced by permission of Overlook Press).

The author wishes to thank Professor Emerita Lorraine Howes, Rhode Island School of Design, for her helpful comments on an earlier version of this essay.

❋

1. Nigel Gosling, *Paris 1900–1914: The Miraculous Years*. London: 1978, p. 124.

2. Gertrude Stein, *Paris, France*. New York: 1970, pp. 11–12.

3. Billy Kluver and Julie Martin, *Kiki's Paris*. New York: 1989, p. 134.

4. Elizabeth Ann Coleman, *The Opulent Era: Fashions of Worth, Doucet, and Pingat*. Brooklyn: 1989, pp. 22, 90–94.

5. Paul Poiret, *En Habillant l'époque*. Paris: 1930, p. 7.

6. *Ibid.*, p. 93.

7. André Dunoyer de Segonzac, "Preface," in Palmer White, *Poiret*. London: 1973, p. 10.

8. Nancy J. Troy, *Modernism and the Decorative Arts in France, Art Nouveau to Le Corbusier*. New Haven: 1991, p. 252, n. 50.

9. Yvonne Deslandres, *Poiret: Paul Poiret 1879–1944*. New York: 1987, p. 50.

10. René Simon Lévy, *The Fabrics of Raoul Dufy: Genesis and Context*. London: 1983, p. 98.

11. Isadora Duncan, *My Life*. New York: 1927, p. 246.

12. Martin Battersby, *Art Deco Fashion: French Designers 1908–1925*. London: 1974, p. 50.

13. *Gazette du Bon Ton: Art, Mode, et Frivolités*, no. 1 (1912), pp. 3–4.

14. Elsa Schiaparelli, *Shocking Life*. London: 1954, p. 90.

15. Roger Shattuck, *The Banquet Years: The Origins of the Avant-Garde in France, 1885 to World War 1*. New York: 1968 (rev. ed.), pp. 168–69.

16. François Chapon, *Jacques Doucet ou l'art du mécénat 1853–1929. Nouvelle édition revue et corrigée*. Paris: 1996, pp. 293–94.

17. Musée Historique des Tissus, *Paquin: une retrospective de 60 ans de haute couture*. Lyon: 1989, pp. 88–89.

18. *Ibid.*, p. 82.

19. Guillaume Garnier, *Paul Poiret et Nicole Groult: maîtres de la mode art deco*. Paris: 1985, p. 120.

20. *Ibid.*, pp. 120–21.

21. *Ibid.*, p. 120.

22. Guillaume Garnier, *Paris couture: les années trente*. Paris: 1987, pp. 247–48.

23. Betty Kirke, *Madeleine Vionnet*. New York: 1998, p. 58.

24. *Ibid.*, p. 137.

25. *Mercure de France* (January 1, 1914), quoted in Jacques Damase, *Sonia Delaunay: mode et tissus imprimés*. Paris: 1991, p. 112.

26. Angela Völker, *Textiles of the Wiener Werkstätte, 1910–1932*. New York: 1994, p. 47.

27. See Troy, *op. cit.*, pp. 79–96, for a discussion of the *coloristes* and the Maison Cubiste.

28. Kirke, *op. cit.*, pp. 34–35.

29. The following has been summarized from Kenneth E. Silver, *Esprit de Corps: The Art of the Parisian Avant-Garde and the First World War, 1914–1925*. Princeton: 1989, pp. 167–85.

30. *Ibid.*, p. 169.

31. *Ibid.*, p. 184.

32. Valerie Steele, *Paris Fashion: A Cultural History*. New York: 1988, p. 247.

33. Anne Hollander, *Seeing Through Clothes*. New York: 1980, pp. 312, 314.

34. Museum of Art, Rhode Island School of Design, *Dynamic Symmetry*. Providence: 1961, *passim*.

35. Kirke, *op. cit.*, pp. 116–17.

36. *Ibid.*, p. 117.

37. Steele, *op. cit.*, p. 246.

38. Richard Martin, ed., *Contemporary Fashion*. New York: 1995, p. 364.

39. Quoted in Madelyn Shaw, "Mainbocher," unpublished typescript, 1994 (courtesy the author).

40. Schiaparelli, *op cit.*, p. 64.

41. *Ibid.*, p. 65.

42. Richard Martin, *Fashion and Surrealism*. New York: 1987, p. 56; Palmer White, *Elsa Schiaparelli: Empress of Paris Fashion*. New York: 1986, pp. 170–71; Schiaparelli, *op.cit.*, *passim*.

43. *Vogue*, vol. 61, no. 1 (January 1, 1923), p. 122.

44. Raymond Loewy, *Industrial Design*. Woodstock (New York): 1988, pp. 74–76; one of several charts illustrating style changes in objects from trains to telephones.

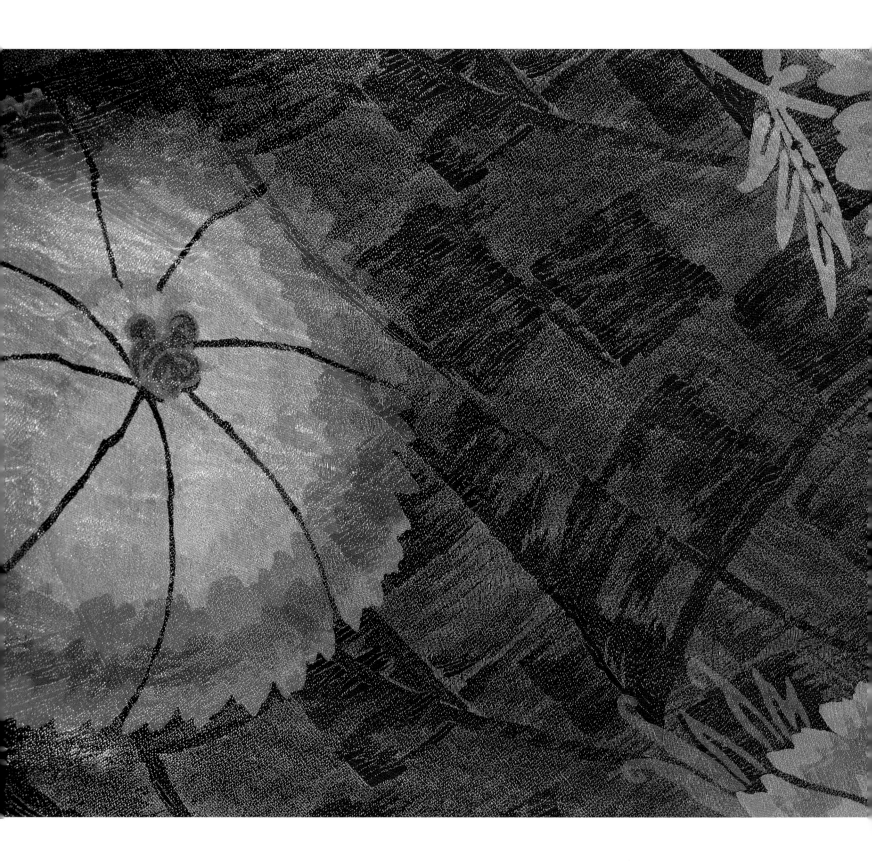

SUSAN HAY
Curator of Costume and Textiles
Museum of Art, Rhode Island School of Design

Modernism in Fabric:

Art and the Tirocchi Textiles

I f the Tirocchi clients coveted and collected the highest quality French fashion, they also demanded the best in textiles. Whether a dress was custom-made, created from a "robe," or purchased ready-to-wear, the finest French fabrics were favored for its construction [fig. 147].

French couture held the allure of Paris and all the status that implied, but French silks were valued because of their long-standing reputation for quality and good design. The Tirocchi sisters knew this from their earlier employment in Italy, where French textiles were widely used. From skirt panels of silk net hand-beaded in French workshops in the 1910s to the sumptuous silk and rayon crepes of the 1930s, each textile from A. & L. Tirocchi now preserved in the RISD Museum bespeaks the luxury that radiated from 514 Broadway and endeared the shop to its clientele.

This was not an accident. As fashion became more simplified, as the transition to ready-made garments proceeded, and as it became possible for nearly everybody to wear up-to-date clothing, the quality of a dressmaker's textiles served more and more to maintain social distinctions that were disappearing with regard to the design of clothing itself. Anna Tirocchi, chief creative spirit in the shop and well aware of this fact, purchased the most luxurious and beautifully designed fabrics she could find from the font of all fashion: France. Whether handwoven on the drawlooms of Lyon, or, with increasing frequency in the 1920s, produced on Jacquard looms, the Tirocchi fabrics were the best that France had to offer. Since the late nineteenth century, professional artists had become increasingly interested in designing both apparel and textiles, collaborating with the couturiers of Paris and the skilled weavers of Lyon, who had long been protected by the

Fig. 147
Textile of silk and silver threads, overprinted in a cubist pattern, demonstrating the ability of the Jacquard loom to lift each warp separately, resulting in a nice "scattering" of silver dots throughout the fabric: this fabric was used by the Tirocchi sisters for an opera coat found in the shop in 1990. Museum of Art, RISD, gift of Dr. Louis J. Cella, Jr.

French government and promoted worldwide for their training and talent.

The selection of fabrics packed away in the A. & L. Tirocchi shop reflects Anna Tirocchi's expert eye for beauty. As with the French couture she sold, the fabrics she chose radiated the excitement of the art world in the early years of the twentieth century, when artists and designers from all over Europe converged on Paris. Painters, printmakers, illustrators, and designers of decorative arts, jewelry, couture, textiles, and theater scenery and costume were often working in all of these areas at once. Also collaborating with literary figures, musicians, composers, dancers, and theatrical entrepreneurs, these artists gave to French design the tremendous burst of creativity and inventive renewal that came to all the arts with the advent of modernism in the early years of the twentieth century.

American admiration of French textiles had been shaped over many years before this creative ferment. Even prior to the American Revolution, when Americans still considered themselves Englishmen, France had been perceived as the capital of luxury, and the English had acquired or copied many Parisian fashions and textiles. A glance at eighteenth-century English terminology gives an idea of the number of fabrics and trims of French origin commonly used in England and America: "French alamode," or black taffeta from Lyon, ordered by Samuel Sewall of Boston in 1690; "serge desoy" for men's coats and waistcoats; "florence légère," fancy silks for sale in the United States in 1797; "jaconot muslin," an inexpensive cotton first made in India but popular in France in the early eighteenth century and ordered by Virginia merchants in 1768 and 1771; "marseilles" for quilted petticoats and coverlets; "siamoises," ordered by Thomas Jefferson as furnishing materials in 1790.[1] Even today, fabrics such as corduroy (*corde du roi*), manufactured in Rhode Island as early as 1789; piqué (*piqué*), first imported to the United States in 1779; organdy (*organdi*), described in a French commercial dictionary of around 1723–30; and the ordinary, but now ubiquitous, denim (*de Nîmes*, originally *serge de Nîmes*), from which Levi Strauss made his work clothes for min-

ers during the nineteenth-century North American Gold Rush; all are so familiar that their French origins have been forgotten.[2]

At first, American colonials acquired these luxuries through London, but by the end of the eighteenth century, merchants in the United States were dealing directly with France. John Holker, whose father had a factory for the production of "siamoises" in Rouen from 1752, as French Consul-General had them imported to Philadelphia in 1779 for use by the U.S. government.[3] In 1792, Providence merchant Welcome Arnold advertised the inexpensive woolens, silks, and cottons that he imported from England, but when it was a question of a special dress for his wife Patience, the brocaded fabric and passementerie trim were ordered from Paris.[4] From the colonial era to the present, Americans have looked to France for innovative fashion and other luxury products. Through fashion plates and ladies' magazines, women in America have stayed in touch with Paris, some even traveling to France themselves in search of high-fashion textiles and apparel made to their measure by its couturiers.

Ever since the late seventeenth century, French producers, supported by their government, have made a commitment to good design, backed by a substantial investment in the education of designers. Schools were established in France in the eighteenth century, and manufacturers paid their graduates twice what they were paid in Britain.[5] Lyon generally purchased its textile designs from Paris. It was superior design that kept French products marketable despite the rapid development of mass production in nineteenth-century England. It was superior design that created some of the most memorable textiles ever woven, such as the legendary French silks used by Worth or the Lyon furnishing silks purchased by the Vanderbilts for their "summer cottage," The Breakers in Newport [fig. 148]. By the early twentieth century, however, critics and producers were concerned that French textiles might not be able to maintain their momentum. French weavers were becoming alarmed as the American industry grew, and they also feared competition from producers in Germany and Austria.[6] Anna Tirocchi's forays into the French textile market therefore took place at a critical time for the fast-expanding industry. The battle for French superiority would be fought against the backdrop of general unease in the French design world, of nationalistic desires to develop a truly modern French style, and of emerging modernism and internationalism in the art world.

At the turn of the century, some French designers of textiles and decorative arts were still producing copies of earlier styles, while at the same time artists and dealers such as Siegfried Bing were promoting art nouveau as the modern French style. In a challenge to art nouveau, German and Viennese workshops were developing their own contemporary styles. Founded in 1897 with a roster of artists in many media, Munich's Vereinigten Werkstätten fur Kunst im Handwerk (United Workshops for Art in Handwork) used machine technology to produce objects in the new German Jugendstil, based on the British arts and crafts movement aesthetic of simplicity and appropriateness. Members of the Vienna Secession movement, also founded in 1897, were influenced by William Morris, Walter Crane, and Charles Voysey and also adopted the British aesthetic for their handcrafted products. Characterized by what the French called an "elegant eclecticism," architects and designers created functional modern buildings that reflected their destined use and employed ordinary materials in judicious ways. In the decorative arts, an interest in pattern, flatness, and abstraction was applied to textile design before 1900 with many striking results.

By May 1903, Koloman Moser and Josef Hoffmann – with funds supplied by Fritz Waerndorfer, Hoffmann's patron, and the advice of Charles Rennie Mackintosh – had founded the Wiener Werkstätte (Vienna Workshops) for "the promotion of the economic interests of its members by training and educating them in handicraft, by the manufacture of craft objects of all sorts in accordance with artistic designs drawn up by Guild members, by the erection of workshops and by the sale of the goods produced."[7] These artists, of similar mind to the founders of the Munich workshops, wanted to institute a particularly Viennese style and to produce ensembles in which all elements would reflect the

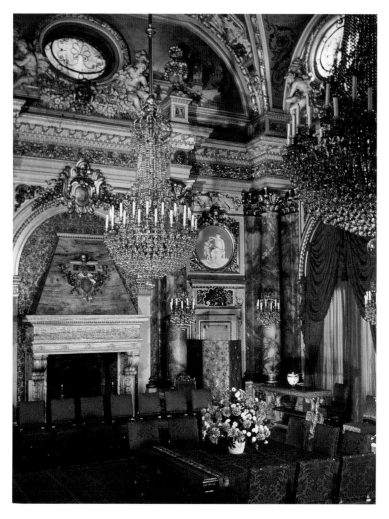

Fig. 148
Dining room of The Breakers, Newport: in the 1890s, its designers selected a dramatic cut- and uncut-velvet upholstery fabric from Lyon. Courtesy Preservation Society of Newport County, Newport.

same aesthetic principles. They looked back to the Biedermeier period of the early nineteenth century as the last great era of genuine Viennese design. Unlike the Munich group, however, the artists of the Wiener Werkstätte regarded the tradition of handcraftsmanship as basic. Machines were used, but the artist maintained complete control over what was produced. Wiener Werkstätte textile and fashion divisions were opened in 1910, and Paris couturier Paul Poiret and Lyon textile manufacturer Charles Bianchini were among the first to visit them.

Critics of French decorative arts urged artists to learn from the effectiveness of the German and Austrian workshops in presenting designs in a single overarching national style. Ironically, French attitudes toward luxury and quality seemed to be part of the problem. French artists, instead of joining to form workshops to produce practical, well-designed objects for the middle class as in Germany and Austria, worked in isolation as fine artists making handcrafted individual pieces aimed at the aristocratic luxury market. French designers decided to band together to form the Société des Artistes Décorateurs in 1901. Artists in many media took part in its exhibitions. Jacques Doucet, Jeanne Paquin, Paul Poiret, Sonia Delaunay, and the American Mainbocher represented fashion over the years, while Émile Jacques Ruhlmann and Louis Süe, among many others, produced ideas for textiles because of their commitment to the decorative arts.[8] This gave designers more visibility through annual exhibitions, but the French still could not agree on a central design philosophy. The debate raged throughout the first decade of the century. What style would be exclusively French and exclusively modern and could compete in the marketplace with industrial creations?

Couturier Paul Poiret, who had been considering these issues even as he looked back to the Empire period for his influential straight loose gowns of 1907, was also acting to develop a new French style in textile design. By 1909, he had already visited Germany, where he showed his collections to great acclaim. There he purchased a group of German and Eastern European decorative arts, which he regarded as akin, in their "primitive" simplicity and

vigor, to all of the various artistic expressions manifested by the Ballets Russes, founded by Serge Diaghilev with painter Léon Bakst and choreographer Michel Fokine and then the toast of Paris. In Vienna, Poiret had been captivated by the Wiener Werkstätte with its cooperative spirit among architects (Josef Hoffmann), decorative artists (Dagobert Pêche, Koloman Moser), and painters (Gustav Klimt, whose companion, Emilie Flöge was herself a fashion designer with a salon in Vienna).

In Germany and Austria, Poiret encountered the new modern styles on their own ground. He purchased textiles. He went to every decorative arts exhibition possible, meeting Hermann Muthesius, the Prussian architect and critic; designer Bruno Paul; and Gustav Klimt. He wandered the streets looking at new buildings and visited every recently completed interior to which he could gain admittance. He was especially struck by the products of the Wiener Werkstätte, and on his return to Paris he decided to adopt the Viennese workshop concept and to strive for the freedom and spontaneity he had observed in both French and Eastern European folk art. Poiret rejected the idea of employing highly trained artists or craftsmen. Thinking of the peasants who had made beautiful objects without any formal art education, he decided to experiment with new designs by untrained artists free of what he called "false principles" learned in school.

Poiret sought out young working-class women of artistic talent who could not afford to continue their education, set up a design program for them in his house, and took them to the country; or the zoo; or the Louvre, where they studied Delacroix's composition; or to Notre-Dame de Paris to look at the bright colors of the stained glass windows.[9] They rewarded him with what he considered to be marvelous results, as fresh and spontaneous as nature itself: fields of wheat, daisies, poppies, forests with bounding tigers. All their designs appeared to him to be charming and completely different from any established style, French or foreign. In 1911, aware of the marketing successes of the German and Viennese workshops, which had established boutiques for the sale of their production, he made a collection of textiles and rugs from his protégées' designs for the opening of his own shop, Martine, which was at its height when Anna Tirocchi visited it in the mid-1920s.

In 1909, Poiret became interested in the work of the young French painter Raoul Dufy, whose first efforts at printmaking he had recently seen. Poiret invited Dufy to a dinner party with Poiret's friends poet Max Jacob, decorative artist Louis Süe, and painter Marie Laurençin, there also introducing him to Guillaume Apollinaire. This celebrated poet was then waiting for Pablo Picasso to produce illustrations for his newest volume of verse, *Le Bestiaire*. Picasso, however, was dragging his feet and had not even begun the work. Apollinaire, who had a printer waiting anxiously for the book, decided to hire Dufy instead.[10]

Dufy's first essays at decorative woodblock prints in large format appealed to Poiret for their echo of German expressionism and for their "primitivism," a quality also instantly apparent to Apollinaire.[11] Dufy and Poiret got along cordially, sharing as they did "the same tendencies in decoration."[12] Dufy, already known as a fauvist painter, was abreast of modernist ideas. He shared with Poiret a profound interest in color, calling it "the creative element of light."[13] Like Poiret, he had traveled in Germany, where he had observed and been impressed by the progress of the decorative arts, particularly as manifested by the Deutscher Werkbund. In 1911, as *Le Bestiaire* went to press, Poiret hired Dufy to make woodcuts for the letterhead of his business stationery and to design a business card for the Martine shop [fig. 149]. Soon the two men were planning a much more extensive project: a joint enterprise to use Dufy's talents to produce textiles for Poiret's couture house. Always insistent on the importance of bright color, they set up a small workshop, which they called the "Petite Usine" ("Little Factory"), where Dufy could experiment with dyes and hues, in the process learning how to print his woodblocks on silks. Some of the designs were reworked from *Le Bestiaire*, others were executed especially for Poiret. Dufy also dealt with the couture house of Doeuillet, for which he provided designs in 1911.[14]

Even before his collaboration with Poiret, Dufy had been interested in textile design. In need of

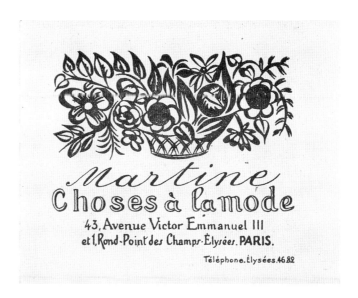

Fig. 149
Business card for Paul Poiret's shop Martine, 1911, designed by Raoul Dufy. Tirocchi Archive.

money to support himself while he produced the illustrations for Apollinaire's *Le Bestiaire*, Dufy approached the Lyon silk manufacturer Charles Bianchini with designs for sale. Bianchini had been anxious for some time to restore the reputation of Lyon silks for artistic excellence and was interested in modern design.

The firm of Atuyer, Bianchini, Férier had been founded in 1888 by Bianchini, François Atuyer, and François Férier. Charles Bianchini was the eye behind the design end of the business. In 1892, he had the idea of opening a store in Paris to market his products at fashion's very heart. He was the first Lyon manufacturer to do so. The address of the shop was 24 bis, avenue de l'Opéra, in the same district as the couture houses. In 1897, Bianchini himself moved to Paris, where he directed the store until his death in 1945. This relocation had the advantage of allowing his firm to sell directly to the end-users, the couturiers, without going through the traditional commission merchants, who had formerly been intermediaries between the Lyon manufacturers and the Paris buyers. In 1900, the parent company moved into a new modernist building in the textile sector of the Croix Rousse, high on a hill overlooking the city of Lyon. In 1902, the partners opened branches in London and Brussels, and in 1909 they established an office in New York at 366 Fifth Avenue.[15]

Before 1910, Bianchini had become interested in Viennese design, traveling to the city to purchase sketches made for him by Austrian artists. Some of these he had printed on silk as early as 1907–08 [fig. 150]. He encouraged artists in his own studio to produce work in the Viennese manner and also to design in the new bold colors favored by fauvist painters after 1905. In 1910, when the firm was at the height of its influence, this forward-looking manufacturer printed the first of Dufy's designs for the firm.[16] On March 1, 1912, with Poiret's permission, Bianchini signed Dufy to an exclusive contract,

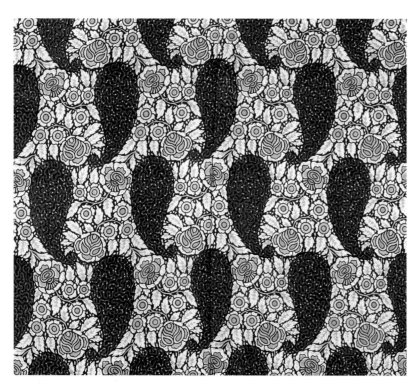

Fig. 150
Silk textile printed by Atuyer, Bianchini, Férier of Lyon, ca. 1907: its pattern of paisley on a background floral in the style of Gustav Klimt represents one of Charles Bianchini's earliest uses of Viennese motifs. Courtesy Musée des Tissus de Lyon; design copyright Bianchini-Férier.

which was to be paid with royalties on sales, an arrangement very unusual for a time when designers normally sold designs to manufacturers outright. This arrangement would continue until Dufy left the company in 1928. In 1912, Dufy was still printing from some of the blocks he had used at the Petite Usine, which came along with him after his work for Poiret; and he was developing many others with the same striking graphic qualities. During the first three years of his contract, Dufy produced more than three hundred sketches, only a few of which were actually produced.[17]

Many of Dufy's most successful patterns employed the new technique of "discharge" printing. The fabric was first dyed "in the piece" after weaving, where formerly the yarn had been dyed before being woven. The richest hues were obtainable only in this manner. Dufy's simple and striking designs were then overprinted onto the ground. The fabric was discharged with bleach to remove the base color wherever necessary, and in the same process bold new dyes were applied according to the patterns cut into the woodblocks [fig. 151]. Dufy's designs had widespread appeal. Paul Poiret continued to use Dufy's patterns, now produced by Bianchini, Férier (the name change occurred upon the death of Atuyer in 1912; the firm today is called Bianchini-Férier). Simple black-and-white prints created by Dufy endured for many years in the company's line. Business records in the Tirocchi Archive show that Anna ordered a printed silk textile with Dufy-like black and white flowers [figs. 151–152] in January of 1923 from a tiny sample sent her by the company. In the same year she purchased a black-and-orange velvet with the same appealing graphic quality [fig. 153]. Neither textile was among those for which Dufy was paid, according to Bianchini, Férier's records, but each demonstrates the power of Dufy's designs to affect the entire line of the company.

In 1951, RISD's Museum purchased a collection of more than four hundred silks from the Lyon firm of Guard Frères, all of which came from Atuyer, Bianchini, Férier and date to its early years. Dufy's hand is evident in a number of them, all but a few of which are printed on plain-weave silk.

Fig. 151
Silk textile, ca. 1912: "discharge" printing, in which the ground color is bleached out and new colors substituted, was important to many of Raoul Dufy's most successful textile designs for Atuyer, Bianchini, Férier. Museum of Art, RISD, Museum Works of Art Reserve Fund; design copyright Bianchini-Férier.

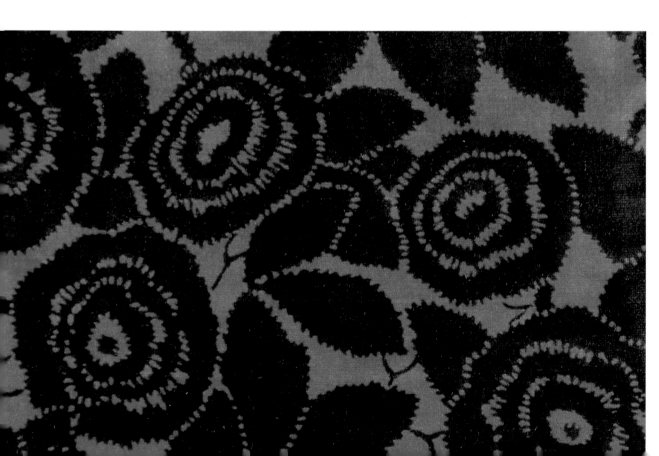

Fig. 152
An order confirmation from Bianchini, Férier to Anna Tirocchi of January 1923 detailing her order of a black-and-white fabric with the graphic qualities that Dufy's textiles made fashionable. Tirocchi Archive; design copyright Bianchini-Férier.

Fig. 153
Silk velvet textile, ca. 1920, purchased by Anna Tirocchi from Bianchini, Férier. Courtesy University of Rhode Island, Kingston, Historic Costume and Textile Collection, gift of Dr. Louis J. Cella, Jr.; design copyright Bianchini-Férier.

Thanks to the survival of the Bianchini, Férier records, many of the RISD textiles have been found to date to the period of Bianchini's first experiments with modern design. The RISD textiles are samples for salesmen, who carried them along as they traversed their territories, or sent them to clients in book form [figs. 154–155]. In Anna Tirocchi's case, her contact (called a "drummer") was J. J. Hannock, who would frequently visit the shop to show his sample swatches or to deliver fabrics by hand from New York. When new sample books came out, Hannock requested that Anna throw the outdated versions away. Unfortunately for this history, she did dispose of something for once in her life, and none were found in the shop when its contents were presented to RISD in 1989.

It is clear that Charles Bianchini's employment of Dufy was an inspiration to other Lyon silk manufacturers. By hiring Dufy, Bianchini pointed to a possible way of restoring Lyon to its former status as the producer of the best-designed silks in the world: the adoption of modernist patterns created by French artists to achieve a contemporary and uniquely French style recognizable to all. Certainly Dufy's creations were unlike anything produced in the workshops of Vienna or Germany, nor could English silks be compared in any way to his designs. Bianchini built on his success with Dufy's textiles by hiring other Parisian artists. All were illustrators or avant-garde painters, and many in addition were fashion illustrators, fashion designers, or theatrical costume designers. Several also exhibited at the salons of the Société des Artistes Décorateurs,

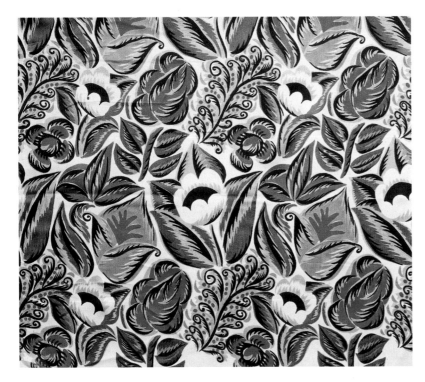

Fig. 154
Printed floral silk for apparel, ca. 1912, designed by Raoul Dufy. Museum of Art, RISD, Museum Works of Art Reserve Fund; design copyright Bianchini-Férier.

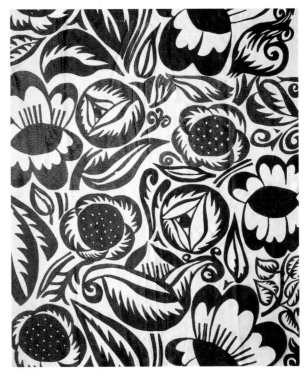

Fig. 155
Printed silk fabric by Raoul Dufy, a variation of which was used by Paul Poiret in a design for a dramatic coat in 1912. Museum of Art, RISD, Museum Works of Art Reserve Fund; design copyright Bianchini-Férier.

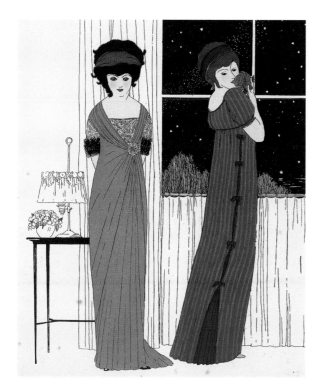

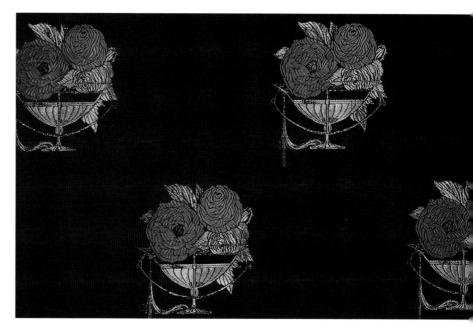

demonstrating once again the close connections between the textile and fashion spheres and the world of early modernist art and design.

Before beginning to design for Bianchini, Férier in 1912, Paul Iribe had been a newspaper typographer and magazine illustrator. In 1906, he founded the satirical journal *Le Témoin*, in which he collaborated with many avant-garde artists, including Jean Cocteau, Marcel Duchamp, André Dunoyer de Segonzac, Lyonel Feininger, and Juan Gris. He continued to produce illustrations throughout his career for the *Gazette du Bon Ton* and other magazines. In 1908, Paul Poiret commissioned the young artist to produce illustrations for a brochure on his collections, *Les Robes des Paul Poiret, racontées par Paul Iribe*, consisting solely of Iribe's plates in the new *pochoir* stencil technique [fig. 156]. Its success made Iribe famous, and the work became a model for subsequent illustrators.[18] After 1910, he designed jewelry, furniture, and other objects, and in 1912, he opened a shop in the Faubourg St. Honoré, where he sold textiles printed to his designs by Bianchini, Férier. From this shop he refurnished the apartment of couturier Jacques Doucet, who, having sold his extensive collection of eighteenth-century furnishings, opted for the ultramodern and began to acquire a collection of Oriental and tribal art and cubist painting. Iribe stopped designing for Bianchini, Ferier after his move to New York following the First World War. In the United States, he became well known for his illustrations in *Vogue* and his costume and set designs for the theater and for Hollywood producer Cecil B. DeMille. On his return to France in 1930, he created a line of jewelry for Gabrielle Chanel.[19] Iribe's textile designs often incorporated his modernistic rose [fig. 157].

Charles Martin had been a friend of artists Georges Lepape, André Marty, and Pierre Brissaud since their student days at the Atelier Cormon in

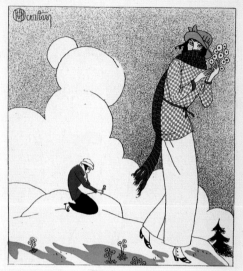

DEUX COSTUMES POUR LES SPORTS D'HIVER

L'un des sweaters, à damier vert et blanc, est de pur cachemire; l'autre, rouge, est en tissu de soie à mailles serrées. Les toques sont assorties et le cache-nez est tricoté en laine des Pyrénées.

Modèles James et Cᵉ.

61

Fig. 158
Illustration by Charles Martin of fashions for Modèles James et Compagnie; published in the *Gazette du Bon Ton,* no. 2 (February 1913), p. 61.

Fig. 159
Charles Martin's silk for Bianchini, Férier, ca. 1920–30, identified by its original design, which still exists in the collection of that company. Museum of Art, RISD, Museum Works of Art Reserve Fund; design copyright Bianchini-Férier.

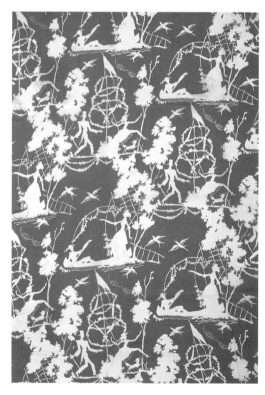

Paris, and he worked with them as one of the creators of *pochoir* illustrations for the fashion magazines that emerged around 1912, particularly the *Gazette du Bon Ton* [fig. 158]. Like these artists, he also designed posters, furniture, and wallpaper. As a member in good standing of the modernist movement, which brought together artists in all media, he collaborated with composer Erik Satie to illustrate Satie's *Sports et Divertissements* of 1914. Martin also designed theatrical sets and costumes. Charles Bianchini printed his design of ladies and gentlemen in a garden on silk [fig. 159].

Bianchini began purchasing designs from Robert Bonfils in 1920. Also an illustrator and exhibitor at the salons of the Société des Artistes Décorateurs from 1912 onwards, Bonfils, like Martin, was a frequent contributor to French fashion magazines, including the *Gazette du Bon Ton* and *Modes et Manières d'Aujourd'hui*. Bonfils designed everything from textiles with exotic and tropical themes to tiny floral prints for Bianchini, Férier. A silk from the Lyon group at RISD bears Bonfils's design of horsemen, printed on a damask designed by Raoul Dufy and dating to about 1920 [fig. 160]. Some of the other artists employed by Bianchini included Russian avant-garde painter Paul Mansouroff; painter/illustrators Georges Barbier, E. A. Seguy, and Henri Gillet; and decorative artists Madeleine Lagrange and Jules Leleu.

Meanwhile, other companies became interested in modernist fabrics. François Ducharne, a merchant who had been selling Lyon silks in Paris and the United States, decided in 1920 to found his own factory and to use modernist methods. He hired the talented weaver Michel Dubost as head of the studio. Dubost was a specialist in brocaded textiles and other patterned weavings and a former professor of design. No doubt inspired by Poiret's school, which Dubost and his students visited annually, this atelier was also structured as a "school for designers," but limited to textile applications.[20] Dubost hired young men and women without formal artistic training and put them in a Paris studio deliberately located in the artists' quarter of Montmartre, where they came in contact with such figures as the writers Gabrielle Colette

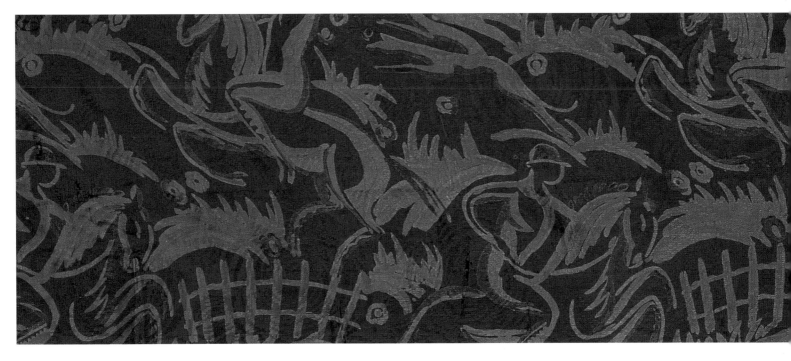

Fig. 160
Robert Bonfils's pattern of horsemen printed on a silk damask designed by Raoul Dufy, ca. 1920.
Museum of Art, RISD, Museum Works of Art Reserve Fund; design copyright Bianchini-Férier.

and Romain Rolland and couturier Madeleine Vionnet, all of whom were brought to the studio by Ducharne. At first Dubost himself did much of the designing for production in Lyon, but the heavy, often stiff silks with large patterns that were his specialty gradually fell out of style in the mid-1920s with the advent of short skirts and the chemise silhouette. Printed silks took on a great importance, and Ducharne was quick to establish the company in this area. By the late 1920s, styles had changed again. Dresses became streamlined, cut on the bias so that they clung to and moved with the body. These required very lightweight fabrics such as crepes, crepes de Chine, and tissue satins. As the 1930s progressed, Soieries F. Ducharne produced more and more prints in medium and small scales, including many for couturieres such as Madeleine Vionnet and Elsa Schiaparelli.

The Tirocchi collection includes several silks that illustrate how these fashion changes affected the Ducharne firm. Anna Tirocchi began buying silks through Ducharne's New York office in 1930, but she visited the company in Paris during either or both of her trips in 1924 and 1926–27. Marginal notes in Ducharne's sample books at the Musée des Tissus de Lyon show that other suppliers with whom Anna dealt were also purchasing designs from this company, so that she may have obtained the earlier examples from Harry Angelo Company or B. Altman in New York. From Ducharne's winter collection of 1922, she purchased a bolt of purple velvet on silver lamé in a large modernist pattern attributed to Dubost and abstracted from a typical Renaisssance velvet design. It was a favorite of François Ducharne, who gave an example in orange and gold to the Musée des Tissus de Lyon in the same year [fig. 161]. This large pattern typifies products of his design studio at this early date and mirrors the production of other Lyon companies. Also found in the Tirocchi shop were a number of Ducharne silks dating to 1930, all of them printed. These silks are fluid, lightweight fabrics, such as a chevron-patterned tissue silk velvet that appeared in a Ducharne sample book of 1930 and a bolt of black silk crepe de Chine with polychrome roses discharge-printed on a black ground [fig. 162], billed to Anna

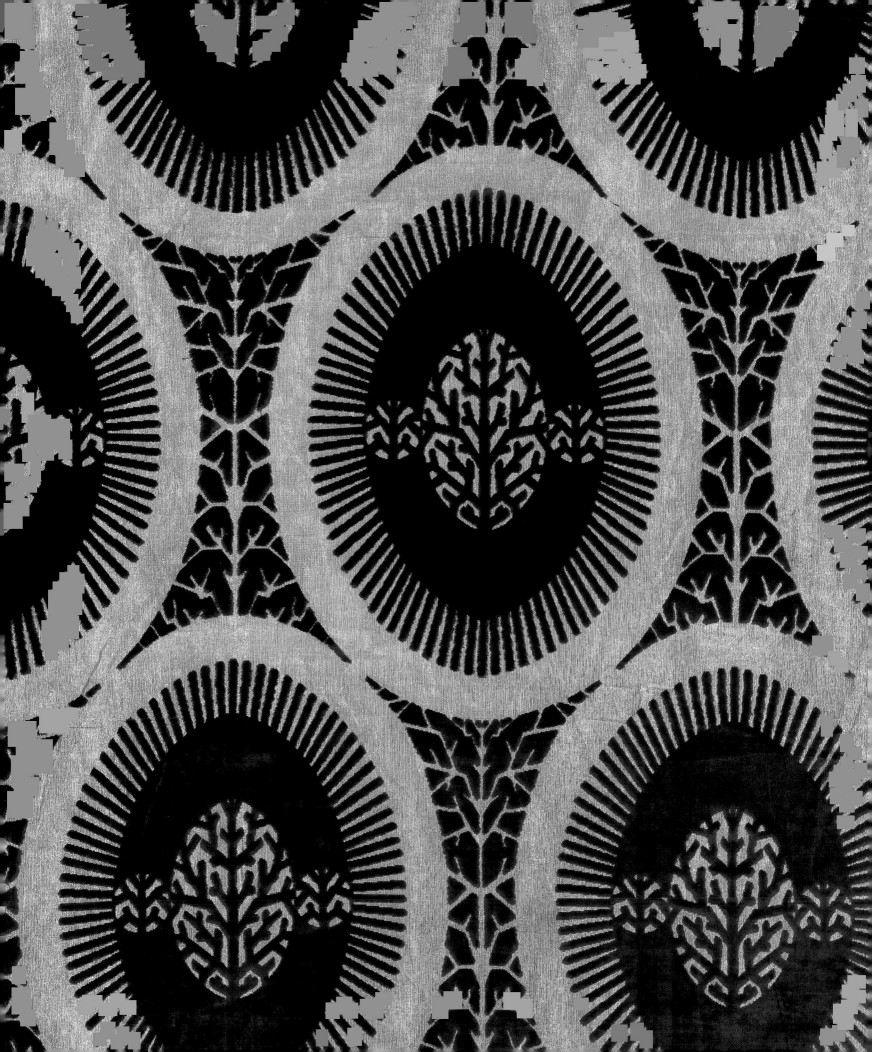

by Ducharne in 1930.[21] The lightness of the fabrics
made them suitable for the new, draped styles, while
their smaller patterns and realistic flowers show a
turning away from the *"moderne"* style that had
appeared in the 1920s.

Rodier, long a household word in France for
its textile production, was another source of modern fabric designs for the Tirocchis. Rodier came
into being in 1810 with the development of a
French version of the fashionable imported Kashmir
shawl. Known for its woolens through the years, but
especially for its brand-name cashmere fabric
"Kasha," Rodier continued to have its woolen cloth
woven on handlooms in villages surrounding its
mechanized factory at Bohain in the north of
France. Although the area was occupied during the
First World War – Lyon was not – and the firm's
production halted, Paul Rodier was able to save his
designs and records and to make a swift recovery
afterward. By February 1924, when Anna Tirocchi
visited its Paris shop, Rodier had become a leader in
the production of woolens with modernist geometric patterns and of couture silk fabrics and scarves
that Gabrielle Colette, always interested in textiles,
described as "gaie, délicate, éclatante." Colette, however, reserved her highest praise for Rodier's woolens:

> Despite the bold, modern design, meticulously pre-
> pared raw material, and complicated dye chemistry of
> such fabrics; inspired by the landscape, impregnated
> with an agrarian poetry, they seem to me like old
> friends…More than that, a touch both humble and
> divine remains upon them: the touch of the hand.[22]

In the 1920s, Anna Tirocchi purchased woolens
embellished with metal threads, wool plaids and
tweeds, and printed silks from Rodier, in addition to
Rodier's "Kasha" cloth bought from B. Altman &
Company. The latter was a favorite of her customers
for winter suits and afternoon dresses. A suit made

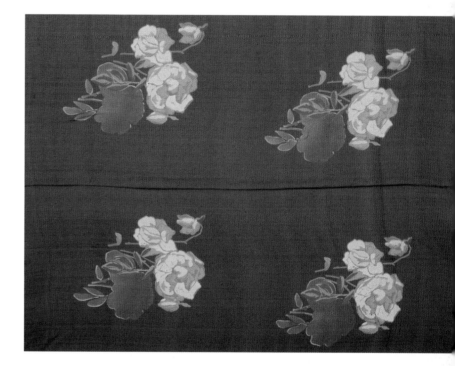

Fig. 162
Black silk crepe de Chine by Soieries F. Ducharne,
1930. Museum of Art, RISD, gift of L. J. Cella III.

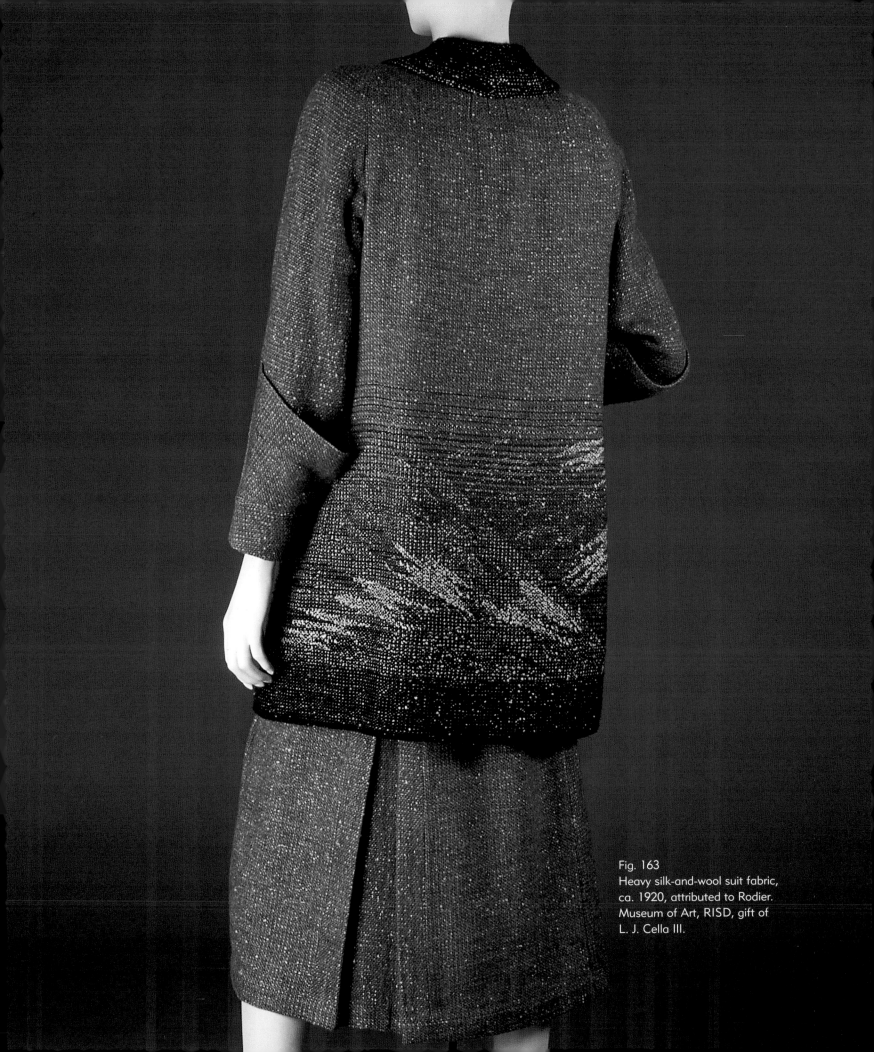

Fig. 163
Heavy silk-and-wool suit fabric,
ca. 1920, attributed to Rodier.
Museum of Art, RISD, gift of
L. J. Cella III.

of heavier tweed attributed to Rodier, found in the shop and now in RISD's collection, represents the earthier, landscape-inspired woolens that impressed Colette [fig. 163].

The Exposition des Arts Décoratifs et Industriels Modernes, sponsored by the French government in 1925, gave worldwide publicity to the *"moderne"* style. In the exhibition, the categories of textiles and wallpaper were combined because of their similar graphic qualities and printing techniques. More than a thousand exhibitors showed their work. The published summary of the exposition credited the high quality of French contributions not only to the fact that French artists were at last being sought out by manufacturers, but also to the production of textiles by many small ateliers, in contrast to the very large mechanized factories in German cities such as Krefeld. In addition, the exigencies of the couture and interior-decoration industries in Paris meant that French products were always changing as the textile industry renewed itself each year.[23]

The writers of the exposition's summary offered a brief definition of the *"moderne"* style. Its principal characteristic, according to them, was the abstraction inspired by Charles Rennie Mackintosh's earlier Glasgow school and by the Viennese and German workshop movements, which had seemed so revolutionary in 1900. By 1920, abstraction was a commonplace, even in floral patterns. Designers had "revived, with a modern accent, the garland, the knot, the rose, the attributes of doves, fans, and cupids, dear to the designers of the eighteenth century." Some had recently adopted the "disassociation of volumes and lines of cubism," creating a "kaleidoscope of lines and colors, richer in decorative possibilities than realistic subjects." The exposition included designs based on cubist concern with the exotic and the "primitive." The summary's authors praised Rodier especially for their textiles based on the art of Cambodia, Vietnam, Guinea, and the Congo. Objects from these cultures had been on view at the Exposition of Marseille in 1922, which presented the indigenous products of the French colonies. Rodier was also the firm that produced fabrics in the brightest, strongest colors, inspiring the authors to marvel that "a dress from their designers is almost a painting."[24] Anna Tirocchi purchased at least two Rodier textiles that reflect this trend [fig. 164].

Exhibitors of textiles included the four largest French firms: Bianchini, Férier, represented by Dufy's works; Soieries F. Ducharne; Coudurier-Fructus-Descher, which displayed lamé shawls and textiles with complicated brocading in gold and silver combined with printing; and Rodier, whose handwoven cottons, rayons, and woolens displayed designs inspired by everything from Hungarian and North African embroideries to the art of the Far East. Many lesser known firms also exhibited, such as Algoud et Joannon, l'Alliance Textile, J. Barret, Blech Frères, Henri Chanée, and Brunet, Meunie et Compagnie.

Some of the new design developments in evidence at the Exposition were credited by its committee to technological advances at the end of the nineteenth and beginning of the twentieth centuries. The dyeing of fabrics in the piece was a major step forward. Earlier, the yarns for textiles had to be dyed before the piece was woven (yarn dyeing), because the technology of vat dyeing lagged behind that of machine weaving: the fifty- or sixty-yard pieces that came off the Jacquard loom were too voluminous to fit into the available vats. By the mid-nineteenth century, larger vats were available and the cloth could be dyed after weaving, making possible brilliant color effects previously unobtainable. Not only did piece dyeing allow the production of the saturated colors preferred by artists such as Dufy, but it also enabled manufacturers to add more twist to their yarns during spinning. Bette Kirke, in her work on couturiere Madeleine Vionnet, explains how this came about. "When dyed after twisting, …yarns tended to untwist. With the development of larger vats, cloth could be piece dyed and the amount of twist of the yarn was no longer limited. It was possible then to twist up to 3,000 turns per meter…The suppleness obtained would replace the previous stiff character of silks."[25] The result was crepe with much more elasticity, or crepe de Chine, whose delicate hand resulted from the alternation of weft threads highly twisted in different directions, allowing the construction of the beautiful bias-cut styles of the 1930s.

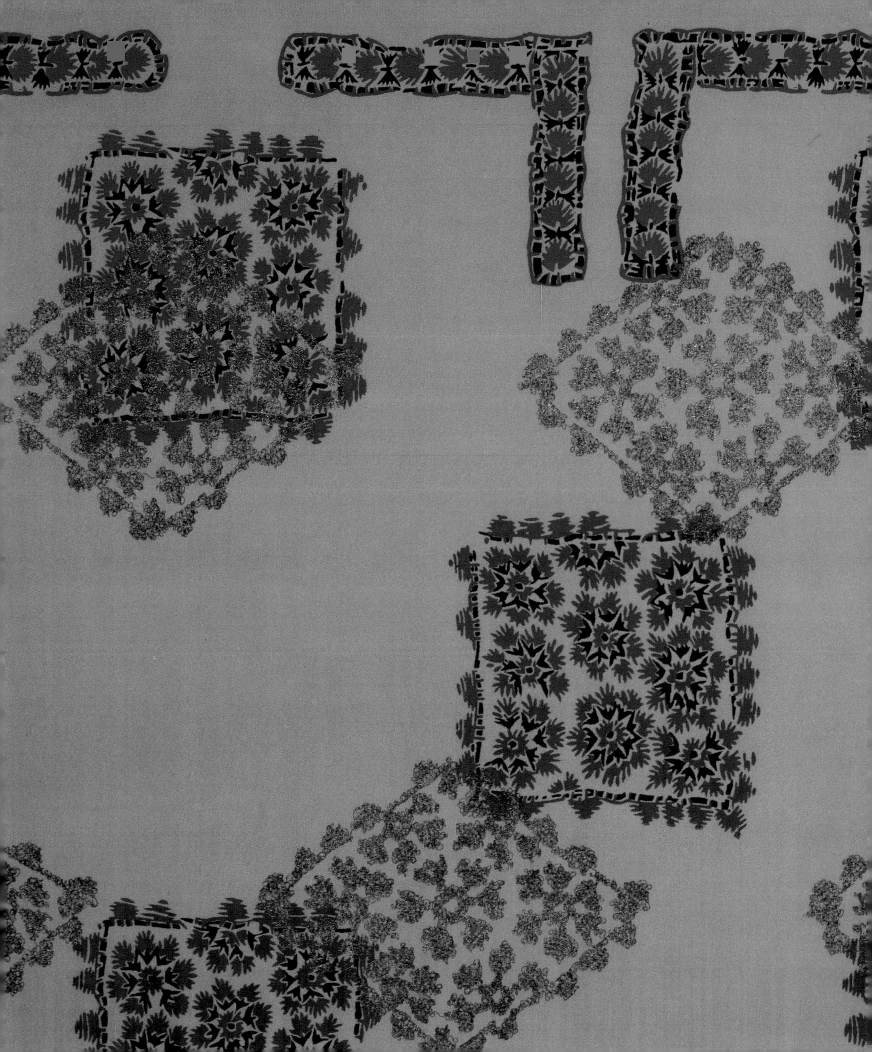

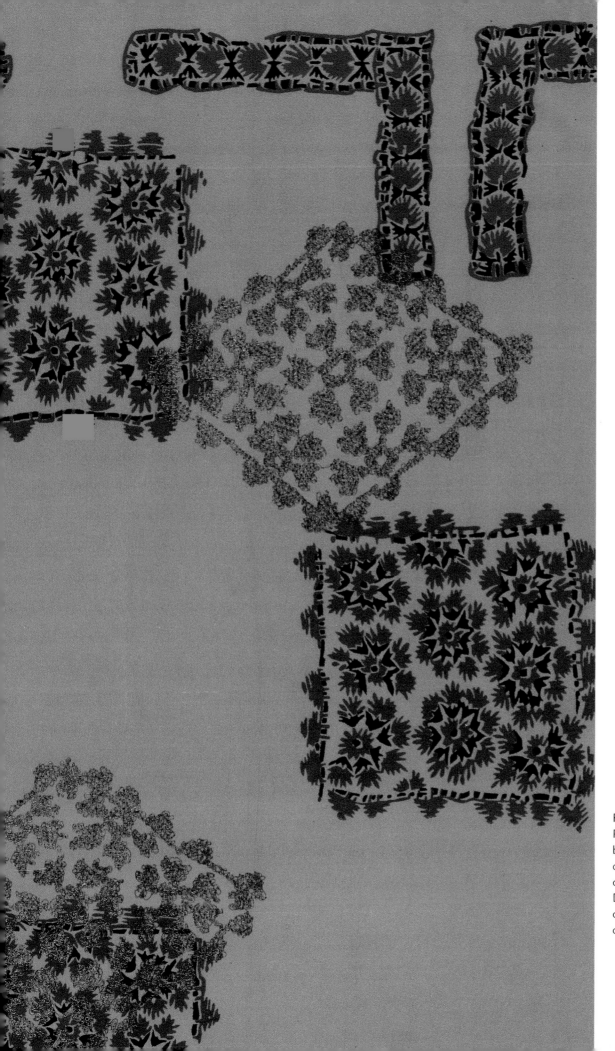

Fig. 164
Rodier silk textile with printed and
brocaded patterns reflecting Persian
art: Rodier produced many like this
one for the Exposition des Arts
Décoratifs et Industriels Modernes
of 1925. Museum of Art, RISD, gift
of L. J. Cella III.

The perfecting of various machine techniques made possible new types of textiles. Refinements to the Jacquard loom resulted in the gauzes, mousse-lines, and ultralight chiffons that became available only in the twentieth century. Panne velvet represented an innovation in a finishing technique: a machine could now flatten the velvet pile in one direction, creating suppleness and a metallic-looking sheen that was especially appealing to contemporary eyes accustomed to the machine aesthetic. The use of metal threads themselves in fabrics was not a new technology. The eighteenth century had brought to perfection "cloth of gold" that glittered and gleamed under the candlelight. The early twentieth century joined metallic threads to the brilliant colors possible with new dyeing and printing techniques to make fluid lamés with gold and silver threads in either weft or warp, another innovation of the 1920s. The chroniclers of the Exposition reserved special praise for designer Michel Dubost at Ducharne for his combinations of printing and brocading. This type of fabric is well represented among the Tirocchi textiles with many spectacular lengths that show off the strengths of the Jacquard loom [cover and fig. 147, p. 172; fig. 172, p. 197; fig. 178, p. 200; fig. 179, p. 201]. A bolt of lace from the period reveals progress in this area as well. The "Leavers" lace machine was a nineteenth-century invention, but the Dognin-Racine company in Lyon, which specialized in machine-made laces, brought the process to new heights with a bolt of rayon lace with many different weaving techniques shaping a pattern of abstract, bizarre poppies. The lace, dyed brown, then discharged and printed in red, orange, and yellow according to each floral motif, is a tour de force [fig. 165].

Anna Tirocchi patronized "the big four" textile manufacturers over the years. In 1916, she was already purchasing silk surahs from Bianchini, Férier through their office in New York. Before the Exposition of 1925, she had purchased matelassés, printed crepes and crepes patterned on the loom, and brocaded lamés. A letter of August 25, 1923, notifies Anna of the dispatch from New York to Providence of sample books for "Chiffon Cascadeuse," "Crêpe

Romain," "Crêpe Éclatante," "Satin Ondoyant," "Fulgurante," "Moiré Mousmée," and "Velours Paradis." This letter reveals how the company was aiming through its product names to indicate the suppleness (cascadeuse, ondoyant) and metallic shine (éclatante, fulgurante) of its fabrics – an example of marketing the "moderne" that was widespread in industry.

Although Anna purchased many textiles directly from the French manufacturers, she also had other sources. B. Altman & Company, the New York department store, was a supplier of yard goods such as cretonne, serge, and lace throughout Anna's career. Anna also patronized John Wanamaker, the fabled Philadelphia department store with a branch in New York. John Wanamaker was the first department store to set up an office for its buyers in Paris, the first to have a resident buyer there, and the first American store to import couture directly for sale in its Philadelphia and New York stores. From 1915, John Wanamaker was a source for silks of all kinds, including pongees, velvets, and brocades, as well as ribbon trims.

A third class of suppliers for the Tirocchi shop was American importing firms with offices in New York and Paris, where they purchased textiles from firms such as Soieries F. Ducharne and Bianchini, Férier for resale in America. Anna's most important source was Harry Angelo Company, from whom she purchased textiles, "robes" (pre-embroidered fabrics for dresses), and Paris imports or copies throughout her career. In 1915, for example, Anna purchased nearly $3,000 worth of laces, trims, skirt panels, chiffons, and other textiles, while her next most important supplier, the venerable Haas Brothers, who had been operating a dry-goods store in New York since 1879, billed her for only half that amount for laces, silks, georgettes, and nets. John Wanamaker was a distant third with only $604 worth of trims, pongees, crepes, and other silks. Anna and Laura Tirocchi traveled to Paris in 1924 and 1926–27 to make purchases directly from the Paris offices of the French firms described above.

Over the years, Anna bought thousands of textiles, most of which she sold to clients and some

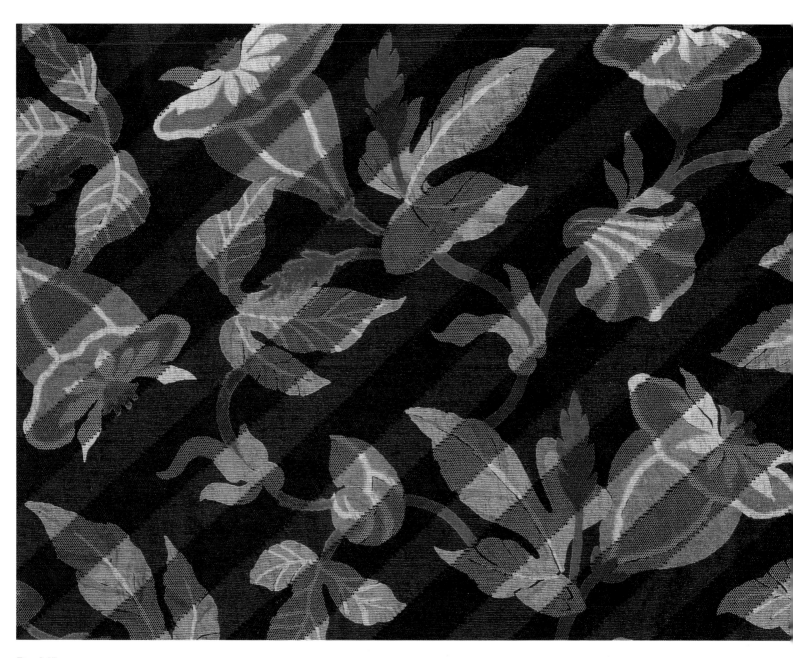

Fig. 165
Rayon Leavers lace, ca. 1930: lace-making technology enabled modernist
designs to be produced with complicated overprinting processes. Museum
of Art, RISD, gift of Dr. Louis J. Cella, Jr.

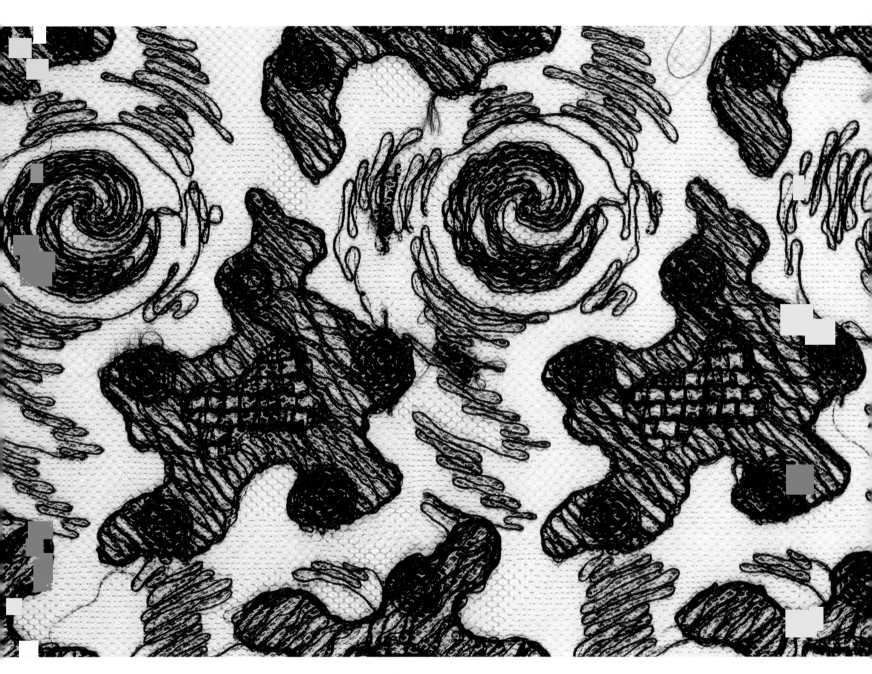

Fig. 166
"Meteor" silk lace, before 1918, with "amoeba" pattern resembling the modernist
imagery of artist Jean Arp. Museum of Art, RISD, gift of Dr. Louis J. Cella, Jr.

of which she returned, although many were still in the shop at her death and are now in RISD's collection. Taken together, they show the design developments of the thirty-odd years of the Tirocchi shop's operation. The textiles reflect not only the development of new technology during the period, but are clear evidence of the advent of modernism and the various styles that it spawned in art as well as decoration. Little remained in the shop from before 1920, but a few pieces are dated by an inventory completed in or about that year. These include several embroidered net borders and lengths patterned with traditional and modern motifs. A length of "Meteor" lace purchased from Maginnis & Thomas has an "amoeba" pattern that suggests the sculptures of Jean Arp and anticipates surrealist designs of the 1930s [fig. 166]. Two cut panels of silk with gold lamé have a stepped motif that foreshadows the "skyscraper" patterns of the late 1920s and 30s [fig. 167]. Geometric patterns also appear among these textiles, while tradition is continued in allover seed beading, florals, and chinoiserie patterns in this inventory, which also includes many examples of machine-made laces, ribbons, and silks.

The 1920s, the heyday of the shop, are represented by hundreds of pieces in the myriad of patterns common to that decade. Many textiles showing an Asian influence reflect artistic trends that predate the early twentieth century. The popularity of chinoiserie (objects or decoration in a "Westernized" Chinese style) in European art dates to the eighteenth century. When Chinese art and decorative objects began to flow into Europe in the sixteenth century, stylized chrysanthemums, Chinese fret patterns, and slim Chinese figures became a recognizable vocabulary in Western decorative arts. Particularly in the eighteenth century, furniture in the Chinese "taste," French wallpapers replete with Chinese scenes, porcelain dining services decorated with Chinese motifs, and silk textiles and ceramics painted in China for the Western market had an important influence in Britain and America, one that has infused and enlivened the decorative arts from that time until this. A "robe" dating to the mid-1920s from the Tirocchi shop is embroidered with pink, green, yellow, and ivory chinoiserie

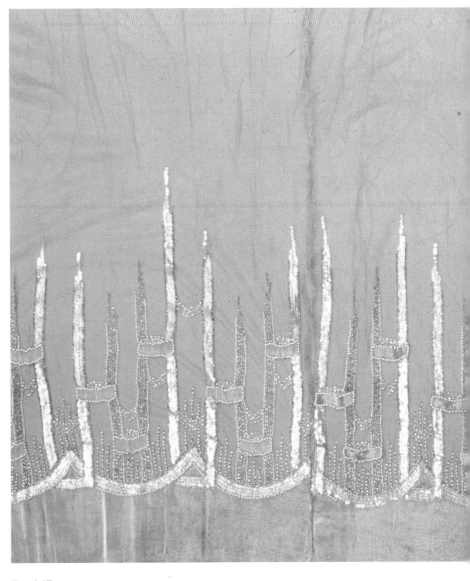

Fig. 167
Stepped, shiny, woven pattern in silk brocaded with gold and silver, ca. 1910–20, that looks forward to "machine-age" designs. Museum of Art, RISD, gift of L. J. Cella III.

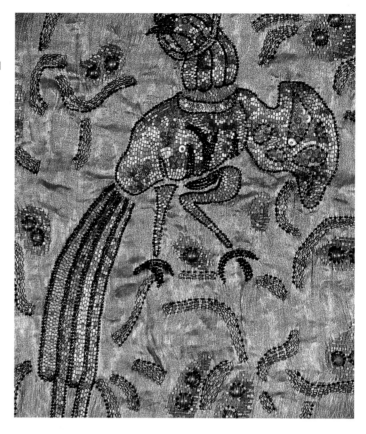

Fig. 168
Fragment of flamboyantly beaded silk fabric in the Chinese style, ca. 1926. Courtesy University of Rhode Island, Kingston, Historic Costume and Textiles Collection, gift of Dr. Louis J. Cella, Jr.

flowers and may even have been embroidered in China for the Western market. This was not a new practice: pre-embroidered pieces of fabric for clothing exist in indigenous Chinese styles from the eighteenth century. These were primarily used for imperial and official robes and may even have been common well before that time. A second chinoiserie found in the Tirocchi shop is but a fragment of what must have been a spectacular chemise dress: its exotic bird is beaded and sequined to create the maximum shine and glitter [fig. 168]. One final example is a supple silk velvet with abstract variations on the Chinese fret pattern in the bright, penetrating colors typical of French art of the time [fig. 169].

Egyptian, Indian, and Persian motifs also appear as decorative elements among the Tirocchi textiles, reflecting an interest in the art of these nations that extends back at least to the early nineteenth century. The arts of Egypt in particular were an important influence on the early nineteenth-century Empire style after Napoleon's conquest of

Egypt in the 1790s, but Persian designs were also part of this vocabulary. Increasingly, Indian elements such as "paisley" patterns came into French design after Napoleon presented his wife Josephine with Kashmir shawls that he had obtained in Egypt. French artists of the early twentieth century looked upon the Empire style as the last great truly French style, and, like couturier Paul Poiret, appropriated it for their own use. The taste for things Egyptian was given further impetus by the discovery and opening in 1922 of the tomb of King Tutankhamen with its rich cache of objects. By the mid-1920s, "Egyptomania" was in full swing. A silk border print in the Tirocchi collection imitates the wall painting, architectural ornament, and decorative art of ancient Egypt with its linear vertical arrangements of plant

Fig. 169
Luxurious silk velvet in abstract motifs based on Chinese fretwork, ca. 1920–30. Museum of Art, RISD, gift of L. J. Cella III.

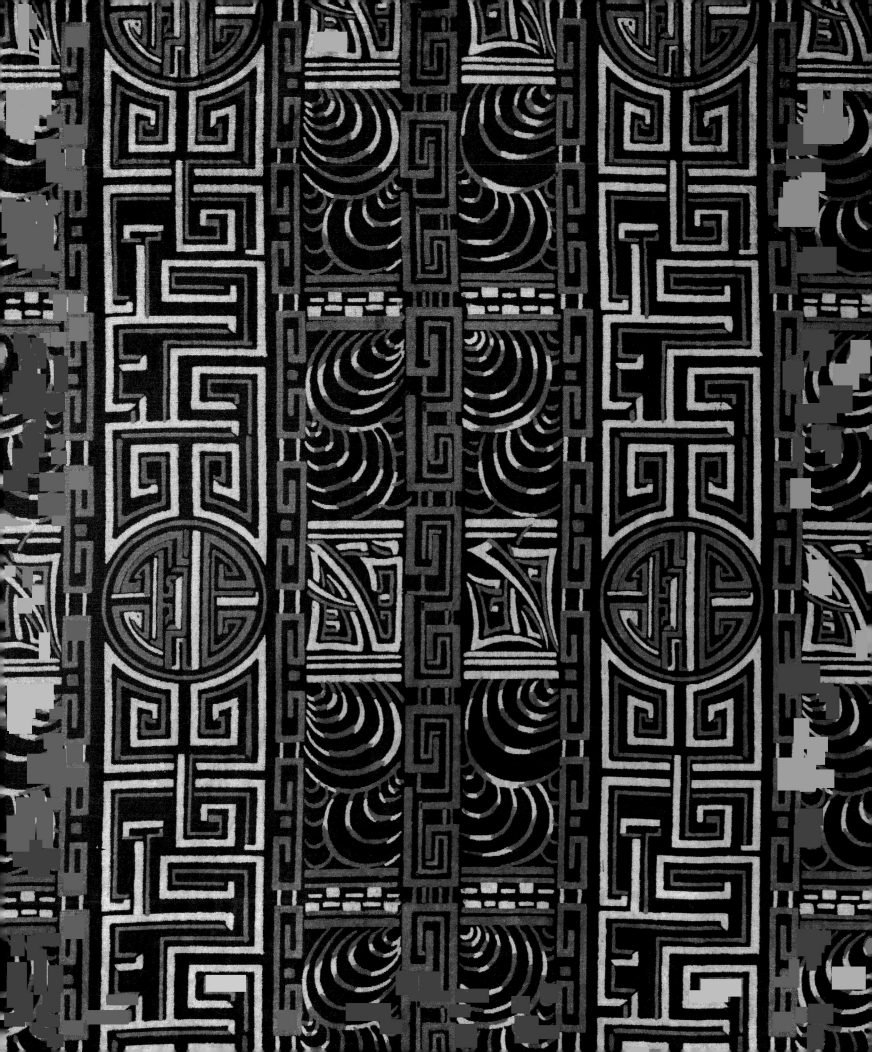

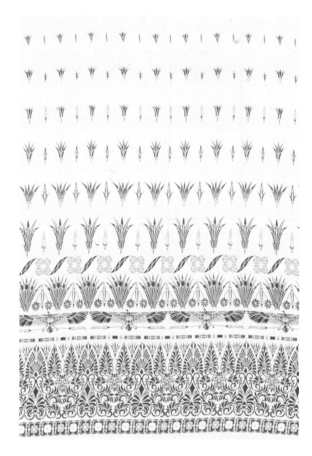

Fig. 170
Silk border print, one of many inspired by the 1922
opening of King Tutankhamen's tomb in Egypt.
Museum of Art, RISD, gift of Louis J. Cella, Jr.

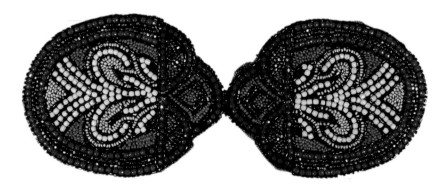

Fig. 171
Beaded dress trim, ca. 1922, with motif based on the
scarab, an ancient Egyptian good-luck charm in the
form of a dung beetle. Museum of Art, RISD, gift of
L. J. Cella III.

elements [fig. 170]. Scarabs (ancient "good-luck"
charms in the form of dung beetles) are common
among the dress trims found in the Tirocchi shop,
sometimes made of paste to be stitched at neck-
lines, formed as belt buckles, or rendered in beading on fabric patches to be sewn down as decorative
devices [fig. 171].

Japanese influence is also evident among the
textiles purchased by Anna and Laura Tirocchi.
Japonism in the Tirocchi holdings reflects a more
recent development in the art world, but still one
that predates the shop's existence. Japanese art began
to filter into the West in the nineteenth century
before 1854, the official opening of Japan to Western
trade after more than two hundred years of self-
enforced isolation. Japanese painting and woodblock prints, in particular, were collected by some
painters and influenced the work of many others in
the second half of the nineteenth century.
Collectors such as Boston's Edward Morse and the
great Parisian art dealer Siegfried Bing brought
Japanese art objects to the attention of the public in
America and France, inspiring the use of Japanese
techniques and motifs – paper parasols, cherry blos-
soms, water lilies, grasses, dragonflies, among others
– in metalwork, printmaking, and the decorative
arts, including textiles. Japanese patterns for sten-
ciled textiles were also copied and adapted by West-
erners. Japanese influence is evident in the *pochoir*
fashion illustrations produced by Paul Iribe and
others after about 1910, with their large, flat expanses
of color; black outlining; lack of perspective; and
other abstract qualities; and is also evident in the
kimono-style dresses produced by couturiers in the
early 1910s.

Among the Tirocchi fabrics is a complex lightweight gold-and-black silk lamé, which has been
dyed, discharged, and printed with a polychrome
floral design in the Japanese taste [fig. 172]. A second textile of shiny brown silk satin has Japanese
weeping willows and rippled pools of water in its
damask patterning [fig. 173]. Several lengths from
the Tirocchi shop were actually made in Japan, an
interesting reminder of Japan's desire to reach
Western markets in this period.

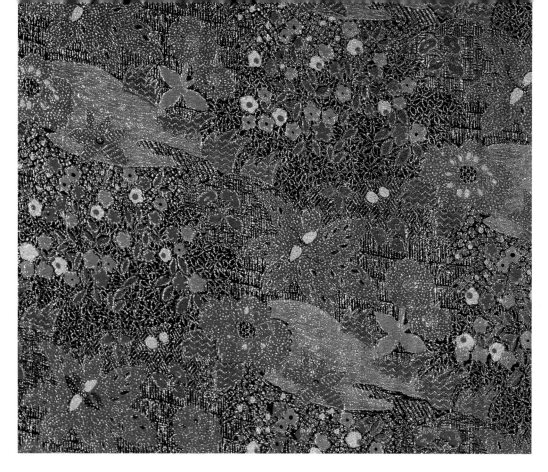

Fig. 172
Silk textile brocaded in gold with a pattern in the Japanese taste, ca. 1920–30. Museum of Art, RISD, gift of L. J. Cella III.

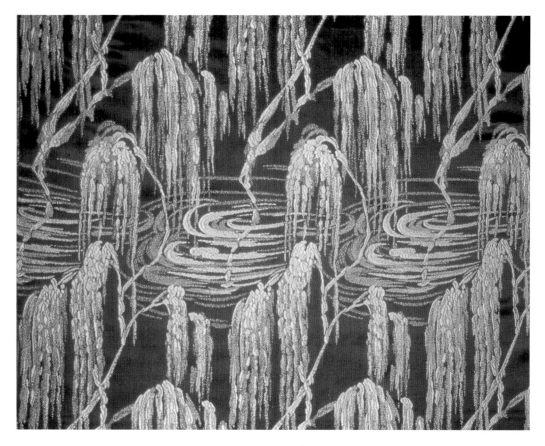

Fig. 173
Silk damask, ca. 1920–30, patterned with Japanese-style weeping willows and rippled pools of water. Museum of Art, RISD, gift of L. J. Cella III.

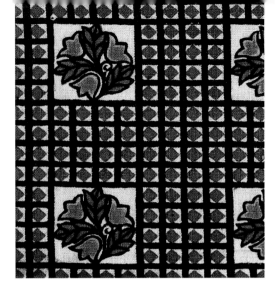

Fig. 174
Gustav Kalhammer's design for a Wiener Werkstätte textile, 1914. Courtesy Musée de l'Impression sur Étoffes, Mulhouse.

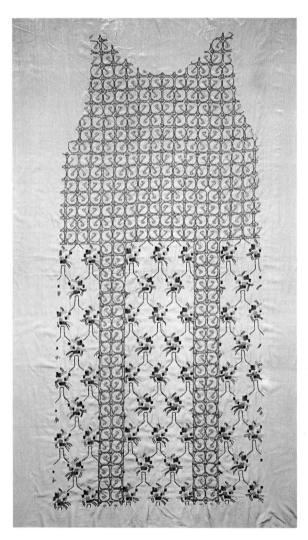

Fig. 175
Silk velvet "robe" with pattern of flowers contained within a grid, ca. 1920. Museum of Art, RISD, gift of L. J. Cella III.

Many textiles in the Tirocchi shop reflect the styles of early modernism. A "robe" of about 1926 shows the strict geometric grid and stylized floral pattern so often seen in designs before 1920 from the Wiener Werkstätte, particularly those of Josef Hoffmann, Kolomon Moser, and Gustav Kalhammer for furniture, textiles, and graphic arts [figs. 174–175]. Cubism also had its influence on fabric design, not only through its relation to modernist design principles, but also through the "primitive" art it drew upon for inspiration. Cubist admiration for the "primitive" emerges in many textiles of African and "exotic" derivation, such as a "robe" from the French embroiderers Maurice Lefranc et Compagnie with an embroidered motif and tassel based on North African patterns [fig. 176]. A bolt of silk velvet shows African shield forms combined with tiger pelts in its wide border [fig. 177]. From Bianchini, Férier came a snakeskin printed fabric with gold threads that Anna purchased in August 1926, one of many reptile-skin patterns made by several companies in the late 1920s. This silk fabric was aptly named "Fluidor" ("Liquid Gold") by Bianchini, Férier to indicate its luxurious quality to customers. A staple of their line, the fabric was still being made in the 1990s.[26]

Also reflecting the cubist preoccupation with the "primitive," textile designers sought new aesthetic elements in European "peasant" cultures in the early years of the century. Paul Poiret was at the forefront of this search in France, having traveled to Germany and Eastern Europe and collected peasant art. Further impetus came in 1909 with the first Paris performances of the Ballets Russes, whose folk costumes, brightly colored scenery, and lusty Russian designs created as much a sensation as the panache of its legendary dancers. (Russia attracted further attention as a source when constructivist artists arrived in Paris after the Russian Revolution in 1917.) Many textiles in RISD's Tirocchi holdings have motifs drawn from peasant art. Several "robes" present such elements of the "primitive" as cut-leather sequins, wooden beads, and brightly colored ribbons. One silk textile displays the onion-domed churches of Moscow in brocaded patterning done on a Jacquard loom in a Lyon studio. Combined in

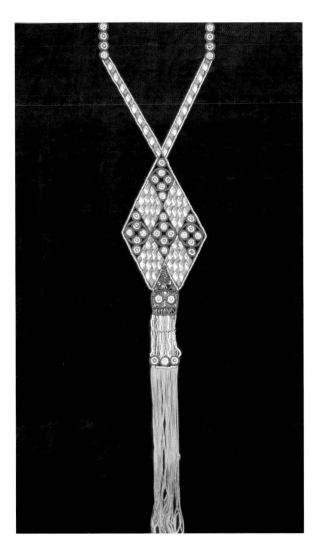

Fig. 176
Detail of an embroidered silk velvet "robe" by Maurice Lefranc et Compagnie of ca. 1926 showing North African influence in its bright colors and tassel. Museum of Art, RISD, gift of L. J. Cella III.

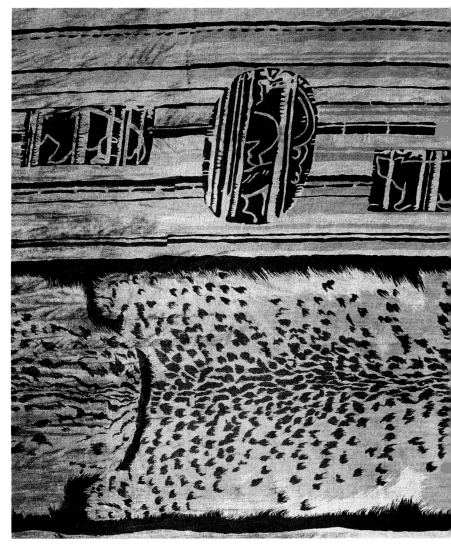

Fig. 177
Silk velvet, ca. 1926, with printed border showing African influence in its shield- and animal pelt motif. Museum of Art, RISD, gift of L. J. Cella III.

a cubist-inspired abstract row, its buildings are flattened and lacking in realistic perspective, an exotic fantasy world of violent color contrasts in orange and green [fig. 178].

Abstract shapes are often seen in the Tirocchi textiles. Perhaps the most beautiful and complex fabric found in the Tirocchi shop is a silver lamé with exquisite "cubist" pattern [cover and fig. 179]. The "leaves" are mere suggestions of natural forms, combined in a manner that denies realistic perspective, but they create a kaleidoscope of shapes and colors, much as do Henri Le Fauconnier's swirls in his *Mountaineers Attacked by Bears* of 1910–12 [fig. 180]. The unknown designer of the fabric has taken advantage of the fact that the Jacquard loom can lift

Fig. 178
Amusing silk textile, probably before 1918, with metallic gold, pink, and yellow silk weft patterning in form of the onion-domed churches of Moscow, reflecting the exoticism of the Ballets Russes. Museum of Art, RISD, gift of Dr. Louis J. Cella, Jr.

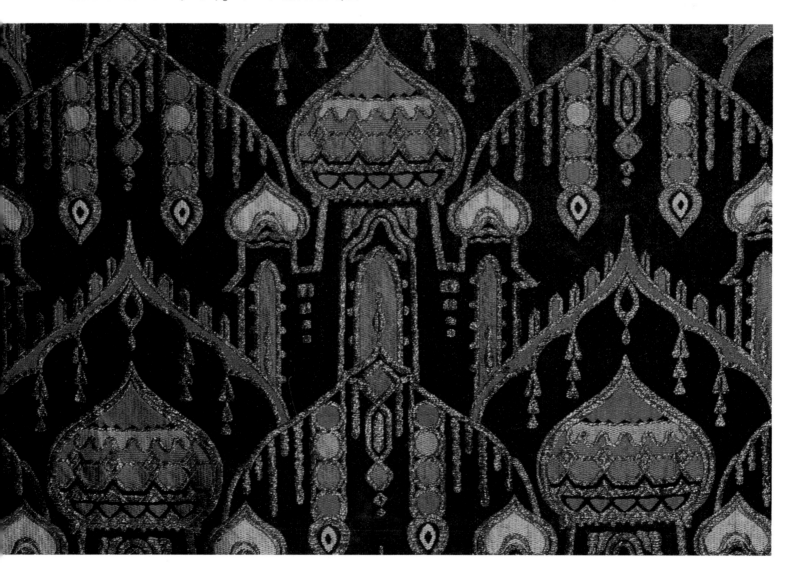

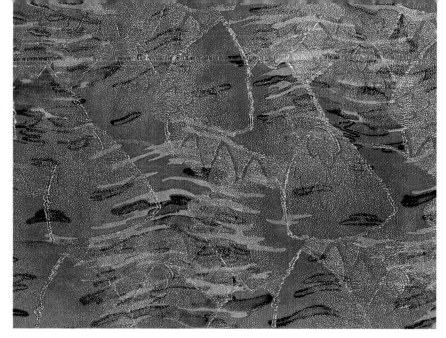

Fig. 179
Silk textile, ca. 1926, with silver
threads and cubist pattern (see
cover). Museum of Art, RISD,
gift of Dr. Louis J. Cella, Jr.

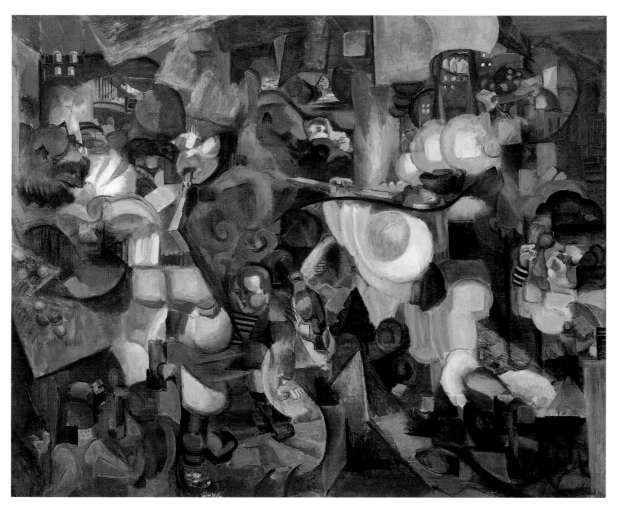

Fig. 180
Henri Le Fauconnier's cubist oil on canvas, *Mountaineers Attacked by Bears,* 1910–12, exhibiting
the abstraction and multiple points of view also employed by modernist textile designers to great
effect. Museum of Art, RISD, gift of the Peau de l'Ours Society II in celebration of Daniel Robbins.

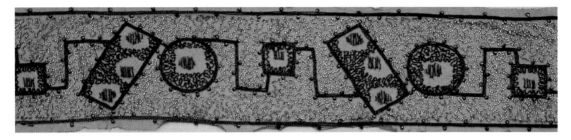

Fig. 181
Dress trim, ca. 1920, of silk lace with abstract pattern.
Museum of Art, RISD, gift of L. J. Cella III.

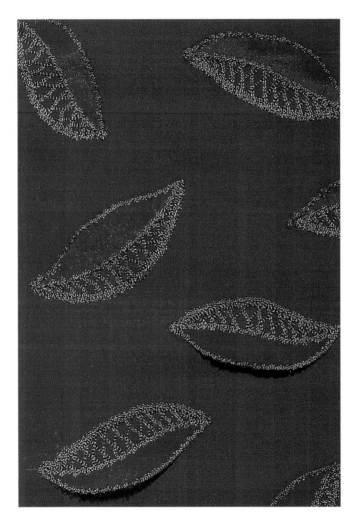

Fig. 182
Detail of a silk chiffon "robe" with applied stylized leaf shapes
that form a collage. Museum of Art, RISD, gift of L. J. Cella III.

each warp independently, creating the effect of scattered pinpoints of light where the silver thread appears on the surface. The blue dye of the ground has then been discharged with bleach and overprinted to create an abstract, modernist pattern. A dress trim based on abstract geometric figures exhibits simple rectangles and circles, which, while oriented in unexpected ways, remain in the band demarcated by the edges of the trim, a flat assemblage of forms [fig. 181]. Collage is the basic reference for a "robe" of red chiffon [fig. 182] with a skirt composed of separate leaves sewn onto a base fabric.

Two textiles based on abstract geometric forms show different ways of treating lines and grids according to cubist principles. A fragment of heavy wool fabric is marked by a linear grid and straight lines, creating an abstract composition in black, gray, and white. Probably from Rodier, it resembles the many identified abstract patterns that were the mainstay of this company in the early to middle 1920s, while its handwoven look is a Rodier trademark [fig. 183]. A printed organdy's patterning might suggest that it had been based on a simple plaid, but the straight lines of the plaid have been displaced and its grid splintered into fragments, which form an intriguing abstraction that nevertheless clings to the flat plane of the fabric [fig. 184], instead of emerging energetically like the optically illusionary Rodier wool. The organdy's abstract forms owe a debt to constructivist art with its painterly yet fanciful devices [fig. 185].

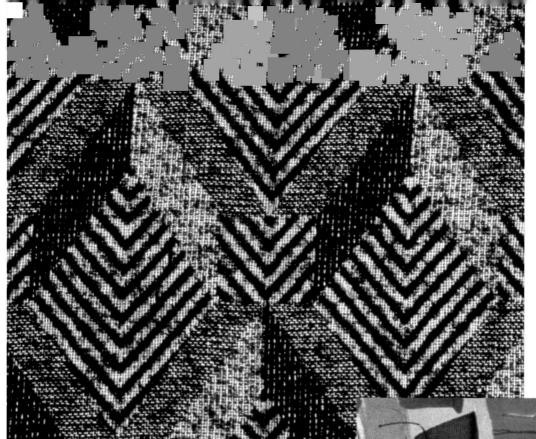

Fig. 183
Heavy wool textile with geometric patterning, ca. 1920–30, probably by Rodier. Museum of Art, RISD, gift of L. J. Cella III.

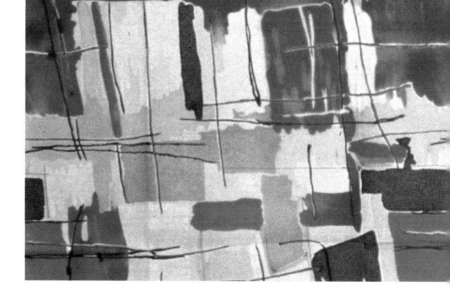

Fig. 184
Silk organdy with a printed abstract plaid, ca. 1920–40. Museum of Art, RISD, gift of L. J. Cella III.

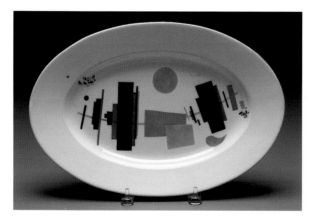

Fig. 185
Constructivist porcelain platter, ca. 1920, with overglaze enamel decoration based on a drawing by Kasimir Malevich. Museum of Art, RISD, gift of Alfred T. Morris, Jr.

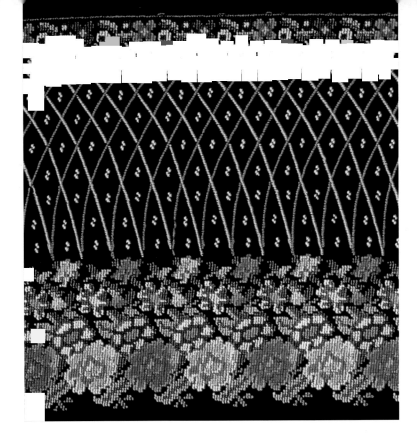

Fig. 186
Detail of a silk-velvet "robe" with "*moderne*" flowers in silk-floss embroidery, ca. 1926. Courtesy University of Rhode Island, Kingston, Historic Costume and Textile Collection, gift of Dr. Louis J. Cella, Jr.

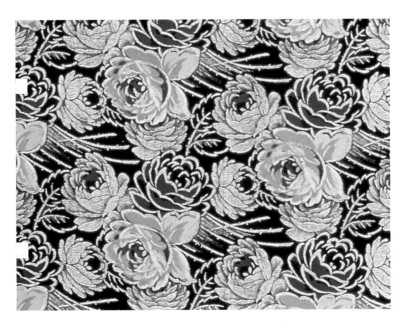

Fig. 187
Plain-weave silk fabric with printed "*moderne*" flower, 1931. Museum of Art, RISD, gift of L. J. Cella III.

By the middle of the 1920s, modernism was firmly established, and French textile artists had adopted abstraction and flat patterning from it. Merging these principles with the intense colors first promoted by Matisse and the fauvists in 1905 and incorporating a taste for the hard-edged shine of a new "machine-age" aesthetic coming from America, French decorative design finally achieved its much desired new national style. The "*moderne*," familiar also by its later sobriquet of "Art Deco," is widely reflected in some of the most spectacular and luxurious textiles found in the Tirocchi shop. The "*moderne*" flower, actually derived from flowers drawn by Scottish artist/architect Charles Rennie Mackintosh in the 1890s, was adopted by French artists before 1910. This flower appears in many Tirocchi textiles, including "robes," laces, and printed fabrics. An unmade black velvet "robe" has not only the "*moderne*" flower, but also shows its debt to peasant art with its brightly colored embroidery of thick silk floss [fig. 186]. Another version exists in a stiff gold lamé cloth of about 1925 with patterning wefts tied into stripes of black, blue, red, white, and green Jacquard twill. By 1931, fabrics had become much lighter in weight, but the "*moderne*" flower was still popular. Another textile, purchased from the New York importing company of Harry Angelo in 1931, bears "*moderne*" flowers with hard edges typical of the more rigidly outlined "machine-age" imagery [fig. 187]. With its supple hand, it would have been appropriate for a draped dress with that year's fluid silhouette.

An outstanding characteristic of "*moderne*" French fabrics is their out-and-out luxury. By this time, the French textile industry had long since reestablished itself worldwide as the primary supplier

Fig. 188
Brocaded silk textile ordered by Anna Tirocchi from Bianchini, Férier in 1929, found in the pattern books of that company at the Musée des Tissus de Lyon: RISD's curator traced it from its order number on the invoice in the Tirocchi Archive. Courtesy Musée des Tissus de Lyon, design copyright Bianchini-Férier (photograph by Pierre Verrier).

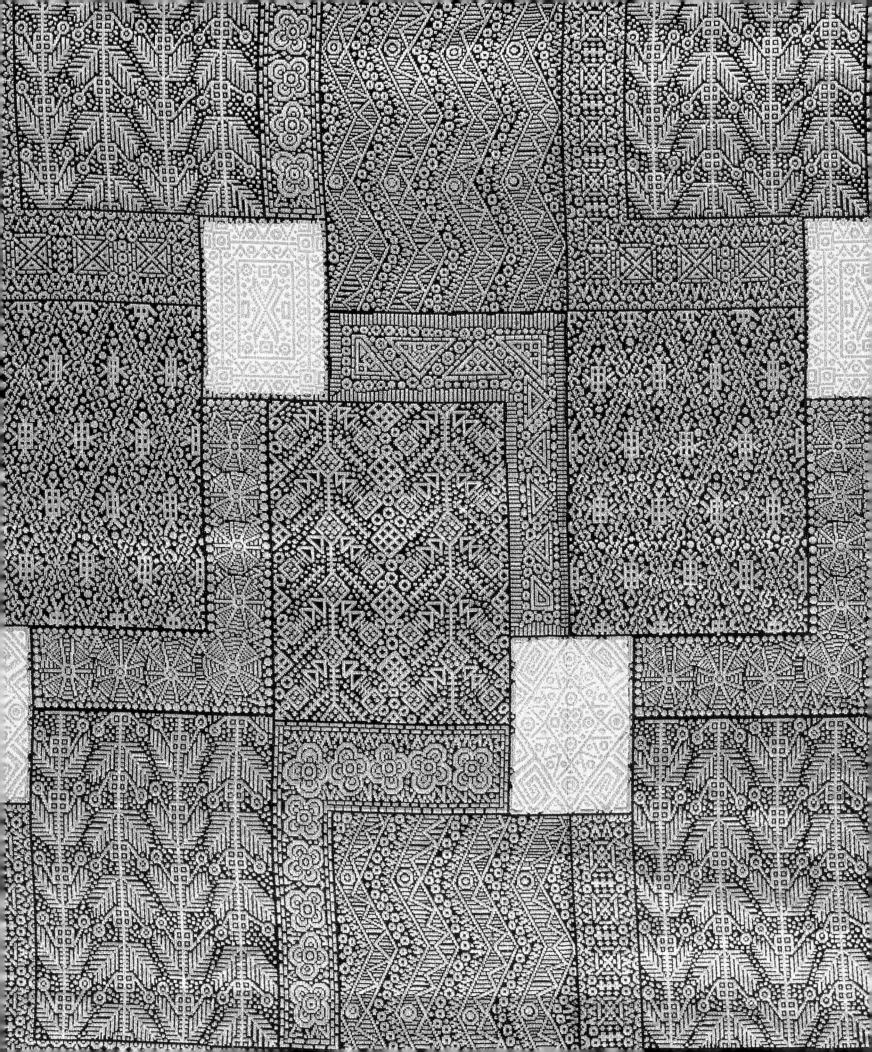

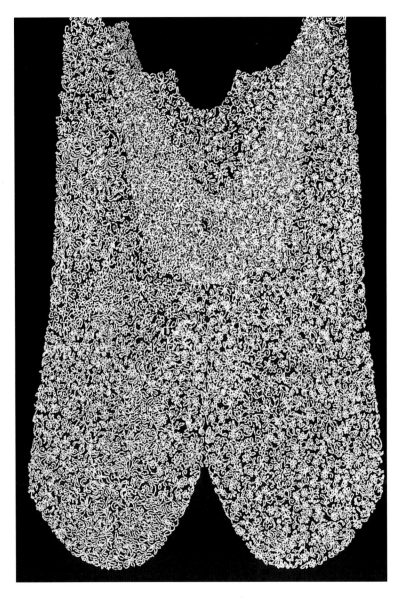

of sumptuous fabrics for fashion. Anna and Laura Tirocchi were quick to profit from this. In 1929, Anna Tirocchi ordered a fabric from Bianchini, Férier that was of unparalleled richness. A black silk chiffon, completely encrusted with brocaded gold threads in a geometric pattern, it was made into a garment and sold immediately to a client [fig. 188]. Another fabric dates from March 1929 and was imported by the Harry Angelo Company. It is a "robe" with a black chiffon bodice, down to tunic length, which is embroidered with thousands of tiny white seed beads in a scroll pattern [fig. 189]. When sewn together, the dress would have had a softly full short skirt of plain black chiffon. The cost to Anna Tirocchi was $39.50. A third example of the French idea of chic luxury is a "robe" dated to fall 1932, also from Harry Angelo Company. By this time, hemlines had descended and the silhouette was closer to the body. This unmade jacket is of a black silk crepe embroidered in stylized roundels reminiscent of Chinese design [fig. 190], a bargain at only $20. The fabric, sewn to a buckram band, was accompanied by a drawing of the jacket the Tirocchis were to produce from it, tight to the body, but with long, full sleeves, the better to show off the large expanses of black and gold. These fabrics form a perfect advertisement for the newly rejuvenated French textile industry and illustrate in an immediate way the reason French textiles were so beloved by the elite Tirocchi clientele.

Fig. 189
Detail of a "robe" of 1929, showing the exquisite luxury of tiny beads sewn to silk chiffon. Museum of Art, RISD, gift of L. J. Cella III.

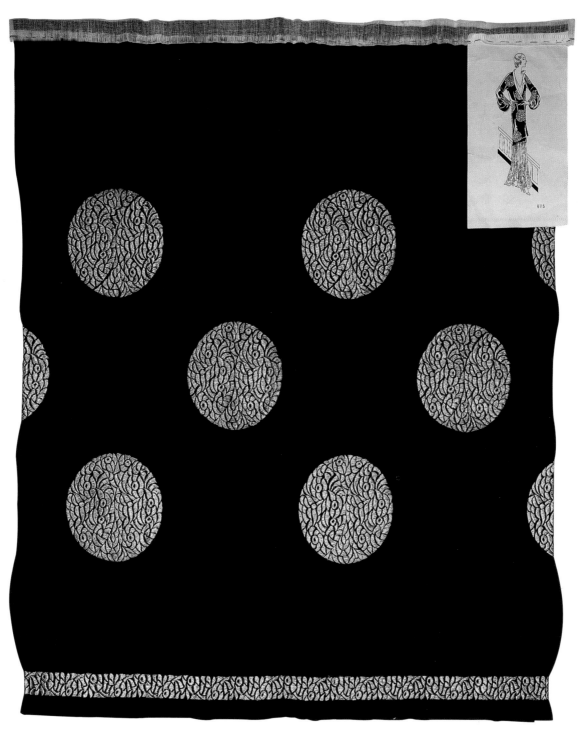

Fig. 190
One part of a silk "robe" of 1932 from Harry Angelo Company with brocaded gold circles: the
sketch, attached to the buckram band that holds the parts of the "robe" together, is meant
to show the dressmaker what the finished garment should look like. Museum of Art, RISD, gift of
L. J. Cella III.

In the 1920s, dress trims, clips, and jewelry echoed textile motifs. They illustrate in a most charmingly miniature form some of the artistic concerns of the era. A Japonist dress ornament with a cream-colored figure of a Japanese woman and child attached to a dark medallion is a particularly appealing detail [fig. 191]. Its tag reveals that Anna patronized other establishments besides suppliers to the couture. According to its attached tag (not shown), she purchased the medallion in Paris on the third floor of the Printemps department store; thus it must date to 1924 or 1926–27, the dates of her two trips to the city. Another ornament, a large plaque with Chinese lettering and a long black silk fringe and lacquered beads, reflects the popularity of Oriental motifs of all kinds.

"Machine-age" motifs of the 1930s seem particularly suited to jeweled trims. The geometric arrangements of rhinestones found in two pieces from the Tirocchi shop reflect this purist aesthetic. Their quintessential Art Deco look is based on the strict alignment of simple components: circles, rectangles, and straight lines. One, a belt buckle, is based on a pattern of interrelated circles and rectangles [fig. 192], while a pin is set with rhinestones in a step-back pattern that echoes skyscraper designs [fig. 193]. They seem especially designed to add sophistication and glitter to a classic streamlined black gown of the 1930s. The Tirocchis kept many of these pieces in small trays covered in black that showed off the modernist designs to perfection [fig. 194]. Among the jewelry is a small pin with steely glitter and purity of line reminiscent of nothing so much as the wheels and struts of America's streamlined locomotives [fig. 195]. Like much of the jewelry from the shop, it is an example of pure "machine-age" inspiration.

By the end of the 1920s, Anna Tirocchi was purchasing fewer and fewer textiles to make up and more and more ready-to-wear. The fabrics in the shop from 1930 on include many plain-colored crepes and satins, appropriate for the new streamlined silhouette that looked to "machine-age" designs, for Anna continued to custom-make some outfits, mainly for older clients. Not all plain-colored

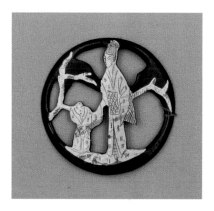

Fig. 191
Charming Japonist dress ornament of 1924 or 1926 in bakelite by an unknown artist for Printemps, Paris; found in the Tirocchi shop, 1990. Museum of Art, RISD, gift of L. J. Cella III (photograph by Cathy Carver).

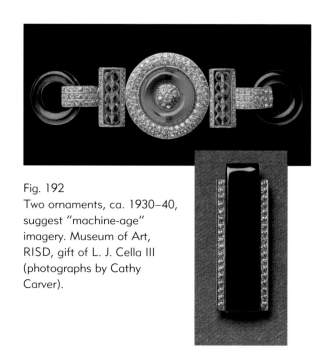

Fig. 192
Two ornaments, ca. 1930–40, suggest "machine-age" imagery. Museum of Art, RISD, gift of L. J. Cella III (photographs by Cathy Carver).

Fig. 193

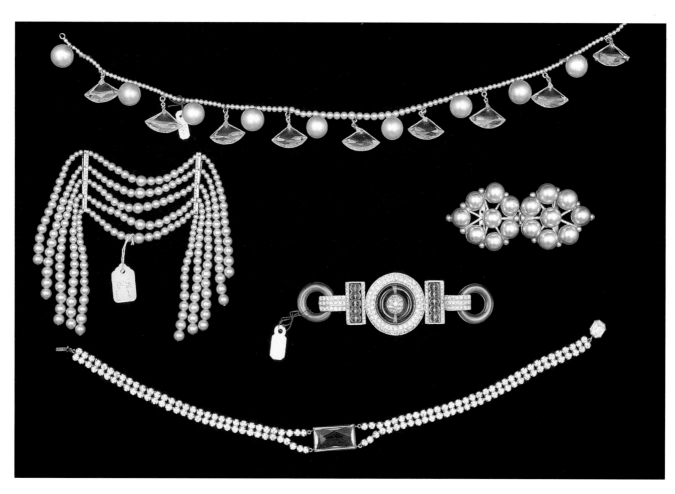

Fig. 194
Jewelry tray just as it was found in the Tirocchi shop in 1990,
displaying an Egyptian-inspired necklace (top), as well as
the buckle in fig. 192, against a stark black background
(photograph by Cathy Carver).

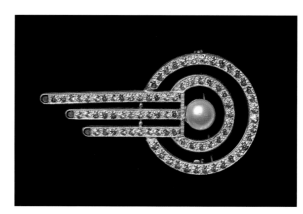

Fig. 195
Rhinestone pin found in the
Tirocchi shop, 1990. Museum of
Art, RISD, gift of L. J. Cella III
(photograph by Cathy Carver).

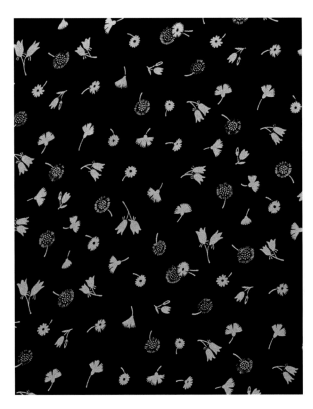

Fig. 197
Printed rayon fabric, ca. 1933, with a smaller, more realistically depicted floral pattern than the *"moderne"* examples it had supplanted by the mid-1930s. Museum of Art, RISD, gift of Dr. Louis J. Cella, Jr.

Fig. 196
Silk damask, ca. 1932, based on a Renaissance textile pattern, imported by Robert Gussaroff. Museum of Art, RISD, gift of L. J. Cella III.

fabrics were unadorned, however. A sumptuous navy silk damask with a large pattern of floral cornucopias that harks back to seventeenth-century textile design came from importer Robert Gussaroff of New York around 1932 [fig. 196].

Printed silks continued to be an important part of Anna's textile purchases, but abstract *"moderne"* florals such as the one illustrated in figure 187 (p. 204) were giving way to traditional, realistic flower prints that had, despite modernism, remained popular all through the 1920s. The change to lighter-weight fabrics brought about an adjustment in pattern size. The large-scale, heavy lamés that prevailed in the early 1920s gave way to smaller designs, a decrease in the use of metallic yarns, and generally more flexible fabrics. Printed plain-weave silks and lightweight crepes were strewn with flowers in small motifs [fig. 197], unlike the elaborate garden effect of some 1920s floral lamés. Anna Tirocchi's selections were right up to the moment, and they paralleled developments in the French textile firms that were the source of most fabrics sold in Europe and New York.

A glance at the records of two of the "big four" textile firms shows how closely Anna followed French design trends over the years and how precisely her choices reflected the advent of modernism in French design. Bianchini, Férier's records have survived, including sample books and sketches from the date of the firm's founding in 1888, and cover the entire period of operation of the Tirocchi shop. From the beginning, Charles Bianchini had shown his interest in novelty. In 1889, one of the most interesting textiles in the Paris Universal Exposition was a design in which he rejected the revivalism that permeated the period, opting for a pattern of chrysanthemums in the Japanese "taste." In 1900, he was still purchasing Japonist designs, but he also chose patterns with English influence that incorporated the stylized plant forms of William Morris, Charles Rennie Mackintosh, and Liberty of London. Modernism was already underway at Atuyer, Bianchini, Férier even at this early date. Charles Bianchini responded quickly to avant-garde design trends. In 1907, his firm's first peasant designs appeared, anticipating the move to bold colors that would be stimulated by the 1909 Paris performances of the Ballets Russes. In 1910, art nouveau was nearly gone from Bianchini's repertoire, with only three patterns in contrast to at least twelve in 1900. At the end of the first decade of the twentieth century, he was interested not only in patterns in Morris and Liberty of London styles, but also in bold geometrics with Wiener Werkstätte influence and equally bold flat-patterned florals.

Bianchini, Férier's "Grands Livres" contain swatches of the textiles that were produced from this early period, showing how modernism blossomed at the company. The company's books of printed designs, "Impression," begin before 1910 and show Charles Bianchini's wonderful eye for graphic patterns that could be used to create elegant and unusual clothing. Printed textiles were his strength, and these record books present one after another in samples measuring about eighteen inches square. The earliest books already display printed Viennese-style patterns derived from his cache of designs purchased in Austria. A floral related to Gustav Klimt's style appears in the very first book [see fig. 150, p. 178], along with patterns derived from exotic batiks from Indonesia, velvets with Persian patterns, and, more traditionally, *indienne* prints that reflected the design of eighteenth-century *toiles de Jouy*, derived from fabrics imported from India in the seventeenth and eighteenth centuries. Flower patterns are the most common, together with Medieval- and Renaissance-revival styles and the occasional Eastern European peasant pattern.

Many realistic flower patterns represent a tradition that does not decline over the years, but as the 1910s advance, more and more abstract "*moderne*" florals appear. Bright and dark jeweled-tone colors arrive in the second book, reflecting the influence of the fauvist painters. Even chinoiserie patterns take on these colorations, giving a modernist look to the most traditional of designs [fig. 198]. In the third book, which encompasses the years 1910–12, designs by both Raoul Dufy and Paul Iribe appear, and "*moderne*" florals roughly equal the number of traditional designs.

Fig. 198
Textile, ca. 1910, printed with modernist dark jewel tones on silk chiffon brocaded with gold threads in a traditional chinoiserie pattern. Courtesy Musée des Tissus de Lyon; design copyright Bianchini-Férier (photograph by Pierre Verrier).

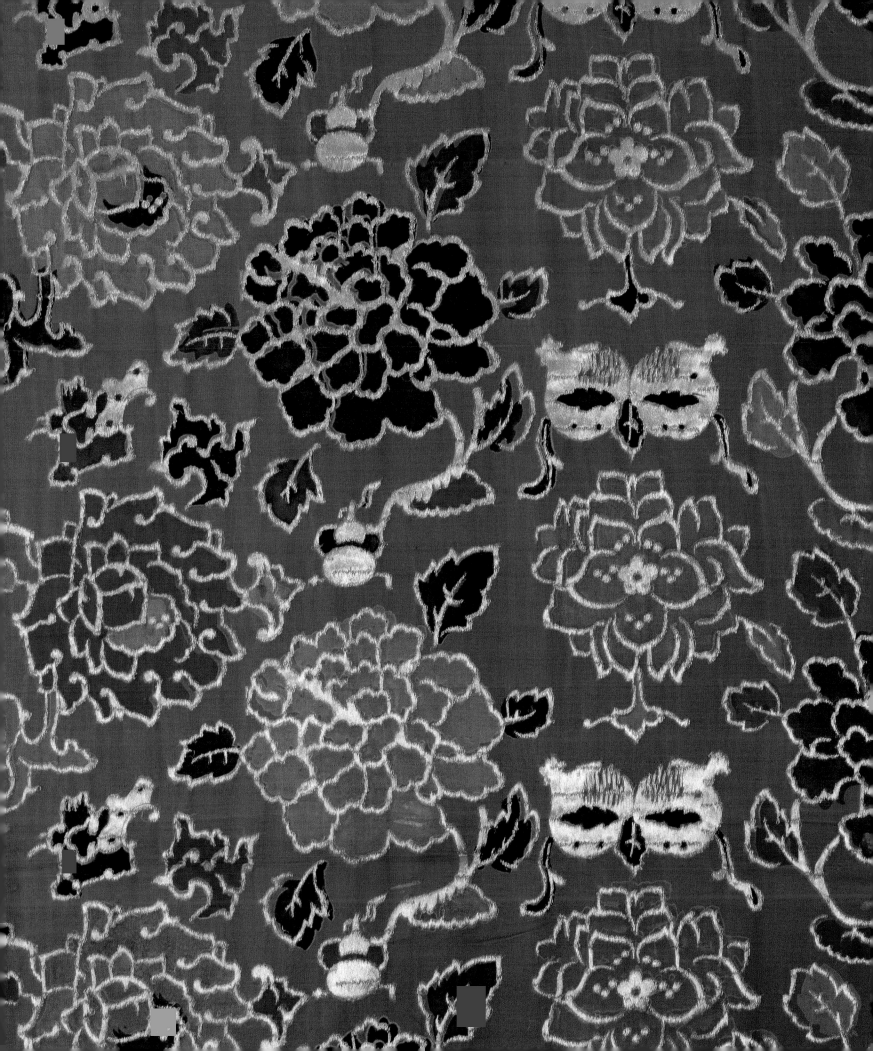

Fig. 199
Large-scale silk voided velvet, ca. 1912, with a chiffon ground, based on a Renaissance velvet pattern: a *"moderne"* floral pattern by Raoul Dufy has been superimposed by discharge printing. Courtesy Musée des Tissus de Lyon; design copyright Bianchini-Férier (photograph by Pierre Verrier).

In the following books, "Viennese" designs continue to appear, but a new and brilliant combination of weaving and printing techniques emerges around 1913. Bianchini had arrived at the idea of chinoiserie patterns printed on velvets with voided Renaissance-revival patterns, large florals printed on damask patterned with "paisley" designs derived from Kashmir shawls, even florals by Raoul Dufy printed on velvets with huge Renaissance-inspired patterns [fig. 199]. These are perhaps Bianchini, Férier's masterpieces, produced only during the 1910s and early 1920s. The imaginative superimposition of patterning creates many levels and points of view, echoing modernist concerns and creating an interesting textile counterpart to the cubist method of collage.

Pattern sample books with textile swatches have also been preserved from the Lyon company of Coudurier-Fructus-Descher in the Musée des Tissus de Lyon. Coudurier-Fructus-Descher, like Atuyer, Bianchini, Férier, responded to developments in the art world, but perhaps less immediately. Its early books reveal many revival designs, from lacy eighteenth-century brocaded silks to Renaissance-revival lamés and realistic florals. Like Atuyer, Bianchini, Férier, Coudurier-Fructus-Descher was a exponent of Japonist and art nouveau patterns in 1900, but it is clear that this house also was responding to textile design influences from abroad, especially Britain. The English influence is explicit, as with the product names that include the famous arts and crafts London department store by name: "Liberty Imprimé," "Liberty Cachemire," or "Satin Liberty," indicating types of woven textiles rather than patterns. Far fewer Coudurier-Fructus-Descher patterns were forward-looking before 1910 than those of Atuyer, Bianchini, Férier.

In 1910, pastel colors predominate, and fabric weights are medium to heavy, even for summer. The modern world begins to creep into Coudurier-Fructus-Descher's products, if only into their names. "Toile auto," "twill flyer," and "moiré radium" all reflect contemporary developments. "Satin Marconi" exhibits an undulating wave pattern that the designer must have thought related to telegraphic transmission or to sound waves. Art nouveau patterns occasionally appear, but there are only two abstract florals or patterns influenced by Charles Rennie Mackintosh [fig. 200]. The following year, 1911, saw a number of modernist changes. In the winter of 1910, four years later than at Atuyer, Bianchini, Férier, bright colors make an entrance: purples, oranges, greens, and reds that reflect the bright unreality of the fauvist painters. Coudurier-Fructus-Descher's metallic lamés now have large areas of glittering gold and silver or patterns in satin weave in stylized floral and Kashmir patterns, reflecting a growing taste for shiny surfaces that previews the coming "machine-age" aesthetic. Abstract motifs also begin to appear. Of 106 patterns produced for winter 1910–11, 14 were decidedly modernistic, ranging from "electric" zig-zags to "Russian" florals in bright peasant colors. In summer 1911, a few small abstract florals reflecting the style of Raoul Dufy's designs for Atuyer, Bianchini, Férier begin to appear in Coudurier-Fructus-Descher's line. The overall predominance of small- and medium-scale traditional patterns continues, however, with only 35 abstract floral patterns out of 198 textiles produced for that season.

By 1915, when the Tirocchi shop opened at 514 Broadway, "moderne" patterns were still the exception rather than the rule. Only 22 of 126 patterns produced by Coudurier-Fructus-Descher for summer 1915 were "moderne," but the abstract, stylized flower was prominent among them. By contrast, the Bianchini, Férier book for 1915 has twice as many "moderne" as traditional florals and includes more than twenty-five abstract geometric designs.

During the late 1910s and after the First World War, French textiles underwent a change in scale. By 1920, both Coudurier-Fructus-Descher and Bianchini, Férier's books included many huge floral, Kashmir, and chinoiserie patterns. The scale of these patterns had expanded greatly since 1915, and the weight of the fabrics had shifted from medium-to-heavy to medium to light. By now, Coudurier-Fructus-Descher had accepted modernist principles, and fully sixty-four patterns represent "moderne" design, including one printed textile with huge

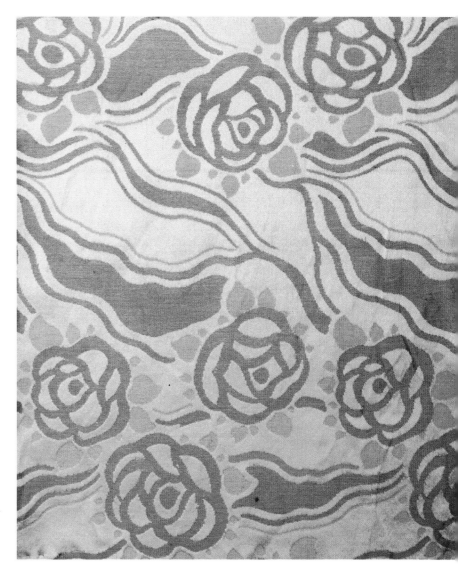

Fig. 200
Coudurier-Fructus-Descher's silk "façonné satin dorure" ("satin brocaded with gold") of 1910–11, one of the first modernist patterns produced by that company. Courtesy Musée des Tissus de Lyon (photograph by Pierre Verrier).

Fig. 201
Modernist silk printed at Coudurier-
Fructus-Descher in 1920 that resembles
the silk and metallic silver textile in fig. 147,
p. 172. Courtesy Musée des Tissus de
Lyon (photograph by Pierre Verrier).

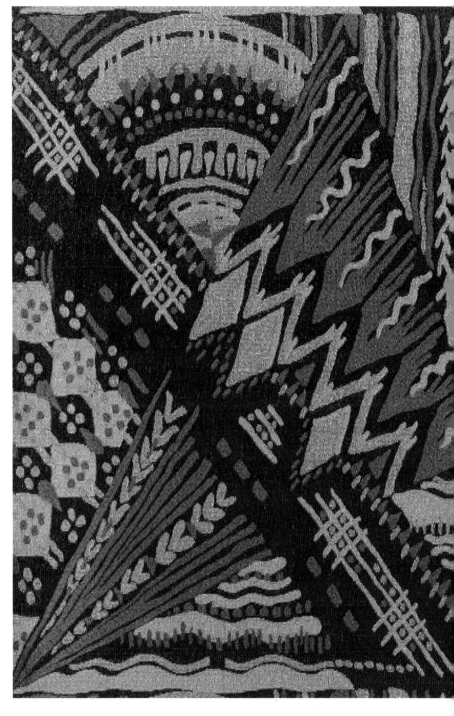

Fig. 202
Complex crepe of 1926, woven by Coudurier-Fructus-
Descher in silk, viscose, and rayon. Courtesy Musée
des Tissus de Lyon (photograph by Pierre Verrier).

flowers [fig. 201] not unlike the fabric used by the Tirocchis for an opera coat [fig. 147, p. 172]. In contrast to Bianchini, Férier, Coudurier-Fructus-Descher was finding its niche in the weaving of extremely complicated brocaded textiles in lampas and double- and triple-cloth techniques with the addition of gold and silver threads. Superimposition of patterning at Coudurier-Fructus-Descher took the form of the combination of weaving techniques: satin stripes with patterned brocade or many-layered woven patterns that fully used the technical potential of the Jacquard loom [fig. 202].

Other patterns reflect the "exotic" inspiration associated with cubist art. Once again, Coudurier-Fructus-Descher's fabric names are revealing. A decided interest in exoticism is evident in "Crêpe Égyptienne," "Crêpe Rajah," "Moiré Saigonnaise," and "Crêpe Muscadin." By 1925, all the depth and breadth of Anna Tirocchi's contemporary taste are reflected in the sample books: modernist Japonist designs; chinoiseries; Kashmir patterns; huge geometric lamés; cubist patterns; exotic designs reflecting the art of Africa or Southeast Asia; and many small-, medium-, and large-scale "moderne" floral patterns.

Textiles manufactured by Bianchini, Férier; Coudurier-Fructus-Descher; and by Soieries F. Ducharne confirm another aspect of French design reflected in the textiles purchased by Anna Tirocchi for her American clients. At the same time that many modernist textiles were being woven in Lyon, other more traditional designs also were being produced by the very same firms. Small geometrics, realistic florals, Renaissance and Medieval motifs continued to be popular throughout the whole period of operation of the Tirocchi shop. They formed an important part of French textile production in 1925 – even at Bianchini, Férier, the leader in modernist design – at what has traditionally been considered to be the height of the *"moderne"*/Art Deco style.

It is often thought that the Exposition des Arts Décoratifs et Industriels Modernes of 1925 popularized *"moderne"* design in America, but textiles in the Tirocchi shop belie this notion. Several modernist designs are documented in the pre-1920s inventory and others can be dated to well before 1925. The early modern design vocabulary had become known in this country first through posters, magazine illustrations, the decorative arts, and other media, and subsequently through painting and sculpture, which were largely seen for the first time at the

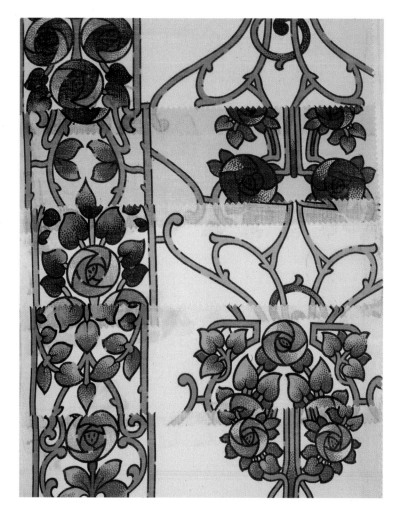

Armory Show in New York in 1913. An examination of American textile samples from as early as 1910 by just one American manufacturer shows that modernism had already arrived in fabric produced for the mass market. In December 1910, at the very time that Paul Poiret and Charles Bianchini were adopting the *"moderne"* rose, the Arnold Printworks of North Adams, Massachusetts, was producing nearly seventy-five thousand yards of a roller print on scrim for curtains with the same flower [fig. 203]. Other stylized florals were also popular, perhaps based on Wiener Werkstätte textiles. That American printworks knew about avant-garde European textile design is certain. Many mills subscribed to pattern services. Claude Frères of Lyon supplied silk and woolen swatches on a monthly basis (many are preserved in the collection of the RISD Museum) to many manufacturers, including Arnold Printworks and the Empire Silk Company in Paterson, New Jersey. Publications such as *Vogue, Harper's Bazaar,* and the *American Silk Journal* also kept American manufacturers abreast of European design.

The skill with which Anna and Laura Tirocchi melded their taste with the already prevailing sense of the modern illustrates once again the reason for the survival of their business beyond the life of many other dressmaking establishments. Just as Anna Tirocchi took advantage of the changeover to ready-to-wear clothing by embracing it, she also adopted modernist French textiles as the basis for her custom trade, which she was able to continue well into the 1930s, although on a declining basis, until she was too old and too ill to sew. The last textiles in the Tirocchi shop date from the early 1940s. Silk and woolen samples, printed rayon textiles, zippers, and a few design folders advertising wartime production constitute a remarkable resource for this period, even as the Tirocchi shop closed and the objects in it were tucked away for posterity.

Fig. 203
Swatches of a cotton curtain scrim, 1910, by the Arnold Printworks of North Adams (Massachusetts), printed on both sides with a *"moderne"* flower pattern, from Arnold Printworks, vol. 83, 1910. Courtesy American Textile History Museum, Lowell (photograph by Kevin Harkins).

1. Florence M. Montgomery, *Textiles in America, 1650–1870.* New York; n.d., pp. 144, 218, 239, 269, 312, 324, and 348.

2. *Ibid.*, pp. 205–06, 312, and 324–25.

3. *Ibid.*, p. 348.

4. Pamela Parmal, "Welcome Arnold and Textiles." Paper presented at the Dublin Seminar, Deerfield, Massachusetts, June 28, 1997.

5. See Susan Hay, "Adolphe Braun and Textile Design," in Maureen O'Brien and Mary Bergstein, eds., *Image and Enterprise: The Photographs of Adolphe Braun.* Providence and London: 1999, pp. 44–65. For an account of Lyon designers, see Florence Charpigny, "Between Tradition and Modernity: Textile Design Education in Lyons at the Beginning of the 20th Century." Paper presented at the Textile Society of America Symposium, Fashion Institute of Technology, New York, September 26, 1998; typescript courtesy of the author.

6. See Yvonne Brunhammer and Suzanne Tise, *The Decorative Arts in France: La Société des Artistes Décorateurs, 1900–1942.* New York: 1990, pp. 12–14.

7. Quoted from the Vienna Trade Register entry of May 12, 1903, in Werner J. Schweiger, *Wiener Werkstätte: Design in Vienna, 1903–1932.* New York: 1984, p. 27.

8. Brunhammer and Tise, *op. cit.*, pp. 269–84.

9. Anne Stauffacher, "L'Évolution stylistique de la fleur dans l'industrie du textile. Un exemple: l'atelier Martine." Mémoire de maîtrise, Sorbonne, Université de Paris, n.d., p. 14; typescript in the Musée des Arts Décoratifs, Paris.

10. Anne Tourlonias and Jack Vidal, *Raoul Dufy, l'oeuvre en soie: logique d'un oeuvre ornemental industriel.* Avignon: 1998, p. 23.

11. Dora Perez-Tibi, *Dufy.* New York: 1989, p. 57.

12. Paul Poiret, *En Habillant l'époque*, Paris: 1930, p. 150.

13. Quoted in Perez-Tibi, *op. cit.*, p. 24.

14. *Ibid.*, p. 70.

15. Pierre Vernus gives the history of this forward-looking company in his unpublished Thèse de doctorat d'histoire, entitled "Bianchini-Férier, fabricant de soieries à Lyon (1888–1973)," Université Lumière Lyon II, 1997. Typescript courtesy of the author.

16. Tourlonias and Vidal, *op. cit.*, p. 27.

17. *Ibid.*, p. 42.

18. Giuliano Ercoli, *Art Deco Prints.* New York: 1989, p. 11.

19. *Ibid.*, pp. 189–91.

20. Charpigny, *op. cit.*, n. 18.

21. Invoice, F. Ducharne Silk Co. Inc., January 29, 1930; Tirocchi Archive.

22. Colette, "Les Tissus de Rodier," in *Art et Industrie*, (December 1926), pp. 51–53, translation by Susan Hay.

23. The entry for "Textiles" in *Encyclopédie des arts décoratifs et industriels modernes au xx siècle, en douze volumes*, vol. xx. New York: 1997 (reprint), p. 9, is the source for the information contained in this paragraph and the following three.

24. *Ibid.*

25. Betty Kirke, *Madeleine Vionnet.* New York: 1998, p. 38.

26. Interview with François Férier, Lyon, conducted by Susan Hay, December 1997.

Baedeker, Karl. *Central Italy and Rome: Handbook for Travellers*. Leipzig, London, and New York: 1909.

————. *Rome and Central Italy: Handbook for Travellers*. Leipzig, London, and New York: 1930.

————. *Southern Italy and Sicily, with Excursions to Malta, Sardinia, Tunis, and Corfu: Handbook for Travellers*. Leipzig, London, and New York: 1930.

Ballard, Bettina. *In My Fashion*. New York: 1960.

Banner, Lois W. *American Beauty*. New York: 1983.

Battersby, Martin. *Art Deco Fashion: French Designers 1908–1925*. London: 1974.

Benson, Susan Porter. *Counter Cultures: Saleswomen, Managers, and Customers in American Department Stores*. Urbana: 1986.

————. "Women, Work, and Family: Industrial Home-work in Rhode Island," in Eileen Boris and Cynthia R. Daniels, eds., *Homework: Historical and Contemporary Perspectives on Paid Labor at Home*. Urbana: 1989.

Blum, Stella, ed. *Everyday Fashions of the Twenties*. New York: 1981.

Blumin, Stuart. *The Emergence of the Middle Class: Social Experience in the American City, 1760–1900*. Cambridge (England) and New York: 1989.

Briggs, John W. *An Italian Passage: Immigrants to Three American Cities, 1890–1930*. New Haven: 1978.

Brunhammer, Yvonne, and Suzanne Tise. *The Decorative Arts in France: La Société des Artistes Décorateurs, 1900–1942*. New York: 1990.

Chapon, François. *Jacques Doucet ou l'art du mécénat 1853–1929: nouvelle édition revue et corrigée*. Paris: 1996.

Charpigny, Florence. "Between Tradition and Modernity: Textile Design Education in Lyons at the Beginning of the 20th Century." Paper presented at the Textile Society of America Symposium, Fashion Institute of Technology, New York, September 26, 1998. Typescript courtesy of the author.

Chase, Edna Woolman. *Always in Vogue*. New York: 1954.

Coleman, Elizabeth Ann. *The Opulent Era: Fashions of Worth, Doucet, and Pingat*. Brooklyn: 1989.

Cooper-Hewitt Museum. *L'Art de Vivre: Decorative Arts and Design in France, 1789–1989*. New York: 1989.

Damase, Jacques. *Sonia Delaunay: mode et tissus imprimés*. Paris: 1991.

Delpierre, Madeleine. *Se Vêtir au XVIIIᵉ siècle*. Paris: 1996.

Deslandres, Yvonne. *Poiret: Paul Poiret 1879–1944*. New York: 1987.

Duncan, Isadora. *My Life*. New York: 1927.

Dunoyer de Segonzac, André. "Preface," in Palmer White, *Poiret*. London: 1973.

Encyclopédie des arts décoratifs et industriels modernes au XXe siècle, en douze volumes. New York: 1997 (reprint).

Ercoli, Giuliano. *Art Deco Prints*. New York: 1989.

Etherington-Smith, Meredith. *Patou*. London: 1983.

Ewing, Elizabeth. *History of 20th Century Fashion*. London: 1992 (3rd ed.).

Franklin Simon Fashion Catalog, Fall 1923. New York: 1993 (reprint).

Gamber, Wendy. *The Female Economy: The Millinery and Dressmaking Trades, 1860–1930*. Urbana: 1997.

Garnier, Guillaume. *Paris couture: les années trente*. Paris: 1987.

————. *Paul Poiret et Nicole Groult: maîtres de la mode art deco*. Paris: 1985.

Gilkeson, John S., Jr. *Middle-Class Providence, 1820–1940*. Princeton: 1986.

Gosling, Nigel. *Paris 1900–1914: The Miraculous Years*. London: 1978.

Hawes, Elizabeth. *Fashion is Spinach*. New York: 1938.

Hay, Susan. "Adolphe Braun and Textile Design," in Maureen O'Brien and Mary Bergstein, eds. *Image and Enterprise: The Photographs of Adolphe Braun*. Providence and London: 1999, pp. 44–65.

Hollander, Anne. *Seeing Through Clothes*. New York: 1980.

————. *Sex and Suits*. New York: 1994.

Jerde, Judith. "Mary Molloy: St. Paul's Extraordinary Dressmaker," *Minnesota History* (Fall 1980).

Katzman, David M. *Seven Days a Week: Women and Domestic Service in Industrializing America*. Urbana: 1981.

Kellner, George H., and J. Stanley Lemons. *Rhode Island: The Independent State*. Woodland Hills (California): 1982.

Kidwell, Claudia B., and Margaret C. Christman. *Suiting Everyone: The Democratization of Clothing in America*. Washington, D.C.: 1974.

Kirke, Betty. *Madeleine Vionnet*. New York: 1998.

Kluver, Billy, and Julie Martin. *Kiki's Paris*. New York: 1989.

Lévy, René Simon. *The Fabrics of Raoul Dufy: Genesis and Context*. London: 1983.

Martin, Richard. *Cubism and Fashion*. New York: 1999.

————. *Fashion and Surrealism*. New York: 1987.

————, ed. *Contemporary Fashion*. New York: 1995.

Mears, Patricia. "Jessie Franklin Turner: American Fashion and 'Exotic' Textile Inspiration," in *Creating Textiles: Makers, Methods, Markets. Proceedings of the 1998 Symposium of the Textile Society of America*. Earleville (Maryland): 1999.

Milbank, Caroline. *New York Fashion: The Evolution of American Style*. New York: 1996.

Montgomery, Florence M. *Textiles in America, 1650–1870*. New York: n.d.

Morelli, Ornella. "The International Success and Domestic Debut of Postwar Italian Fashion," in Gloria Bianchini et. al., trans. Paul Blanchard. *Italian Fashion*. New York: 1987.

Musée Historique des Tissus. *Paquin: une rétrospective de 60 ans de haute couture*. Lyon: 1989.

Museum of Art, Rhode Island School of Design. *Dynamic Symmetry*. Providence: 1961.

Parmal, Pamela A. "Welcome Arnold and Textiles." Paper presented at the Dublin Seminar, Deerfield, Massachusetts, June 28, 1997. Typescript courtesy of the author.

Peiss, Kathy. *Cheap Amusements: Working Women and Leisure in Turn-of-the-Century New York*. Philadelphia: 1986.

Perez-Tibi, Dora. *Dufy*. New York: 1989.

Pesaturo, Ubaldo U. M. *Italo-Americans in Rhode Island*. Providence: 1936, 1940.

Poiret, Paul. *En Habillant l'époque*. Paris: 1930.

Ribiero, Aileen. *Dress in Eighteenth-Century Europe, 1715–1789*. New York: 1985.

Roshco, Bernard. *The Rag Race: How New York and Paris Run the Breakneck Business of Dressing American Women*. New York: 1963.

Schiaparelli, Elsa. *Shocking Life*. London: 1954.

Schneider, Dorothy and Carl J. *American Women in the Progressive Era, 1900–1920*. New York: 1993.

Schweiger, Werner J. *Wiener Werkstätte: Design in Vienna, 1903–1932*. New York: 1984.

Scranton, Philip. "The Transition from Custom to Ready-to-Wear Clothing in Philadelphia, 1890–1930," *Textile History*, vol. 25, no. 2 (Autumn 1994), pp. 243–73.

Shattuck, Roger. *The Banquet Years: The Origins of the Avant-Garde in France, 1885 to World War I*. New York: 1968 (rev. ed.).

Silver, Kenneth E. *Esprit de Corps: The Art of the Parisian Avant-Garde and the First World War, 1914–1925*. Princeton: 1989.

Smith, Judith E. *Family Connections: A History of Italian and Jewish Immigrant Lives in Providence, Rhode Island 1900–1940*. Albany: 1985.

Stauffacher, Anne. "L'Évolution stylistique de la fleur dans l'industrie du textile. Un exemple: l'Atelier Martine." Mémoire de maîtrise, Sorbonne, Université de Paris, n.d. Typescript in the Musée des Arts Décoratifs, Paris.

Steele, Valerie. *Paris Fashion: A Cultural History.* New York: 1988.

Stein, Gertrude. *Paris, France.* New York: 1970.

Tentler, Leslie Woodcock. *Wage-Earning Women: Industrial Work and Family Life in the United States, 1900–1930.* New York: 1979.

Tétart-Vittu, Françoise. *Au Paradis des dames: nouveautés, modes et confections, 1810–1870.* Paris: 1992.

Tomasek, Kathryn Manson. "Irrepressible Women, Work, and Benevolence in Providence, Rhode Island, 1860–1936." Paper presented at the conference "Rhode Island Reconsidered," John Nicholas Brown Center, Brown University, Providence, November 15, 1997.

Tourlonias, Anne, and Jack Vidal. *Raoul Dufy, l'oeuvre en soie: logique d'un oeuvre ornemental industriel.* Avignon: 1998.

Trautman, Pat. "Personal Clothiers: A Demographic Study of Dressmakers, Seamstresses and Tailors, 1880–1920," *Dress,* vol. 5 (1979), pp. 74–95.

Trautmann, Julieanne. "'Sizing up' the Client: Minneapolis Dressmaker Madame Rose Boyd." MA thesis, University of Minnesota, 1997.

Troy, Nancy J. *Modernism and the Decorative Arts in France, Art Nouveau to Le Corbusier.* New Haven: 1991.

Vernus, Pierre. "Bianchini-Férier, fabricant de soieries à Lyon (1888–1973)." Thèse de doctorat d'histoire, Université Lumière Lyon II, 1997. Typescript courtesy of the author.

Völker, Angela. *Textiles of the Wiener Werkstätte, 1910–1932.* New York: 1994.

White, Palmer. *Elsa Schiaparelli: Empress of Paris Fashion.* New York: 1986.

————. *Poiret.* London: 1973.

Wilson, Elizabeth. *Adorned in Dreams.* Berkeley and Los Angeles: 1985.

Wilson, Robert Forrest. *Paris on Parade.* New York: 1932 (3rd ed.).

Yans-McLaughlin, Virginia. *Family and Community: Italian Immigrants in Buffalo, 1880–1930.* Ithaca: 1997.

This book was designed
and set into type by
Gilbert Design Associates,
Providence,
Rhode Island.

The typefaces used in this book
were designed by
William Addison Dwiggins.
The sans serif, Metro, appeared in 1930
and Electra in 1935.

The book was printed and bound
in Hong Kong.

4500 copies for the Museum of Art,
Rhode Island School of Design,
on the occasion of the exhibition
January 2001